Novel Health Interprofessional Education and Collaborative Practice Program: Strategy and Implementation

Mohammed Yahya Alnaami
Dalal Abdullah Alqahtani
Eiad Abdelmohsen Alfaris
Hamza Mohammad Abdulghani
Ciraj Ali Mohammed
Editors

Novel Health Interprofessional Education and Collaborative Practice Program: Strategy and Implementation

Springer

Editors
Mohammed Yahya Alnaami
Department of Surgery, College of Medicine
King Saud University
Riyadh, Saudi Arabia

Eiad Abdelmohsen Alfaris
Department of Family and Community Medicine
College of Medicine, King Saud University
Riyadh, Saudi Arabia

Ciraj Ali Mohammed
Medical Education, College of Medicine and Health Sciences,
National University of Science & Technology,
Sohar, Oman

Dalal Abdullah Alqahtani
Oral Medicine and Diagnostic Sciences
College of Dentistry, King Saud University
Riyadh, Saudi Arabia

Hamza Mohammad Abdulghani
Department of Medical Education
College of Medicine, King Saud University
Riyadh, Saudi Arabia

https://doi.org/10.1007/978-981-99-3420-1

This Springer imprint is published by the registered company Springer Nature Singapore Pte Ltd.
The registered company address is: 152 Beach Road, #21-01/04 Gateway East, Singapore 189721, Singapore

"To health professional faculty eager for excellence in pedagogy and educational scholarship; to our students who are striving for successful learning and training experiences; to our universities aiming for higher ranks among other world-class universities; and to our society looking for trustful and quality health professional graduates."

Foreword

The World Health Organization Framework for Action on Interprofessional Education and Collaborative Practice [1] defines interprofessional collaboration in education and practice as an innovative strategy that plays an important role in mitigating the global health workforce crises. Interprofessional Education and Collaborative Practice (IPECP) is collective by nature, emerging as it does at the intersection of a wide variety of professional knowledge and scopes of practice. Many studies of IPECP focus on the determinants or inputs of collaborative practice as well as on the results, outputs, or outcomes. This is echoed methodologically, as a preponderance of IPECP teamwork studies that primarily employ interview and survey data. However, close observations are also necessary to build an understanding of the collective behavioral processes of interprofessional collaboration. Many authors point out the need for more studies of the actual practices of collaboration. In many senses, IPECP represents what Rittel and Webber [2] have called a "wicked problem." Wicked problems are "difficult or impossible to solve. Their solutions depend on incomplete, contradictory, and changing requirements that are often difficult to recognize. And they are confounded by complex interdependencies between actors and agents." If ever there was a wicked problem, innovation in IPECP is surely one.

Learning to become a competent health professional has always been a two-part process—that focuses on "classroom" teaching and that engages students in an apprenticeship with qualified professionals in real-world settings. Universities, colleges, and institutes depend upon practice settings for the apprenticeship education of their health professional students. Clinical training, or more accurately practice education (PE) settings, requires competent healthcare professionals to deliver quality care to patients. Until recently, delivery of health professions education has been almost entirely discipline based, with each discipline educating their own students in isolation—whether on campus or in the community. There is now increasing emphasis on all healthcare professions to learn how to be competent collaborators. This emerging shift in education has led to a new interest in different approaches to the delivery of health professional education, approaches that embrace more opportunities for interactions among and between learners across health and human service/social care professions. PE settings are being recognized as ideal environments for IPECP, in which students can witness and practice how to work interprofessionally with others in healthcare teams, that is to learn about, with and from each other, for the purpose of collaboration to improve quality of care and health and social care services.

The term practice tends to occupy a black box in the interprofessional literature. Although it is frequently invoked in considerations of collaboration, teamwork, and team working, it is seldom explicitly defined. One exception is Thistlethwaite et al. [3] who suggest that practice can be understood in three ways: (a) as the enactment of a role or profession, (b) as a moment of collective unity or performance, and (c) as a "socially institutionalized and socially acceptable form of interaction requiring cognitive understanding and reflection." These three ideas provide a better understanding of the term "practice" by removing it from a black box and placing it within our concept of a partnership between a team of healthcare providers.

It is now recognized that effective IPECP requires the active engagement of students from different professions using interactive learning methodologies to develop health professional students' knowledge, skills, attitudes, perceptions, and behaviors. IPECP requires a complex adult learning (andragogy) approach that is most effective when integrated throughout a program of study moving from simple to more complex learning activities that bridge from post-secondary to PE settings. This program at King Saud University (KSU) reflects most of these principles that if implemented correctly, it should produce well-equipped professional graduates and better IPECP outcomes.

Accreditation standards, now being developed to stimulate the advancement of IPECP, have an impact on policies in both academic and clinical settings, and on the development of continuing professional development (CPD) programs for IPECP are recognized as integral parts of the learning continuum particularly when built on a theory-informed base and sustained in changing health and social care environments. IPECP is now an established discipline and field of research. Its current and future development holds promise for urgent changes needed in health and social care education and in health and social care practice.

University of British Columbia
and WHO Collaborating Centre
on Health Workforce Planning & Research
Dalhousie University
Vancouver, BC, Canada

John H. V. Gilbert

References

1. Gilbert J, Yan J, Hoffman SJ. A WHO report: framework for action on interprofessional education and collaborative practice. J Allied Health. 2010;39 Suppl 1:196–7.
2. Rittel HWJ, Webber MM. Dilemmas in a general theory of planning. Policy Sci. 1973;4:155–69.
3. Thistlethwaite J, Jackson A, Moran M. Interprofessional collaborative practice: a deconstruction. J Interpr Care. 2013;27(1);50–6.

Preface

Globally, health professional education has not kept pace with the current changes and challenges of the twenty-first century healthcare systems and needs; most curricula are outdated and often created in isolation, producing under-equipped graduates for today's healthcare environment. Interprofessional education and collaborative practice (IPECP) is one of the recommended strategies to improve healthcare systems as they are becoming more complex and costly, relying on care delivered by teams, institutions, and systems. Our aim is to improve health sciences educational programs and their graduates through collaborative, interprofessional co-education and practice through the creation of the Center of Excellence in Interprofessional Education and Collaborative Practice (CEIPE-CP). In 2010, King Saud University in Riyadh, Kingdom of Saudi Arabia (KSA), launched a new program to support the development of learning, teaching, and assessment in health sciences education across all specialties and professions. A leadership group of health educators representing the health colleges that educate more than 7000 students and have about 2000 faculty staff was involved in the development of the strategic plan and structure of the "Center." This project was planned in collaboration with Partners Harvard Medical International (PHMI) over the course of 1 year. Based on student surveys; strengths, weaknesses, opportunities, and threats (SWOT) analysis; internal and external program accreditation reviews for health sciences colleges; and other evaluation initiatives for graduate health education programs; the need to improve health professional education became apparent in all health sciences colleges (medicine, dentistry, pharmacy, applied medical sciences, nursing, and emergency medical services). Aside from planning sessions, the leadership group was involved in six faculty development exercises, three workshops in Riyadh, KSA, and three courses in Boston, USA, at the Harvard Macy Institute (HMI) focusing on various aspects of the project. A strategic plan was developed for the "Center" that includes a vision, mission, values, short-term strategies (initiatives) that are usually accomplished within 1–2 years, long-term goals that may take several years to achieve, and action steps with key performance indicators to guard the quality and fulfillment of the strategies. The governance structure of the Center was designed to include the Vice-Rector for Health Specialties, later changed to the Vice-Rector for Educational and Academic Affairs; Deans of all Health Science Colleges (HSCs) as an internal advisory board; an external advisory board from well-known health professions educational institutes and individual experts; leadership of the "Center" represented by educational leaders from all health science colleges; and an administrative arm that deals with IT, communications, budget, and scheduling. The leadership group is now responsible for implementing the various functions of the "Center Units," which include curriculum development, assessment and evaluation, educational and IT resources management, faculty skills development, quality and accreditation, educational research support, and consultation/outreach support in a phased approach. The proposed center is an innovative approach to improve health professional education and practice across all health sciences colleges at KSU, developed with the involvement of all stakeholders and supported by outside facilitation and structured programs and exercises. The university will move quickly to implement the Center using a phased approach, starting with strategies and structure of the program, followed by the implementation.

Riyadh, Saudi Arabia — Mohammed Yahya Alnaami

Part III: Preface

King Saud University (KSU) witnessed a bold transformation journey that started in 2008, led by its Rector, Professor Abdullah Alothman. This signaled the start of an important transformation of higher education in Saudi Arabia in general. A new strategic plan was established, and wide restructuring of the university was well underway. A new vice-rectorship for health specialties was established at that time with the undertaking to promote the development of health professional education in KSU.

Health professional education in Saudi Arabia is relatively new. The first pharmacy and medical colleges were established at KSU, Riyadh, at the end of the 1960s. Colleges of dentistry, applied medical sciences, and nursing were established later. These colleges introduced a cadre of trained Saudi health professionals to the local healthcare workforce. These professionals shared in the predominantly expatriate workforce. In general, the Saudi health sector is facing many challenges in its quest to build up its healthcare-related human resources, which has become a major concern of the government in recent years.

An example of these challenges is related to health professional education. By the mid-1990s, 13% of the medical, 11.2% of the nursing, and 38% of other health professions workforce had become local nationals. Thus, the government adopted a policy of increasing its health professions training capacity. As a result, by 2021, 24 medical, 17 dentistry, 19 pharmacy, 13 nursing, 23 applied medical sciences, and 12 other health-related public colleges are in existence nowadays. The establishment of these new health professional colleges was not a "smooth sailing." The rapid expansion led to an acute shortage of trained health professional educators, which, in turn, posed a new set of challenges.

In addition to recruiting and retaining qualified faculty, health professional educators faced additional challenges dealing with curricular design, teaching and learning, assessment, instructional material development, and educational strategies. A leadership steering committee was formed by colleagues from medical, dental, pharmacy, applied medical, and nursing colleges. Partners Harvard Medical International (PHMI) healthcare company was recruited as a consultant of the project. The committee held regular meetings, workshops, and symposia both in Riyadh and in Boston in the USA. The Center of Excellence in Interprofessional Education (CEIPE) was proposed. This section represents the planning and structure of the program with emphasis on the strategies for successful learning and training experiences, excellence in pedagogy and educational scholarship, and utilization of best assessment and evaluation systems. The strategic plan framework presented in all tables of this section was derived from KSU general strategic plan template, which was also recommended for our project strategic planning. It is hoped that this case study at KSU will represent an example of a local initiative that can be helpful to other universities and higher education institutions. It was understood from the beginning that this would be a major change effort, which needed to be carefully planned and executed in order to be effective. The next part presents a case study summary of our endeavor and the lessons learned in launching such a university-wide change program.

Riyadh, Saudi Arabia Mohammed Alshehri

Acknowledgments

The editors and contributors of this book would like to thank his Royal Highness Crown Prince Mohammed Bin Salman for his continuous support and enthusiasm to develop and motivate King Saud University (KSU) to rank as one of, or at least near, the top 10 world-class universities in his vision for the Kingdom by 2030. Accordingly, we also thank H.E. Badran Alomar, Rector of KSU, and Mohammed Alnumy, Vice-Rector for Educational and Academic Affairs, who took this initiative seriously to support and develop KSU educational and academic achievements. This work would have not been made possible without the support of H.E. Abdullah Alothman, former Rector of KSU; the leadership of H.E. Mohammed Alshehri, former Vice-Rector for Health Specialties (VRHSs); Thomas Aretz from Partners Harvard Medical International, Boston, USA, who initiated and launched this program in KSU. Credit also goes to Abdulrahman Almuammar, the former CEO of KSU Medical City, and Deans of HSCs who continued to support all subsequent activities of this program. We also acknowledge the great work of the expert groups (themes) at the VRHSs, representing all HSCs, namely Colleges of Medicine, Dentistry, Nursing, Applied Medical Sciences, Pharmacy, and Emergency Medical Services. The Teaching & Learning Theme Steering Committee includes Dalal Abdullah Alqahtani, Awatif Alam, Basil Amarneh, Sahar Albarakati, Ahmad Mitwalli, Amal Fatani, Tawfeq Alhowairiny, Kelechi Ogbuehi, and Naghma Naeem. The Assessment Theme Steering Committee includes Einas Aleisa, Hazar Yacoub, Salwa Elsobkey, Asma Faden, Olfat Salem, Eqbal Darandari, and Hamza Mohammad Abdulghani. The Leadership Committee Members include Mohammed Yahya Alnaami, Eiad Abdelmohsen Alfaris, Hisham Aljadhey, Fahad Almoqbel, Omar Gazi, Raed Alsadhan, Sami Alnassar, Abdulmajeed Aldrees, Nehal Khamis, Abdullah Alhwaimel, Abdullah Aldahmash, Abdulaziz Alomar, and Saud Alkhatheri. We especially thank those who shared in the milestones of the program planning and activities including Mohamed Zahedi, Sulaiman Alhadlaq, Khalid Alwazzan, Khalid Alharbi, Abdullah Alzahrani, and Sainaa Alaqeel. We appreciate the unlimited administrative support of Essam Mattar, Saad Alammar, Mohammad Alobaid, Nasser Alshehri, and Agung Prasetijo. Gratitude is extended to the great secretarial assistance of Saad Abdulsabour, Fahad Almowenes, Saad Alamri, Mohammed Abdulghani, Abdullah Alghamdi, and Dalal Alsaleh. We highly appreciate the contribution of Rafik Abdelmoati for revising and editing Part III of this manual. We appreciate the valuable contributions of Sir John Gilbert who actually made the road map for this work. Special thanks to Jill Thistlethwaite who made the framework of Part I; Alla El-Awaisi for connecting contributors from the different IPECP-research groups and countries to share in writing this book; and the Leaders of Manipal Academy of Higher Education—Foundation for Advancement of International Medical Education and Research (MAHE-FAIMER) International Institute for Leadership in IPE in India. Special thanks also to Fatimah Alnaami for her contribution in graphics and multimedia works of this book.

Finally, the editors and contributors of this book would like to thank the reviewers and administrators of **Springer Nature** for their guidance and support.

Contents

Editors and Contributors

About the Editors

Mohammed Yahya Alnaami is currently a professor of surgery and medical education at King Saud University (KSU), Riyadh, Saudi Arabia. He works as a consultant general and bariatric surgeon, and a board member of the Saudi Society of Medical Education (SSME). He is a graduate fellow in interprofessional education leadership certified by Manipal University and the Foundation for Advancement of International Medical Education and Research (FAIMER). Mohammed is interested in teaching and training undergraduate and postgraduate health professional students, residents, and fellows. He is heavily involved in health professional education development activities. Mohammed has published more than 45 articles and three books in surgery and medical education research.

Dalal Abdullah Alqahtani is an assistant professor in oral pathology in the Department of Oral Medicine and Diagnostic Sciences at the College of Dentistry, King Saud University (KSU), Riyadh, Saudi Arabia. Besides teaching oral pathology to undergraduate and postgraduate students, she practices oral pathology, and she is the Head of the Oral Histopathology Laboratory at a dental university hospital. She is involved in the curriculum reform project of the undergraduate dental curriculum at KSU, as she is directing the project. She has received awards and grants in education, giving lectures and workshops in medical education, and published several papers.

Eiad Abdelmohsen Alfaris is a professor of family medicine and medical education. He has been a family medicine consultant and a member of the Royal College of General Practitioners (London) since 1989. He is the supervisor of the King Saud University (KSU) chair for medical education and development. He had completed a Master's degree in Medical Education (MMed) from the University of Dundee, UK. He has contributed substantially to the development of medical education in Saudi Arabia and has published around 65 articles in national and international journals. His main research areas are health professional students' well-being, psychiatric disorders in family medicine, learning environment, and epidemiological studies on different health issues. He has run various workshops for the Saudi Commission for Health Specialties, KSU health schools, and national and international symposia.

Hamza Mohammad Abdulghani is a medical education and family medicine professor, and the head of the assessment and evaluation center, College of Medicine, KSU. He has organized and conducted many faculty development workshops in medical colleges at the national and international levels. He is an invited speaker for many national and international conferences and scientific gatherings, consultations, and workshops focused on clinical teaching and learning, feedback skills, and different types of assessment. He is on the editorial boards of many peer-reviewed journals. He has published extensively in reputed peer-reviewed journals in the field of medical education and family medicine.

Ciraj Ali Mohammed is currently a professor and head of medical education at the College of Medicine and Health Sciences, National University, Oman. He is a fellow and global faculty of the Foundation for the Advancement of International Medical Education and Research (FAIMER) Institute, Philadelphia, USA. He is a Fulbright visiting scholar at the Department of Molecular Biology and Infectious Diseases. He is a recipient of the international fellowship in medical education (IFME), Florida International University, Miami, USA. He has authored articles and chapters in medical education and microbiology and served on the editorial board of many journals. Ciraj is the director of the MAHE-FAIMER fellowship program that focuses on leadership in interprofessional education organized in collaboration with FAIMER. He is currently the secretary of the Academy of Health Professions Educators, India, Chair of the Indian interprofessional education network (IndiPEN), and a member of the global confederation for interprofessional education and collaborative practice. Ciraj also serves on the Network's Advisory Board—Towards Unity for Health.

Contributors

Hamza Mohammad Abdulghani, MD, MMEd, PhD Department of Medical Education, College of Medicine, King Saud University, Riyadh, Saudi Arabia

Eiad Abdelmohsen Alfaris, MBBS, MSc, MRCGP, MMed Department of Family and Community Medicine, College of Medicine, King Saud University, Riyadh, Saudi Arabia

Hani Alghamdi, MBBS, MPH, PhD College of Medicine, King Saud University, Riyadh, Saudi Arabia

Mohammed Almansour, MD Department of Medical Education, College of Medicine, King Saud University, Riyadh, Saudi Arabia

Mohammed Yahya Alnaami, MBBS, FRCSC, MEd, FIPE Department of Surgery, College of Medicine, King Saud University, Riyadh, Saudi Arabia

Dalal Abdullah Alqahtani, BDS, MSc, MMEd, PhD Oral Medicine and Diagnostic Sciences, College of Dentistry, King Saud University, Riyadh, Saudi Arabia

Nouf Alrumaihi, MBBS, MSc, MedEd, PMP Health Academy in the Saudi Commission for Health Specialties (SCFHS), Riyadh, Saudi Arabia

Mohammed Al Shafaee, MD, PhD, MRCGP Family Medicine, College of Medicine and Health Sciences, National University of Science and Technology, Sohar, Oman

Mohammed Alshehri, MBBS, FRCSC, MEd Vice-Rectorship for Health Specialties, Department of Surgery, College of Medicine, King Saud University, Riyadh, Saudi Arabia

Mona Alsheikh, MBBS, PhD, MHPE Physiology Department, College of Medicine, Imam Abdulrahman Bin Faisal University, Dammam, Saudi Arabia

Osama Alshogran, PhD Department of Clinical Pharmacy, Faculty of Pharmacy, Jordan University of Science and Technology, Irbid, Jordan

Abdullah Alzahrani, BA, MD, PhD Department of Health Management, College of Applied Medical Sciences, King Saud University, Riyadh, Saudi Arabia

Hana Alzamil, MBBS, MSc, PhD Physiology Department, College of Medicine, King Saud University, Riyadh, Saudi Arabia

Basil Amarneh, RN, MSc, PhD College of Nursing, King Saud University, Riyadh, Saudi Arabia

Anand R., MD Pulmonary Medicine, Kasturba Medical College, Mangalore, India

Mohammad Azzam, MD Curriculum Studies and Studies in Applied Linguistics, Faculty of Education, Western University, London, ON, Canada

Lubna Baig, MBBS, FCPS, PhD APPNA Institute of Public Health, Jinnah Sindh Medical University, Karachi, Pakistan

Gulam Begum, MD College of Medicine and Health Sciences, National University of Science and Technology, Sohar, Oman

Anthony Breitbach, PhD, ATC, FASAHP, FNAP Doisy College of Health Sciences, Saint Louis University, St. Louis, MO, USA

Sunitha Calvin, MSc Manipal College of Nursing, Manipal Academy of Higher Education, Manipal, India

Abhishek Chaturvedi, MSc Department of Basic Medical Sciences, Manipal Academy of Higher Education, Manipal, India

Eqbal Darandari, BEd, MSc, PhD College of Education, King Saud University, Riyadh, Saudi Arabia

Alla El-Awaisi, MPharm, MSc, PhD Department of Clinical Pharmacy and Practice, College of Pharmacy, QU Health, Qatar University, Doha, Qatar

Salwa Elsobkey, BSc, MSc, PhD College of Applied Medical Sciences, King Saud University, Riyadh, Saudi Arabia

Asma Faden, BDS, MSc, PhD College of Dentistry, King Saud University, Riyadh, Saudi Arabia

Marie-Andree Girard, MD, FRCPC, LLD Faculty of Medicine, University of Montreal, Montreal, QC, Canada

Nighat Huda, MS, MSED, MPhil Liaquat National Hospital & Medical College, Karachi, Pakistan

Ganesh Kamath, MSc, PhD Manipal University College Malaysia (MUCM), Melaka, Malaysia

Farah Mansuri, MBBS, MCPS, HPE, FCPS College of Medicine, Taibah University, Almadina Almunawwara, Saudi Arabia

Nichola McLarnon, BMedSc, PhD Glasgow Caledonian University, Glasgow, UK

Ciraj Ali Mohammed, MSc (Med), PhD, MHPE Medical Education, College of Medicine and Health Sciences, National University of Science and Technology, Sohar, Oman

Naghma Naeem, MBBS, MMEd, PhD College of Medicine, King Saud University, Riyadh, Saudi Arabia

Prajna Nayak, MDS Manipal College of Dental Sciences, Manipal Academy of Higher Education, Manipal, India

Kelechi Ogbuehi, MSc, PhD College of Applied Medical Sciences, King Saud University, Riyadh, Kingdom of Saudi Arabia

Olfat Salem, RN, MSc, PhD College of Nursing, King Saud University, Riyadh, Saudi Arabia

Jill Thistlethwaite, BSc, MBBS, PhD, MMed, FRCGP University of Technology Sydney, Sydney, Australia

Ramprasad Vasthare, BDS, MDS Manipal College of Dental Sciences, Manipal Academy of Higher Education, Manipal, India

Saleena Velladath, MSc, PhD Biochemistry Department, College of Medicine and Health Sciences, National University of Science and Technology, Sohar, Oman

Susan Waller, MPhty, PhD Department of Medical Education, College of Medicine and Health Sciences, UAE University, Al Ain, United Arab Emirates

Hazar Yacoub, PhD College of Pharmacy, King Saud University, Riyadh, Saudi Arabia

Part I

Interprofessional Education for Collaborative Practice: Background, Theory, and Context

Interprofessional Education: Defining and Developing Centers of Excellence

1

Mohammed Yahya Alnaami, Farah Mansuri, and Nighat Huda

1.1 Introduction

Interprofessional education (IPE) is an educational concept that imposed itself when the Centre for the Advancement of Interprofessional Education (CAIPE), established in the United Kingdom in 1987, published its statement on the definition and principles of IPE as *"occasions when two or more professions learn together intending to cultivate collaborative practice"* [1]. In 2002, CAIPE amended its definition of IPE to *"occasions when two or more professions learn with, from, and about each other to improve collaboration and the quality of care"* [2]. In 2016, CAIPE extended the definition of IPE further to *"occasions when members or students of two or more professions learn with, from, and about each other to improve collaboration and the quality of care and services"* [3].

Health Interprofessional Education (HIPE) is one of the novel philosophies of delivering medical knowledge, with a focus to facilitate collective learning among various relevant medical and allied disciplines. In its framework for action on interprofessional education and collaborative practice, the World Health Organization (WHO) defines interprofessional education and collaborative practice (IPECP) as "*occurs when two or more professional students, residents, and health workers learn with, about, and from each other to enable effective collaboration and to improve the health outcomes*" [4]. Other terms used for Interprofessional education are "multi-profession education,"

M. Y. Alnaami (✉)
Department of Surgery, College of Medicine, King Saud University, Riyadh, Saudi Arabia

F. Mansuri
College of Medicine, Taibah University, Al Madinah Al Munawwarah, Saudi Arabia

N. Huda
Liaquat National Hospital & Medical College, Karachi, Pakistan

M. Y. Alnaami et al. (eds.), *Novel Health Interprofessional Education and Collaborative Practice Program: Strategy and Implementation*,
https://doi.org/10.1007/978-981-99-3420-1_1

"collaborative learning," and "shared learning," or "interdisciplinary education." Lately, its scope also has been broadened to apply Continuing Professional Development (CPD) besides undergraduate and postgraduate medical education [5].

The philosophy of IPE gets embodied as the functional frame of IPECP along with certain standards of teamwork woven into it. Teamwork requires a person's openness and willingness to work together to achieve the greater benefit of patient care. Several studies have been published in the last couple of decades endorsing positive outcomes in specific clinical and educational settings where an interdisciplinary approach is required like emergency medicine, primary care, public health, etc. Interprofessional communication claims to be improved and higher quality of patient-centered care is ensured when medical students learn with seniors, share their basic science knowledge, and escalate their clinical understanding in a team.

1.2 Evolution of IPE in Global and Regional Perspectives

Interprofessional education (IPE) is a recurring old term that has evolved since the early 1970s [6]. The Institute of Medicine (IOM) of the USA produced the first report on *"Educating for the Health Team,"* which emphasizes improved healthcare delivery by educating health professional students in teams [7]. Then, CAIPE was the first IPE center established in 1987 to generate, synthesize, and translate the evidence base for best practices in interprofessional education (IPE) and collaborative practice (CP) [8].

In 2010, IPE was taken further by the WHO and produced a new framework for IPE and collaborative practice (IPECP) among health professionals [4]. This was followed shortly by the Lancet Commission Report [9], which provides a vision for the twenty-first century that calls for a new era of professional education that advances transformative learning and harnesses the power of interdependence in education. Then in 2011, the famous report of the "Interprofessional Education Collaborative Expert Panel" was issued describing the four core competencies for interprofessional collaborative practice [10].

Another global confederation in IPECP (Interprofessional.Global) [11] was founded in 2018, which also provides a forum for the growing number of national and international IPECP networks to share their work and debate on common issues and has been a proving ground for the development of a global network. It also facilitates support and exchange between regional interprofessional education and collaborative practice (IPECP) networks, establishes relationships with other like-minded organizations and welcomes and supports new networks sharing the same aims and values. IPECP networks will be discussed in more detail in "Chap. 6."

In 2019, the InterprofessionalResearch.Global (IPR.Global), a special interest group that provides global leadership in IPECP research, published a guidance on interprofessional education and collaborative practice as a discussion paper [12]. The discussion paper offers perspectives to inform discussions around the global research agenda for IPECP by identifying research priorities and providing guidance on theoretical frameworks, research methodologies, and composition of research teams.

1.3 Strategic Planning for IPE

Introducing IPE usually starts with faculty and students' awareness through conducting workshops and symposia explaining IPE definition and concepts, needs assessment, rationale, goals, design, and assessment and evaluation [13]. As a first step towards quality need-based care, strategic mechanism and cooperation among health professions deans, administrators, staff, and students is required to ensure the quality and sustainability of the IPE program. Stimulators for educators include real-world experience and insight by the learners, input into program development by different professionals, and learning about other professions and practitioners in a single educational setting. For health policymakers, the motivators include improved workplace practices and productivity, improved patient outcomes, raised staff morale, and improved patient safety with better access to healthcare. To ensure interprofessional activities, and initiatives are developed, delivered, and evaluated under internationally recognized best practices.

Developing an IPE program in a recent context seems attainable because problem-based and case-based learning cultures are prevalent globally in medical schools and other health professions. Interprofessional education programs can be twined in the same spiral curriculum with predefined tasks and competencies with appropriate research and utilization. The efforts for IPE are driven to ensure collaborative practice while later leading to the transformation of a fragmented health system into a more cohesive system. The main components of IPE include defined learning outcomes and shared competencies among various related disciplines along with training of staff and determined leadership in health sciences colleges. An important feature of IPE is the common competencies in those interactive disciplines and also the team spirit required to ensure patient safety and effective healthcare delivery.

Also, developing IPE programs require consensus on terminology and definitions for IPE and related concepts, involving institutional leaders to develop a systematic approach to foster IPE in their institutions, collaborating with academic institutions, health systems, and community partners, and providing a framework similar to the WHO framework for IPECP [4] for program leaders and faculty to develop a plan for quality IPE [14].

McKinsey, Deloitte, and BCG Management Consultants [15], world's best strategic planners, have introduced a toolkit to improve the institutional strategic planning capability with a simple and comprehensive four-phase strategic planning approach:

Phase I: Setting up the strategic planning project through the following steps:

1. Formulation of the strategic planning team.
2. Setting guiding principles.
3. Forming a strategic plan structure.
4. Listing strategic plan key inputs.
5. Writing the strategic planning project plan.

Phase II: Gather and analyze data and provide key insights through:

1. Market analysis.
2. Competitor analysis.
3. Customer feedback.
4. Company data analytics team.
5. Employee feedback.
6. Executive feedback.
7. SWOT summary of the key business insights.

Phase III: Define the strategic plan considering the following aspects:

1. Mission, vision, and values.
2. Strategy map including the strategic objectives to reach our vision.
3. Balanced scorecard including the key performance indicators linked to the strategic objectives.
4. List of potential initiatives to reach our strategic objectives.
5. Business cases and financial models to help us prioritize our list of potential projects.
6. Project prioritization.
7. Business roadmap including our prioritized projects.

Phase VI: Implement, track, and manage progress through the following steps:

1. Governance structure.
2. Dashboards.
3. Projects plans.
4. Project implementation: Agile, Design Thinking, and Traditional methodologies.
5. Quarterly update of the strategic plan based on new data.
6. Post projects evaluation and lessons learned.
7. Post-strategic planning evaluation and lessons learned.

Although McKinsey's toolkit for strategic planning is more business-oriented; however, educational strategic planning may benefit from their four-phase strategy, with adjustments in the details under each phase. The ideal strategy must include a clear mission and vision of the program, leadership and faculty suitability, attached values, learning activities with its settings, learning outcomes, and the student's evaluation plan according to the defined core competencies. Competencies are the abilities of an individual to integrate knowledge, skills, and attitudes, demonstrated through behaviors, in performing their tasks. The competencies are considered a basic determinant in health professional education and practice that can easily be replicated in different settings and objectives. Competencies can be defined and grouped according to the level of learners while the "Competence" of the practitioners per se is assessed in real practice by evaluating the quality of care and patient satisfaction.

In the provision of IP collaborative healthcare, skills, and professional knowledge need to be augmented by, but not exclusively, the following core competencies:

- Effective communication.
- Teamwork and collaboration.
- Roles and responsibilities.
- Ethical practices.
- Conflict resolution.
- Patient/community-centered care.

Interprofessional practice (IPP) has established itself as an articulation of those models of competencies as proposed by Brewer and Jones, Canadian IPH collaborative, IPEC, WHO, Institute of Medicine, etc. [16]

There are three levels of competency:

1. Common (to be shared between multiple professions).
2. Complementary (to bc specific for each profession).
3. Collaborative (to be shared between professionals).

Sub-competencies identification is dependent on the demand of the course/profession and requires vigilant faculty commitment to developing it according to the structure of the team.

Training of educators is mandatory to help them facilitate educational activities with diverse professional backgrounds. The flipped classroom approach, acquaintance with the role of other professions, reviewing, and reflection skills are to be nurtured into those of typical educators' profiles [17].

Implementation of IPE will be ensured according to its design for the courses and disciplines together. Then, formative evaluation is needed for possible modifications in the design and conduct to identify the lapses in standards and procedures if any; while process and outcome evaluation are included as part of the plan to measure the achievement of competencies at all levels.

Problems may arise during the implementation process of IPE, however, the students need to be encouraged to adapt to experiential learning in a positive manner that may be well-matched to this generation of the digital era. Therefore, this may be a good time to bring some twists to the PBL system with few modifications in the conduct of multidisciplinary learning through IPE principles.

To assess the best approach for interprofessional competencies, the following criteria can be used [18]:

- Provision of clear general aims/goals to share an understanding of the objectives/initiatives.
- Clarity of the integration process of knowledge, effective communication, conflict management, and appropriate roles of the team members.
- Proactive leadership and adequacy of skilled academic and managerial staff.
- Documentation of effectiveness of team meetings and utility of resources.

Table 1.1 Sample of KSU strategic planning template

Goal			
Objective (initiative)	Responsible	Accountable	Partners
Initiative description			
Requirements and interdependencies			Stakeholders
Action plan			Estimated time
KPIs			Estimated budget

The spectrum of IPE-CP extends from simple to complex structures depending on competencies and contextual issues that demand careful planning along with quality assurance. For example, emergency care IP teams may be diverse and not constant over some time as compared to community IP teams for their comprehensive services to the person, family, and communities. Similarly, chronic disease-integrated teams usually grow as service organizations in themselves over a long period.

Succinctly, IPE would be serving as a basic educational strategy to deliver a competency-based curriculum as a future approach to universal health coverage in this decade [19].

King Saud University (KSU), in collaboration with Monash University-Australia, adopted a strategic plan template that could apply to all educational programs' strategic planning (Table 1.1).

This template involves the general goals, specific objectives (initiatives), responsible agencies, accountable departments, partners, stakeholders involved, timeline to achieve the initiative, required budget if needed, initiative's description, initiative's requirements and interdependencies, achievement actions, and key performance indicators (KPIs) for monitoring and evaluation of the strategy.

1.4 Developing IPE Centers of Excellence

A center of excellence (CoE) refers to a group or team with subject matter expertise that supports the organizational environment to conduct high-standard research, education, and training [20]. A CoE is established by the organization with a mandate to develop future leaders of specialized experts who constantly pursue progress and advancement to generate new knowledge; sustain innovation, standardize best practices in the provision of outstanding healthcare, education, information technology, industry, and business; and leveraging internal and external resources in a blended manner is a critical aspect of CoE. In recent decades across different countries, numerous research and higher education institutions and healthcare institutions have established centers of excellence with a common belief in excellence and intention to meet the requirements associated with excellence.

The basic determinants of a CoE are identified as the following features [20]:

- Outstanding visionary leadership with diverse specialized teams,
- Well-defined objectives,
- Exceptional communication within and outside,
- Participative decision-making,
- An excellent research environment, and,
- Planned staff recruitment.

Moreover, CoE's infrastructure and robust governance are among the other determinants that provide international visibility and recognition of high research quality and output. In this respect, exceptional leadership qualities are of critical importance for creating a true research culture and environment that inspire high-performance experts to further the higher-order strategic goals in areas of innovation or related social impact.

1.5 Scope of Centers of Excellence for IPE

Leadership commitment to excellence is critical to inspire the overall functions and long-term visions of the CoE. The leadership challenge is to explore resources for financially sustainable mechanisms which can be from government institutions, lending agencies, and public–private partnerships, or create capacity for the generation of revenues through consultancy or services in areas of training or research. Moreover, the participatory approach to decision-making is of significant importance for staff retention, motivation, and ambition.

The mission of most CoE proposals aims at academic and socio-economic outcomes creating scientific excellence, educational, technological, and learning innovations, policy direction, or development at regional levels. Therefore, academic CoEs should progress constantly with a drive to be high-quality performers and develop an academic environment that can nurture and retain high-performer students and researchers with exceptional attributes, that can form the basis of a dynamic society.

In the developing world, the concept of CoE is emerging in research and higher education sectors with senior professors' concentration on specific areas of scholarly work and expertise. International organizations assist in particular higher education institutions of developing countries in the development of CoE to fill in the knowledge gaps and build research capacity through strengthening higher education and collaborative research in priority areas of the region [21].

The commitment to interprofessional education and collaborative practice is increasing worldwide. Therefore, educational and health systems are implementing a variety of curricula and organizational models to support the advancement of interprofessional education and collaboration across classroom and practice-based experiences. Many CoE in IPE and IPECP are in existence nowadays utilizing different organizational strategy and governance that meet local and global needs. For establishing a novel CoE in IPE and CP, institutional experts can benefit from an established center with similar needs and use it as a reference or even a benchmark.

1.6 The Proposed Center of Excellence for IPE at KSU

Recent years have witnessed major changes in health professional education, which comes in response to the changes in the system of working in the health field. Most healthcare systems nowadays are characterized by high and rising costs as well as gaps in quality, safety, equity, and access. Health professional education (HPE) has not kept pace with these challenges because of fragmented, outdated, and static curricula that produce ill-equipped graduates. Moreover, there is a considerable mismatch of competencies to patient and population needs, poor teamwork, hospital-based more than primary care and community training, quantitative and qualitative imbalances in the professional labor market, and weak leadership to improve the health-system performance [22].

Studies of regional and many international initiatives stressed the need to improve HPE beyond the acquisition of knowledge and skills, to learning that emphasizes professionalism and the development of leadership attributes as a change agent. In addition, HPE programs should develop from working in isolation to more interprofessional education and collaboration, local and global networking, alliances, and consortia. The twenty-first century's HPE programs are expected to graduate professionals who can cope with modern practices by adapting competencies that match developing healthcare systems and public health needs [9].

Educational reforms require comprehensive strategic planning based on needs assessment and healthcare problem identification. Reforms, whether instructional or institutional, require enabling actions to achieve the overall goals of the strategic plan.

Instructional reforms may include competency-based curricula matching local contexts and needs, teamwork through the promotion of interprofessional education, adoption of new pedagogic instruments and IT, addressing changing local contexts, global education, addressing current health problems, outreach programs, and anticipating emerging health problems. *Institutional reforms* may include the promotion of professionalism and leadership, strengthening local resources, aligning institutional reform with national efforts and involving all stakeholders, extending education to primary care and community, linking together with national and international networks, and nurturing a culture of critical inquiry.

Pursuit of these reforms will naturally face some challenges and barriers that require some *enabling actions* such as the engagement of experts and leaders at all levels (local, national, and international); financial support from multi resources including government, private sectors, foundations, donations, research grants, etc.; alignment with national and international accreditation bodies; involvement of all stakeholders; and enrichment of educational research as supporting evidence. Educational and institutional goals for health vary from one university to another based on local contexts and needs. In general, the ultimate goal is to promote transformative and interdependent professional education for equity in health [9, 23, 24].

Transformative learning as an outcome implies leadership attributes that can make three educational shifts; first, from fact memorization to critical reasoning, searching, analysis and synthesis of information, and decision making; second, from seeking professional credentialing to achieving core competencies for effective team working in complex healthcare systems; and third, from non-critical adoption of educational models to creative adaptation of global resources to address local priorities. *Interdependence* in education is a key element in the systemic approach to health problems, in which systems' components and disciplines interact with each other to make three shifts in education; first, from isolation to harmonized education and health systems; second, from standalone institutions to networks, alliances, and consortia; and third, from self-regulated and self-controlled institutional assets to harnessing global flows of educational content and resources and innovations.

In the last couple of decades, IT advancements have revolutionized student-teacher roles and shifted the focus of learning from basic to transformative learning at the undergraduate and postgraduate levels. Therein, IPE provides the opportunity to learn across medical disciplines and amid different levels of learning, with varying roles of the team members involved in a particular task.

The concept of IPE in the Arab world is relatively new and the medical schools are preparing to adopt it with presumably enough required means. The challenges that may be confronted are, extensive curriculum changes according to the need assessment of professions and training of the faculty to switch to much more complex transformative learning demands as compared to previous informative or formative learning.

Vocational education is not ignored, and the Kingdom of Saudi Arabia is part of this global movement. Perhaps the most important evidence is the spread of centers concerned with continuing HPE in hospitals and health cities. This is in addition to the large expansion in the establishment of colleges of health professions disciplines. However, these efforts need to be more efficient by a systems approach that is controlled by expert educational and healthcare leaders who will fix the bolts and nuts of the educational framework through the provision of graduates who are knowledgeable, skillful, professional, and leaders as change agents. The purpose is to enhance the performance of the health systems for meeting the needs of patients and the population equitably and efficiently.

Based on its responsibility, the vice-rector ship for health specialties (VRHSs) at KSU carried out an analytical study of the educational system and health services at the university as they take advantage of the available information on the level of health services and developmental mobility in the corridors of the national health system, regional and global level. In light of this study [25], the VRHSs have the honor to raise a proposal to establish the CoE in IPE (CEIPE).

1.7 Needs Assessment

Needs assessment included:

- Reviewing selected and relevant student and faculty surveys conducted before the NCAAA visits [26].
- Performing extensive SWOT analysis.
- Reviewing program accreditation preparedness reports carried out by external reviewers for HSCs.
- Reviewing other evaluations of initiatives for graduate health education programs by external academic and commercial consulting groups.

1.8 Summary of the Main Results of the Study

The result of these reviews and analyses indicated an obvious need to improve health professions education in all HSCs, especially in the areas of teaching, learning, and most importantly, assessment and evaluation. The core project group conducted a 1-day strategic workshop at KSU during which the group discussed the various issues related to the programs and developed a preliminary strategic plan and set of goals focusing on these aspects, thereby providing the basis for the planning and implementation of the center.

Perhaps one of the most important conclusions of this study is that the proposed center is an innovative approach to improve and foster IPECP across all health science colleges (HSCs) at KSU, developed with the involvement of all stakeholders, and supported by experts' facilitation and structured programs and exercises. The university will move quickly to implement the strategic plan and "the center" using a phased approach. The most important aspects to be considered for the implementation process may include the following:

- Supporting the project by the state health service and education.
- The presence of a large number of health professions schools with a variety of specialties is a step towards providing effective national cadres as a tributary of strong healthcare.
- Availability of infrastructure and financial resources and human talent.
- Cognition and higher awareness of the importance of change and development of educational and training programs provided to keep pace with modern trends in learning health professions in terms of preparation and development of curricula, teaching methods, and assessment.
- Creation of quality management modules in health professional schools and the readiness of all HSCs to adopt the National Commission for Academic Accreditation and Assessment (NCAAA) standards [27].
- Creation of medical education departments/units in health professions schools.
- Curriculum development: obviously, most health science curricula need comprehensive development to keep pace with changes in informatics and successive

technical developments in the field of healthcare, with a focus on integration among HSCs adopting interdisciplinary education.

- Creating new mechanisms for education and training: Because of the omission of the importance of providing the ideal environment and basic tools and techniques, there has been a wide gap between the content and educational experiences for students and the training competencies and skills required to carry out the role of effective and safe practice in the healthcare system. This is in addition to the weakness that the health system is suffering at the level of integrative mechanisms that guarantee the achievement of the goal for integrated education, thus ensuring the spirit of working in teams that include many disciplines.
- Developing evaluation mechanisms: Methods of assessment of students and programs are mostly traditional that often don't guarantee credibility and stability, and they also suffer a lack of tools and capabilities needed to analyze assessment results.
- Scarcity of scientific research for HPE: There is reluctance and a lack of significant scientific research in the field of HPE, especially research related to the assessment of program outputs and measuring the results of developmental mobility. Although there are efforts to develop assessment and evaluation methods in a lot of health professional colleges, most of these efforts are done individually and do not achieve the goal of integrated education.
- Poor interprofessional cooperation among HSCs: Despite the conviction inherent to all employees of the health sector to the health system integrity starting from the educational process and through the process of training, research, and finally the service, it is noticed that there is a lack of genuine cooperation among colleges of health professions. Therefore, the potential of financial, material, and human resources is not exploited optimally.

Extrapolating from the previous analysis results, it is clear to us that there is a need to establish a center of excellence in the field of health professions education and training to deal with the activities of educational and related health facilities as a single integrated system. This includes the provision of technical support, training, and consultations for colleges and faculty members to be able to prepare curricula compatible with modern health practices; to be one of the most important merits of integration among the various HSCs; to provide an enabling environment that stimulates innovative thinking to enhance the ability to solve problems; to communicate and work as one team; to provide learning and teaching methods and innovative technology that make the educational process attractive to students; and to make practical and clinical training closely linked to the real role expected from graduates in the framework of the health team. Therefore, they will not get shocked by real practice after graduation by an educational program that does not prepare them for safe and effective practice.

In addition, there is a preparation of cadres capable of assessing students in ways that credibly measure the extent of achieving the educational process goals and targeted output of the program as a whole.

1.9 Strategy for the Proposed Center

It became obvious that the nature of the healthcare system is characterized by change and continuous development. The scope of change includes the development of roles and adding new members of the health team such as physician assistants and advanced nursing practitioners. This resulted in continuous improvement in health systems over the years to provide healthcare by more complex teams, which lead to the need to focus on the process of preparing graduates of the health professions on the ability to work in a team to ensure better results and improve the rates of safe practice and quality of care provided. Therefore, we find that international recommendations in the field of HPE focus on the necessity of integration, and almost all advocate interprofessional and multidisciplinary education. For example, "The Future of Medical Education in Canada" project [28], recommends a cultural change in faculties of medicine and other health professions to create positive attitudes towards the adoption of interprofessional and interdisciplinary and professionalism among the members of faculty and students.

The establishment of such a center is a unique orientation of its kind in the Gulf region and the Arab world as it is one of the strategies resorted to by American and Canadian universities to improve health professions education based on previous recommendations. It is also the center that will contribute directly to the achievement of KSU strategic goals, especially the second goal that aims at reaching "for faculty distinguished by improving the level of support for faculty members," as well as the fourth goal for "strengthening the capacity of graduates by supporting skills faculty members and upgrade them in addition to employ creative teaching methods in academic programs" as it is stipulated in the strategic plan of the University. As KSU has a leading role in the region, we see the CEIPE plays its role in this unique area to become a scientific guide for health professional colleges and lead to healthcare system improvement through preparing national and regional cadres ready for competitiveness.

1.10 Vision

To become a leading referral center for global excellence in health professional education, training, and collaboration.

1.11 Mission Statement

To develop education and provide modern training; and to foster interprofessional collaboration to enhance the performance of modern healthcare systems for meeting the needs of patients and population equitably and efficiently.

1.12 Values

Interprofessional education and collaboration among HSCs professionals to share, but not exclusively, the following common values:

- Leadership.
- Teamwork.
- Scientific inquiry.
- Critical analysis.
- Coping with uncertainty.
- Anticipating and planning for the future.

1.13 Goals

- Creating a common education and training reference for health science colleges at KSU.
- Implementing, monitoring, and evaluating the strategic plan for the achievement of successful learning, excellent teaching, and effective assessment in HPE.
- Applying interprofessional education and interdisciplinary collaboration among HSCs and healthcare facilities.
- Providing educational resources for faculty and students for best educational practices.
- Providing training and support for faculty members to develop their activities and research in the field of HPE.
- Developing management and leadership qualities among faculty members in healthcare professions to cope with the speed of global changes in the educational environment.

1.14 Recipes for the CoE in IPE

The following qualities are considered mandatory for supporting the center to reach excellence in HPE:

- Strong administrative support of the Rector and Vice-Rector for Educational and Academic Affairs.
- Strong support of all Deans of HSCs.
- Interprofessional coordination and collaboration among health colleges at the university.
- The necessity for the quality management unit at the center to be established.
- Full-time professional staff and qualified instructors in the clinical skills center.
- Presence of qualified faculty, statisticians and research assistants, administrative personnel, secretaries, and a treasurer in the "health professional education center."

- Providing educational opportunities for all faculty members in HSCs with the help of local and international experts through courses and workshops.
- Presence of national or international benchmarks and networking to provide advice when needed.
- A new building for the center that holds offices, a main auditorium, lecture halls, small group learning rooms, a library, and clinical skills lab.
- IT support from the university for processing an autonomous database unit related to the center for electronic transactions, e-learning resources, distant learning and training, and webinars.
- Developing the center's website further.

1.15 Steps in Planning

Project launch and Core Project Team:

This project was originally launched in May 2010 following the directives of the VRHSs of KSU in Riyadh, Saudi Arabia to improve HPE in all HSCs. A Project Director was appointed and a group of experts in HPE representing all HSCs were chosen and officially appointed to lead and manage this program (the leadership committee). The core planning team was thereby officially established and began working with key stakeholders at KSU.

Stakeholders include the Vice-Rector for Educational and Academic Affairs and related educational section heads; the Dean of Quality and Development; the Dean of Skills Development; the Dean of e-Learning and Distance Learning; the Dean of Faculty Affairs; Dean of Students Affairs; Dean of Admission and Registration Affairs; Dean of Library Affairs; and Deans and Vice-Deans for Academic and Quality Affairs of the various HSCs. HSCs include medicine, dentistry, pharmacy, applied medical sciences, nursing, and emergency medical services. There are upwards of 2000 faculty members across the HSCs responsible for the education of more than 7000 graduate and undergraduate students. In addition, educational consultants from outside KSU were invited and participated in the planning process.

The next stage of the project was to design strategic, business, and program plans (Fig. 1.1), and an initial governance structure. During this project planning phase, the VRHSs oversaw all aspects of the project, and the director of the program managed the project. This includes leading all the program workshops, attending all pertinent committee meetings, presenting the project to all relevant stakeholders, and acting as a liaison among the different working groups. To complete the rest of the strategic plan tasks on time, the Core Project Group was divided into three committees:

- The Teaching and Learning (T&L) Steering Committee which comprised six members representing all HSCs, has the task to complete all action plans for the teaching and learning goals and initiatives and corresponding KPIs.

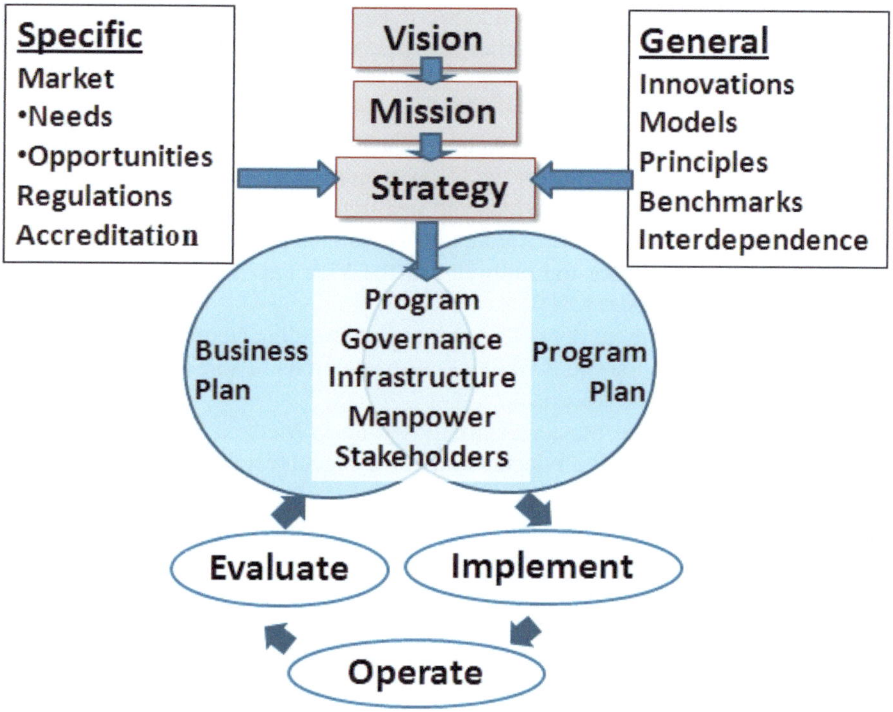

Fig. 1.1 Strategic, business, and program plans

- The Assessment and Evaluation (A&E) Steering Committee consisted of the same number of members and college representation, having the same tasks as the T&L committee but as related to A&E.
- The Leadership Committee for Health Sciences Education comprised the heads of the T&L units that were established in the meantime in each HSC as agreed upon and recommended by the various Deans and the VRHS. The heads of these units were carefully chosen based on their educational background, interest, and commitment to the program in particular, and the promotion of HPE at KSU in general. The committee members representing all HSCs, supported by other consultants from the college of education and educational psychology at KSU, had the responsibility for reviewing and analyzing all recommendations presented by the T&L and A&E committees and liaising with their corresponding HSCs as necessary to obtain feedback. They also had the responsibility for providing all necessary documents and data needed from the HSCs and more widely across KSU including information requested by the other two committees. A significant role was to facilitate the conduct of the program activities in the various HSCs. The Assistant Vice-Rector for Development Affairs in the VRHS office provided support for this program in IT, quality assurance, finance, personnel, and communication including educational endeavors outside KSU.

Other multiple activities were conducted during the 2-year development period, which aided the buy-in from all parties and the creation of an acceptable product. These other activities included:

- Faculty development workshops were conducted upon the request of HSCs.
- Collaboration with the Chair for the Development of Medical Education at KSU in its faculty development activities and research.
- Liaison and dialogue with the Center for Distinguished Teaching and Learning activities, working under the umbrella of the Vice-Rectorship for Educational and Academic Affairs at KSU.
- Consultation with the Student Guidance and Counseling Center at KSU.
- Review of some courses and faculty staff evaluations in some HSCs providing honest and confidential feedback.
- Collaboration with the Master Degree Program in Medical Education at KSU, including an agreement to educate and certify faculty members from this program every 2 years.

1.16 Overall Approach

Given that the proposed Center represented a major change at KSU, we employed a three-stage process that was used successfully in the past to affect curriculum reform as well as the creation of new programs, curricula, and institutions [29].

Stage 1 Create a distinct vision and mission and translate this into a strategy that combines specific needs, regulatory requirements, and opportunities, with institutional values and general goals based on models and benchmarks. The template of KSU strategic planning was used for that purpose. It includes the main goal that includes the specific objective (initiative), description of the initiative, responsible, accountability, partners, stakeholders, requirements and interdependencies, action plan, KPIs, timeframe, and estimated budget.

Stage 2 Make the desirable doable by ensuring that the program plan is based on a solid business plan addressing not only program elements, but also the appropriate governance, necessary resources, and a concrete plan to address professional development needs. At this stage, KSU decided to enter into a consultative relationship with PHMI, and then PHI conducted a 2-day strategic workshop in Riyadh attended by all internal stakeholders. The goal of this facilitated workshop was to explore commonalities and differences between the HSCs at KSU in their visions, missions, goals, competencies, and existing strategies for Teaching, Learning, and Assessment.

The workshop accomplished the following:

- It initiated the creation of a community of practice involving educators from all related colleges.
- It defined the topics and projects for near-term work.

- It created a common understanding of the issues and the necessary early steps in moving forward.
- It outlined long-term goals.

These long-term goals included the following:

- Refinement of the vision, missions, and goals of various colleges.
- Alignment of their strategic plans with the overall strategic plan of the university.
- Creation of a governance structure for the Center in the long run.
- Definition of the common competencies for all health sciences graduates of KSU, i.e., "the trademark of a KSU graduate."
- Career opportunities (including promotion) in education for the change teams as well as the faculty at large.

Shortly after the workshop outlined above, the VRHS and members of the core project group representing all themes attended a 6-day course at Harvard Macy Institute (HMI) in Boston, entitled *Leading Innovations in Health Care and Education*. One of the course requirements was that participants worked on a change project important to their home institution. During the previous workshop in Riyadh, teaching, learning, and assessment-themed projects were chosen to be worked on by different teams.

About 6 months after this key workshop, some of the leading group members and the Deans of the HSCs attended a 16-day course at HMI entitled *Program for Educators in Health Professions* to discuss and complete their assigned project tasks. After the course, the core project group synthesized all tasks and projects into a unified vision, mission statements, strategic goals, and corresponding objectives (initiatives) in a 2-day workshop in Riyadh.

The final intensive 6-day course at HMI entitled *A System Approach to Assessment in Health Professions Education* was attended by the program director to finalize the strategic plan and structure of the program with consultation from HMI faculty and scholars. Throughout all Boston-based activities at HMI, PHI conducted special sessions and meetings to aid in the further development of the KSU project.

Stage 3 Implement, monitor, and evaluate the strategic and business plans with quality assurance in mind by addressing success metrics from the outset.

1.17 Governance Structure of "The Center"

The Vice-Rector for Educational and Academic Affairs will be on top of the governance pyramid of this center, as the VRHSs has been merged with KSU Medical City, assisted by two advisory boards, an internal advisory board represented by the deans of HSCs, and external advisory board represented by external consultations and benchmarks. This is followed by the director of the center and supported by the assistant director for administrative affairs and the assistant director for academic

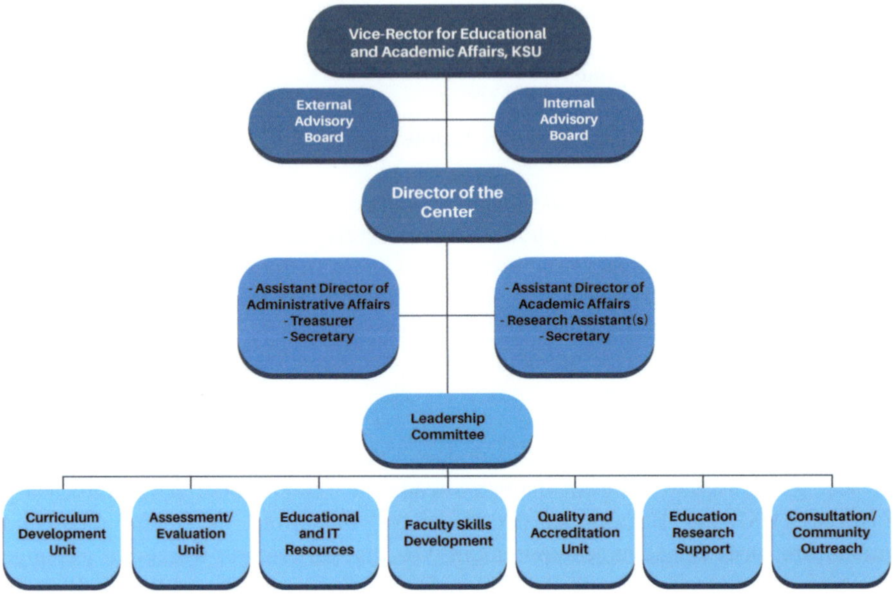

Fig. 1.2 The governance structure of "the center"

affairs. The center will be run by two experienced secretaries who will help each other to execute all related administrative and academic works of the center. Ideally, the center should have its financial treasurer and research assistant(s). Under the director of the center comes the leadership committee that is represented by the heads of health professional education units/medical education departments of HSCs and seven functional units (Fig. 1.2).

The *Vice-Rector for Education and Academic Affairs* will have the following responsibilities:

- General supervision of the performance and activities of the center.
- Consultation of the Deans of HSCs on the progress and issues related to the center in the presence of the director of the center, who will present quarterly updates.
- Annual consultation of external experts in the field of HPE and/or educational institute(s) representatives to discuss the annual report of the center in the presence of HSCs deans and the debriefing presentation by the director of the center.

The *Internal Advisory Board* represented by *Deans* of HSCs will:

- Attend the quarterly meetings of the center's updates with the Vice-Rector for Education and Academic Affairs and share the center's impact and issues on professional education developments in each HSC.

- Attend the annual report debriefing with the Vice-Rector for Education and Academic Affairs and the External Advisory Board, and share HSC's experience of the center's impact and issues on HPE.
- Give their feedback and advice for further improvement and development of the center's functions.

The *External Advisory Board* represented by educational institutes and experts from outside KSU will:

- Study the annual report,
- Attend the annual debriefing workshop and share feedback for further improvement and development of the center,
- Contribute to educational expertise,
- Share programs,
- Exchange experience.

The *Director of the Center* will be responsible for:

- The leadership of the center.
- Liaison with the Vice-Rector for Education and Academic Affairs and Advisory Boards.
- Networking with local and global health professional education institutes.
- Chairing the monthly meeting of the leadership committee of the center.
- Development of the various units of the center.

The *Assistant Director for Academic Affairs* will be responsible for:

- Management of the academic affairs of the center.
- Assistance in the development of the various units of the center.
- Management of academic meetings, workshops, seminars, etc.
- Liaison with HSCs and all academic and educational centers at KSU.
- Assistance in all works of the research assistant.
- Assistance in all works of the academic secretary.

The *Assistant Director for Administrative Affairs* will be responsible for:

- Management of the administrative affairs of the center.
- Assistance in the development of the various units of the center.
- Liaison with the various departments and sections inside and outside KSU.
- Assistance in all works of the administrative secretary.
- Supervision and assistance of the Treasurer.

The *Research Assistant(s)* will be responsible for:

- Management of the center's database.
- Data collection, analysis, and reporting.

- Liaison with the various research centers and institutes inside and outside KSU.
- Assistance in the conduct, production, and publication of research.

The *Treasurer* will be responsible for:

- Management of all financial affairs of the center.
- Liaising with financial suppliers, beneficiaries, and all other stakeholders.
- Production of the quarterly financial report.

The *secretaries* will be responsible for:

- All secretarial works of the center and IT affairs.
- Arrangement for meetings, workshops, and events.

1.18 The Leadership Committee and Functional Units of the Center

The *Leadership Committee* will:

- Make the general strategies of the center in alignment with KSU educational strategies.
- Facilitate their implementation, monitoring, and evaluation at all levels.
- Foster education and training of the personnel needed for the aforementioned processes.
- Facilitate the exchange of expertise and resources among HSCs.
- Support and develop the various functional units of the center.
- Liaise between the central leadership and health professional units/medical education departments at all HSCs.
- Supervise all educational and academic activities of the center.
- Support and develop all research activities of the center.

1.19 Curriculum Development Unit

Curriculum as an educational model is a sensitive subject when it comes to the discussion by some HSCs. Each HSC is following a curricular model that has been developed over many years of adjustment and refinement. Any major disruption of such a model may lead to resistance and extreme rejection of any change. That is why we started our strategic plan for HPE development by the development of learning, teaching, and assessment to avoid curriculum change sensitivity. Once this plan has been developed and implemented, then all HSCs may be ready to discuss the development of their curricula and eventually its development. However, each HSC must come out of its silo and get involved in an interprofessional exchange of knowledge and experience of modern curricula that match local and global healthcare demands, and patients and population needs. The following discussion highlights updated knowledge and research on *curriculum development* that need to be considered by all HSCs.

Curriculum development has undergone several transitions and forms through the last century. The *Flexner era* at the beginning of the twentieth century was noted for the idea of teaching basic sciences as the basis of clinical sciences and practice [30]. In the 1970s, *problem-based learning* was strongly promoted in an attempt to integrate basic, clinical, and social sciences through the use of problem scenarios [31]. *Competency/outcomes-based curricula* became popular around the turn of this century [32]. The key competencies focus on demonstrable professional outcomes guided by local and global needs [33]. *Curriculum mapping* is an essential tool for curriculum development [34] when educators can align all aspects of the program that include the expected learning outcomes; curriculum content or areas of expertise covered; assessment; learning opportunities; learning location; learning resources; timetable; curriculum management; and educators and learners. Harden's SPICES model [35] [15] is another innovation for curriculum development that recommends some curricular components' shift from one traditional extreme to another developed one (Fig. 1.3).

On the other hand, Kern et al. [36] highlighted a six-step approach for curricular development (Fig. 1.4).

Harden's SPICES model addressed six curricular component shifts that need to be considered seriously by educators for curricular development. The degree of the shift, however, may be different from one component to another according to needs and available resources and expertise in the program. The six-step curriculum development approach described by Kern et al. [36] includes performing a general and specific needs assessment, writing goals and objectives, determining content,

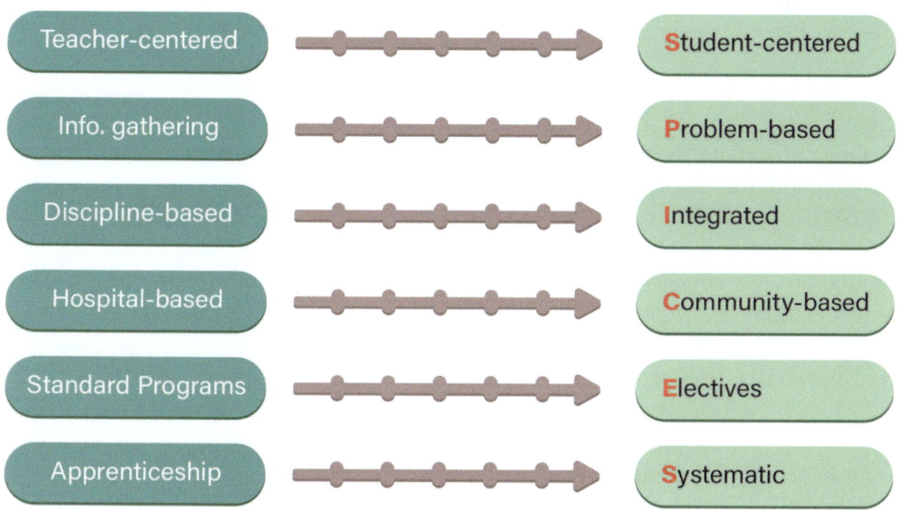

Fig. 1.3 Harden's SPICES Model

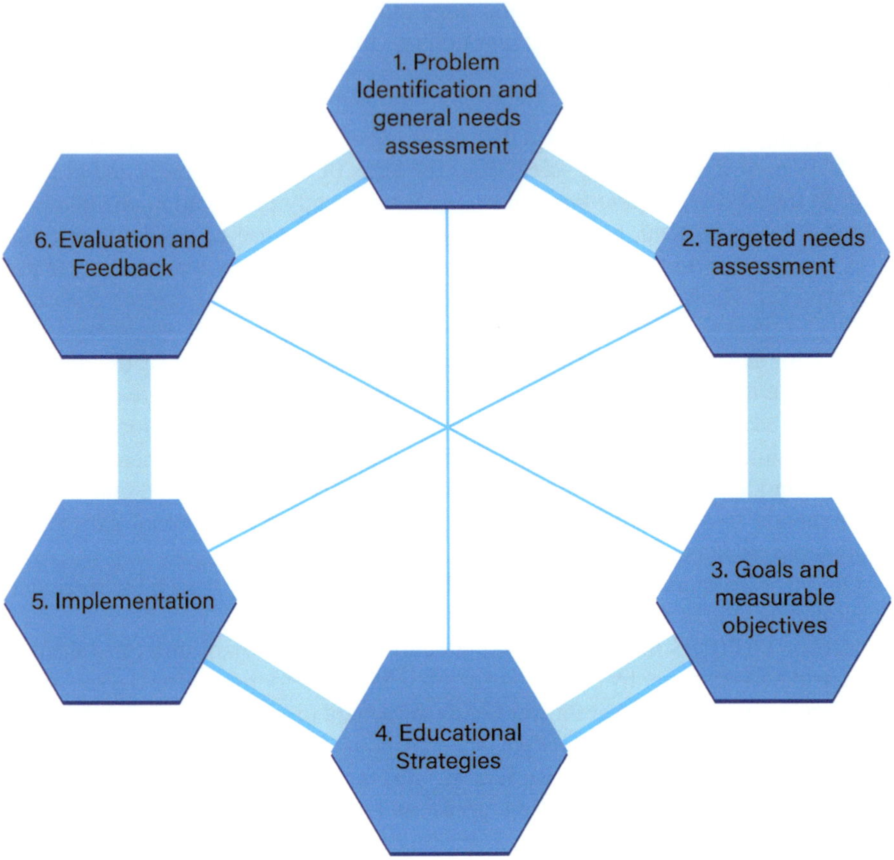
1. Problem Identification and general needs assessment
2. Targeted needs assessment
3. Goals and measurable objectives
4. Educational Strategies
5. Implementation
6. Evaluation and Feedback

Fig. 1.4 Kern's six-steps framework

selecting educational strategies, implementing the curriculum, and finally evaluating the curriculum for feedback and further improvement.

Once this center is approved, supported, and started to operate, the curriculum development unit should formulate a *curriculum development steering committee (CDSC)*, represented by the heads of HSCs curriculum committees. This committee will replace the *teaching and learning steering committee.* The *CDSC* will be chaired by a nominated member whose term is 4 years, and preferably each period will be led by a different HSC representative at a time unless the corresponding nominee declines for any reason. The *curriculum development steering committee* is expected to follow modern curricular development approaches and start to:

- Implement, monitor, and evaluate the strategic plan pertinent to Learning (Chaps. 9–12) and Teaching (Chaps. 13–16).
- Review and update health science curricula so that they will continue to evolve to become of high quality in line with the healthcare systems demands, patients, and population needs.

- Develop health professional education and participation through innovations in the curriculum that reflects education based on evidence.
- Evaluate the courses through students' feedback according to approved models.
- Monitor management and analysis of the results of approved evaluation models for courses and faculty members.
- Provide professional advice that is evidence-based to HSCs and faculty members.
- Be directly engaged in the development, implementation, and monitoring of various programs during the evaluation of the curriculum.
- Participate in the development of the HSC program to assess the quality of education.
- Facilitate the access of faculty members to international experts and gain experience in HPE.
- Ensure and facilitate students' participation in the management of the curriculum and the assessment process.
- Conduct educational research in curriculum development processes and outcomes.

1.20 Students' Assessment and Programs Evaluation Unit

Students' assessment and program evaluation have been discussed thoroughly in (Chaps. 17–19). Once this center is approved and becomes operational, the Assessment Steering Committee will change to the *Assessment & Evaluation Steering Committee (AESC)*. Similar to the *CDSC*, this new committee will be represented by the heads of HSCs assessment units. The AESC will be chaired by a nominated member whose term is 4 years, and preferably each period will be led by a different HSC representative each term unless the corresponding nominee declines for any reason. The *Assessment & Evaluation Steering Committee* will:

- Implement, monitor, and evaluate the strategic plan pertinent to the Assessment and Evaluation.
- Ensure the use of strong and effective students' assessment that is valid, reliable, and feasible when assessing HSCs students.
- Assure the use of assessment tools appropriate for corresponding tasks and context.
- Make use of the interface and analysis of difficulty indicators.
- Provide expertise and advice to ensure the orderly conduct of examinations.
- Conduct appropriate educational research in students' assessment and program evaluation and make use of results for proper feedback and further improvement.

1.21 Educational and IT Resources Unit

Educational and IT resources have developed exponentially over the last few decades to involve digital libraries, general and specific e-learning resources, articles and databases, literature reviews, images and videos, web citations, and mobile apps. Although most of these resources are costly and provided by different competitive companies, universities usually have good deals in the long run. For the institutes that cannot provide such expensive resources, the government may solve this issue through the Ministry of Education, private donations, or networking with other universities and institutes. Such resources will be necessary to facilitate bridging the gap between education and real clinical practice [17]. This unit can form a group of educational resources recruitment experts at HSCs or KSU that can manage and facilitate the use of state-of-the-art resources by faculty and students. This committee will be responsible for:

- Developing, implementing, monitoring, and evaluating the strategic goals and objectives for educational resources pertinent to learning, teaching, and assessment themes of this manual.
- Developing a learning environment and effective teaching based on the Internet.
- Assisting in the development of a comprehensive strategy for IT.
- Adopting systems for course management and schedule depending on IT.
- Helping to improve communication levels among staff and students who use methods that depend on IT.
- Creating a unified electronic library for HSCs in the center.
- Creating a unified database for HSCs at the Vice-Rectorship for Educational and Academic Affairs.
- Cooperating with other experts inside and outside the university who can help to improve the functions of this unit further.

1.22 Faculty Skills Development Unit

Training and skills development for postgraduates and faculty staff encompasses a wide range of activities including seminars, workshops, courses, and hands-on training in wet and dry laboratories. Currently, the *Clinical Skills & Simulation Center (CSSC)* is conducting several undergraduate and postgraduate courses for healthcare workers under the umbrella of *King Saud University Medical City (KSUMC)*. These courses include skills laboratory, medical simulation, and life-support and trauma courses. On the other hand, the Faculty Skills Development Unit in this center will concentrate on the "teaching" aspect; research involving teaching practice and student learning; and the professionalism and leadership skills of the faculty staff. This has been covered to some extent in (Chaps. 13–16). Moreover, the faculty skills development unit can partner with the *CSSC* for the exchange of some courses, as well as sharing some activities and resources. As described by McLean et al. [37], faculty skills development requires tremendous efforts and strategies to make them voluntarily attracted to develop their teaching and research skills. Therefore, the Faculty Skills Development Unit will be obliged to formulate the *Faculty Skills Development Committee (FSDC)* to plan, implement, monitor, and evaluate faculty skills development activities in collaboration with both the Deanship for Skills Development at KSU and the CSSC at KSUMC. The FSDC will be then responsible for:

- Further developing, implementing, monitoring, and evaluating the strategic plan pertinent to faculty development.
- Conducting needs assessment, similar to the work published by Algahtani et al. [38], and analysis of feedback from the participants to evaluate the results of each activity and use the information to improve future activities.
- Focusing on the development of training programs among health disciplines that include various health professions and promoting the concept of interprofessional education and collaboration.
- Participating in activities of the multidisciplinary health professions such as the "Medical Education Master's Degree Program" at the College of Medicine, and other similar programs in HSCs to promote their recognition as high-level qualifications [39].

1.23 Quality and Accreditation Unit

Although quality management (QM) is widely recognized as a management philosophy for improving customer satisfaction and institutional performance, its use in higher education literature has been limited to some areas such as "leadership," "vision," "measurement and analysis," "process control and evaluation," "programs design and resources allocation," and "stakeholder focus" at different levels [40]. Over the past few decades or so, growing drivers and demands for higher education institutes were noticed to adopt and apply quality management systems (QMSs) to be recognized and accredited. Some of these drivers may include governmental forces and accreditation, economic forces, and socio-cultural forces [41]. There are many QM models available for commercial use, but an institute should choose whatever matches their needs and areas of interest. In HSCs, particularly HPE, areas that need to be qualified and accredited internally by the Quality and Accreditation Unit, and externally by the NCAAA and other international bodies may include learning outcomes, instruction, and training, assessment at all levels, program evaluation, resources utilization, implementation of the strategic objectives of this manual, the satisfaction of stakeholders, costs containment, and data analysis and accuracy.

The HSCs need to establish their own QMS (*see* Chap. 17, *initiative 9: design a comprehensive quality management system [QMS] that dovetails with the university [QMS]),* that can be applied to educational activities, policies, programs' efficiency, etc., for purposes of quality assessment and further improvement, as well as the accreditation by the NCAAA and other authorities. After completing their task for the above initiative, the assessment steering committee can merge with the quality and accreditation unit to work together for its implementation, monitoring, and evaluation. Therefore, a new committee represented by the vice deans for quality and development from all HSCs would be the ideal authority to:

- Provide consultancy and technical support for all HSCs and academic quality units concerning the development, implementation, monitoring, and evaluation of quality management systems and the improvement of their efficiency.
- Assist health professions colleges to meet the elements of quality and accreditation set by national or international authorities in cooperation and coordination with other units of the center.
- Develop and implement a program of continuous quality improvement of the performance of all other units of "the center."
- Partner with scientific institution's counterparts to research the development of quality standards and practices.
- Confirm the commitment of HSC staff to work towards the success of its quality improvement plans.
- Promote quality culture across all HSCs to increase their academic and administrative productivity.

1.24 Educational Research Support Unit

Medical education is traditionally known among medical educators who have an interest or qualification in this field. However, not all teachers in health professional schools are educators, or interested or qualified in medical education. Few teachers resist and antagonize innovations in health professional education claiming that "what they have been doing is still efficient" and prefer to continue "the status quo!"

To generate more teachers' buy-in, to be interested and qualified in health professional education, educators have to "make strange" [41]. This implies bringing (e.g. transformative learning, flip classes, interprofessional education, etc.), that make teachers ponder and wonder. Once they reach this stage of critical thinking, they will most likely ask for more information and data, which is the product of the "educational research." Therefore, most changes happen when innovative strategies in HPE are substantiated by data and evidence.

In health science programs, most of the research published in medical/health professional education has been limited in amount and quality compared to basic sciences and clinical research, and mostly championed by highly qualified educators and experts who are known in this field. Training and certification of more educators will increase the production of more research in this field. Furthermore, more funding and recognition of educational research in faculty promotion would also foster more interest and enthusiasm.

Faculty need a research-supporting environment that encompasses the provision of educational resources, research assistants and statisticians, regular symposia and workshops, and the creation of the proposed *Educational Research Unit*. (*See* Chap. 13*: faculty development and educational research, initiative 5–6: provide support for educational research*).

Like the other units of the center, elite educational research experts from HSCs and other non-health colleges at KSU would formulate a research expert group/committee led by a nominated leader who will be elected and appointed by voting for a term of 4 years, renewable for another term when necessary. This committee will form the backbone of the Educational Research Unit. Supported by the aforementioned *initiative*, the research expert group will:

- Develop, monitor, and evaluate (Chap. 13, initiative 5–6: provide support for educational research).
- Encourage and support scientific research activities in the field of HPE through submitted and published research.
- Provide secretarial and translation services for researchers in the field of health professional education.
- Provide editing services in the field of scientific research, statisticians, data management, and literature review services for researchers in the field of HPE.
- Establish ties of cooperation and networking with other research groups locally and internationally.
- Develop a program for activities that promote further educational research.
- Seek research grants and donations to support health professional research in general and research related to the unit in particular.

1.25 Consultations and Community Outreach Unit

Once "the center" becomes operational and experienced, it can expand its functions and services outside KSU boundaries by providing studies and consolatory services to develop and promote HPE in other universities and institutes. This work can be shared by all units under the umbrella of the center's leadership as a business unit that will make use of its revenues for ongoing expenditures and incentives of all units of the center. This business will not only help in solving some financial issues of the center only, but it will also enrich its experience and networking locally and globally. Therefore, an ad hoc committee will be formulated for each project to:

- Provide consultancy services at all educational levels.
- Create a unified reference supported by a detailed database of excellence at KSU in the areas of HPE.
- Provide studies and scientific and technical support for the establishment and development of educational institutions and health educational centers at the national and regional levels.
- Identify health problems in the Kingdom and put mechanisms and systems to deal with priorities in the areas of education, training, and certification.
- Actively get involved with organizations and institutions that are directly and indirectly related to health professional education products. For example, but not limited to, the Saudi Commission for Health Specialties.
- Support further partnership with the Saudi Society for Medical Education (SSME).

- Participate in a wide spectrum of society's activities including patients and their families, governors of students, the labor market, and government agencies concerned, and communicate with them and benefit from their feedback in the formulation and revision of plans and curricula.

1.26 Progression of Governance

In order to maintain and improve a quality performance of the governance and operational units, we have to ensure gradual implementation and progression of the strategies, policies, guidelines, budgets and oversight, with a continuous monitoring by the internal advisory board (e.g., The leadership committee that represent all HSCs) and periodical monitoring by an external review committee (e.g., outside advisory board and benchmarks), continuous institutional resources support, involvement of the middle management level (e.g., Deans, vice-deans and heads of the departments) as authoritative people, and the courses' directors/faculty/students as operational executives. Data collection and feedback from the operational units would help in maintaining and actually improving their quality with time, so the strategies and policies can be updated for improvement every 5 years or so (Fig. 1.5).

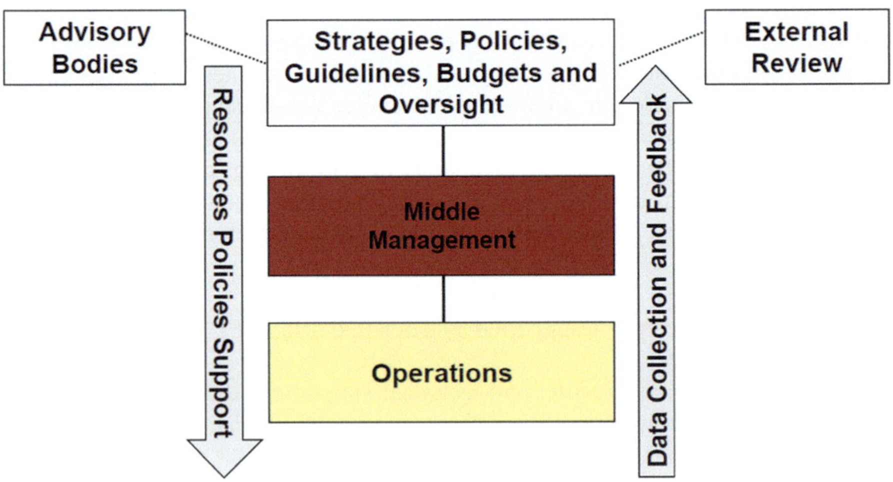

Fig. 1.5 Progression of governance

1.27 Implementation Action Steps

Of course, once the program (center) is established a careful implementation strategy should be considered to decrease the burden on faculty and students, absorb and manage challenges and obstacles efficiently, and avoid implementation resistance. Below are some of the suggested action steps for the implementation process:

- Decide on organizational structure and initiate implementation group.
- Decide on priorities (match need with feasibility and impact) and design pilot projects.
- Develop overall timeline.
- Develop pro forma business plan.
- Create initial physical and IT infrastructure.
- Create communications strategy (webpage, newsletter, list serves).
- Roll out pilot projects.
- Conduct faculty development workshop to promote and demonstrate capabilities and plans and enlist interested faculty.
- Evaluate pilots and adjust timeline and roll-out of the center.

In conclusion, the proposed Center is an innovative approach to improve and foster health professions educational development across all HSCs at KSU, developed with the involvement of all stakeholders, and supported by outside facilitation and structured programs and exercises. The University will move quickly to implement the Center using a phased approach. The toolkit for successful implementation of "the center" includes a pro forma business plan, implementation groups' training, matching needs with feasibility and impact on HSCs, initiation of pilot projects starting with the implementation of some interprofessional courses, establishment of an initial physical and IT infrastructure of the center, development of the webpage and newsletter and list serves, and improvement of faculty development programs further at HSCs in specific and KSU in general.

1.28 Summary

HPE has undergone dramatic changes over the last century through many stages of innovation. Driving forces included increasing demands by the ever-developing healthcare systems, patients, and society. On the other hand, educational programs are becoming under continuous pressure by global and local demands for development and accreditation to match the healthcare demands of the twenty-first century. KSU is taking up the challenge of enacting these recommendations by studying needs assessment results of students and faculty surveys, reports of readiness for accreditation, and accredited programs. It became obvious that KSU and HSCs are enthusiastic and willing to develop their programs further through a planned strategy to address the learning, teaching, and assessment, and create a center of excellence in IPE-CP.

References

1. Interprofessional education: what, how & when? CAIPE Bulletin; 1997;13:19. https://www.caipe.org/resources/publications/archived-publications/caipe-bulletin-nos-13-1997-interprofessional-education-what-how-when.
2. Barr H. Interprofessional education—today, yesterday and tomorrow: a review. Commissioned by The Learning and Teaching Support Network for Health Sciences & Practice from The UK Centre for the Advancement of Interprofessional Education. https://www.caipe.org/resources/publications/caipe-publications/caipe-2002-interprofessional-education-today-yesterday-tomorrow-barr-h.
3. https://www.caipe.org/resource/CAIPE-Statement-of-Purpose-2016.pdf.
4. Gilbert J, Yan J, Hoffman SJ. A WHO report: a framework for action on interprofessional education and collaborative practice. J Allied Health. 2010;39(Suppl 1):196–7.
5. Global competency and outcomes framework for universal health coverage. World Health Organization. 2022. https://www.who.int/publications/i/item/9789240034662.
6. Brandt BF. Interprofessional education and collaborative practice: welcome to the "new" forty-year-old field. Advisor. 2015;3:9–17.
7. Institute of Medicine. Educating for the Health Team. Washington, DC: National Academy of Sciences; 1972.
8. CAIPE strategy; 2022–2027. https://www.caipe.org/strategy#1.
9. Frenk J, Chen L, Bhutta ZA, Cohen J, Crisp N, Evans T, et al. Health professionals for a new century: transforming education to strengthen health systems in an interdependent world. Lancet. 2010;376(9756):1923–58.
10. Schmitt M, Blue A, Aschenbrener C, Viggiano T. Core competencies for interprofessional collaborative practice: reforming health care by transforming health professionals' education. Acad Med. 2011;86(11):1351.
11. Interprofessional. Global Confederation. 2018. https://interprofessional.global/confederation/.
12. Khalili H, Thistlethwaite J, El-Awaisi A, Pfeifle A, Gilbert J, Lising D, Xyrichis A. Guidance on global interprofessional education and collaborative practice research: a discussion paper, 2019;29.
13. Alruthia Y, Bashatah A, Batis A, Alradhi S, Almohammed O, Sales I, et al. Exploring the opportunities and challenges to implementing interprofessional education in Saudi Arabia: a qualitative study among faculty. J Interprof Care. 2022;37:1–11.
14. Health Professions Accreditors Collaborative. Guidance on developing quality interprofessional education for the health professions. Chicago, IL: Health Professions Accreditors Collaborative; 2019. https://www.cpme.org/files/CPME/Guidance%20on%20Developing%20Quality%20Interprofessional%20Education%20for%20the%20Health%20Professions.pdf.
15. Business & Consulting Toolkits created by ex-McKinsey, Deloitte & BCG Management Consultants, free sample, 2023. https://www.domontconsulting.com.
16. Van Diggele C, Roberts C, Burgess A, Mellis C. Interprofessional education: tips for design and implementation. BMC Med Educ. 2020;20(Suppl 2):455.
17. Global Forum on Innovation in Health Professional Education, Board on Global Health, Institute of Medicine. Interprofessional education for collaboration: learning how to improve health from interprofessional models across the continuum of education to practice: workshop summary. Interprofessional education, vol. 2. Washington, DC: National Academies Press; 2013. https://www.ncbi.nlm.nih.gov/books/NBK207102/.
18. Hammick M, Freeth D, Koppel I, Reeves S, Barr H. A best evidence systematic review of interprofessional education: BEME Guide no. 9. Med Teach. 2007;29(8):735–51.
19. Global competency and outcomes framework for universal health coverage. Washington, DC: World Health Organization, 2022. https://www.who.int/publications/i/item/9789240034686.
20. Balderston FE. Managing today's university: strategies for viability, change, and excellence. 2nd ed. New York: Wiley; 1995.

21. Sulistyowati E, Walker L. Interprofessional education (IPE) in developing countries: challenges and lessons learnt from its implementation in the United Kingdom: a systematic review. Nurse Media J Nurs. 2019;9(2):197–209.
22. Dzau VJ, Ackerly DC, Sutton-Wallace P, Merson MH, Williams RS, Krishnan KR, et al. The role of academic health science systems in the transformation of medicine. Lancet. 2010;375(9718):949–53.
23. Mezirow J. Learning as transformation: critical perspectives on a theory in progress. San Francisco: Jossy Bass; 2000.
24. Palsdottir B, Neusy AJ. Transforming medical education: lessons learned from THEnet. 2010. Commission paper. http://www.globalommehp.com.
25. Alnaami M, Aretz T, Alshehri M, Daud MZ, Al-Muammar A. A novel interdisciplinary health professions education program at King Saud University: strategy and structure (Phase I). Southeast Asian J Med Educ. 2015;9:26.
26. Zahedi M, Alshehri M, Al-Hadlaq SM, Jarallah N, Alnaami M, Alzahrani AM. Faculty perception and readiness to engage in initiatives towards excellence. South East Asian J Med Educ. 2015;9(1):35–40.
27. National Commission for Academic Accreditation and Assessment (NCAAA). Standards for Program Accreditation. 2018. https://etec.gov.sa/en/productsandservices/NCAAA/AccreditationProgrammatic/Pages/insprogdeve.aspx.
28. Busing N, Harris K, MacLellan AM, Moineau G, Oandasan I, Rourke J, et al. The future of postgraduate medical education in Canada. Acad Med. 2015;90(9):1258–63.
29. Aretz HT, Armstrong EL. Undergraduate medical education. In: Walsh K, editor. The Oxford textbook of medical education. Oxford: Oxford University Press; 2013.
30. Flexner A. Medical education in the United States and Canada. From the Carnegie Foundation for the advancement of teaching, Bulletin Number Four, 1910. Bull World Health Organ. 2002;80(7):594–602.
31. Schmidt HG. Problem-based learning: rationale and description. Med Educ. 1983;17:11–6.
32. Albanese MA, Mejicano G, Mullan P, Kokotailo P, Gruppen L. Defining characteristics of educational competencies. Med Educ. 2008;42(3):248–55.
33. Zaini RG, Bin Abdulrahman KA, Al-Khotani AA, Al-Hayani AM, Al-Alwan IA, Jastaniah SD. Saudi Meds: a competence specification for Saudi medical graduates. Med Teach. 2011;33(7):582–4.
34. Holycross J. Curriculum mapping: an essential tool for curriculum development. J Physician Assist Educ. 2006;17:61–4.
35. Harden RM, Sowden S. Educational strategies in curriculum development: the SPICES model. Med Educ. 1984;18(1):284–97.
36. Kern DE, Thomas PA, Hughes MT. Curriculum development for medical education: a six-step approach. 2nd ed. Baltimore, MD: The Johns Hopkins University Press; 2009.
37. McLean M, Cilliers FJ, Van Wyk J. Faculty development: yesterday, today and tomorrow. Med Teach. 2008;30:555–84.
38. Algahtani H, Shirah B, Subahi A. Effectiveness and needs assessment of faculty development programme for medical education: experience from Saudi Arabia. Sultan Qaboos Univ Med J. 2020;20(1):e83–9.
39. Asif M, Awan MU, Khan MK, Ahmad N. A model for total quality management in higher education. Qual Quant. 2013;47:1883–904.
40. Brookes M, Becket N. Quality management in higher education: a review of international issues and practice. Int J Qual Serv Sci. 2007;1:1–37.
41. Kuper A, Whitehead C, Hodges B. Looking back to move forward: using history, discourse and text in medical education research: AMEE Guide No. 7. Med Teach. 2013;35:e849–60.

2 Interprofessional Collaborative Practice in Contemporary Health Care: Defining and Exploring the Meaning of Practice

Mona Alsheikh and Hana Alzamil

2.1 Introduction

What is Interprofessional collaborative practice? What are the levels of its implementation? What are the components and enablers of this practice? How is it represented in the World Health Organization (WHO) and Canadian models?

In the modern times, the healthcare team is challenged with ever rising expectations from the global community [1]. These expectations were augmented by the evidence that conflict and poor communication within the health care team increases the chance of medical error [2], jeopardizes the quality of patient outcome, patient safety [3], and leads to burnout [4, 5]. High quality patient care requires among other things effective interprofessional teamwork [6, 7]. There is compelling evidence that effective teamwork interaction and health care team collaboration affects the quality of patient outcome [8–12].

Team performance is defined as "a multilevel process that results from team members' engagement to accomplish individual-level and team-level task work and teamwork" [13] (Fig. 2.1). The level and quality of interprofessional collaboration practice (ICP) can be improved by team training programs, structured communication protocols, effective organizational care pathways and interprofessional education [7, 8]. Care pathways are defined as "a complex intervention for the mutual decision making and organization of care for a well-defined group of patients during a well-defined period" [14]. In other words, care pathways are high-performance

M. Alsheikh (✉)
Physiology Department, College of Medicine, Imam Abdulrahman Bin Faisal University, Dammam, Saudi Arabia

H. Alzamil
Physiology Department, College of Medicine, King Saud University, Riyadh, Saudi Arabia

M. Y. Alnaami et al. (eds.), *Novel Health Interprofessional Education and Collaborative Practice Program: Strategy and Implementation*,
https://doi.org/10.1007/978-981-99-3420-1_2

Fig. 2.1 Levels of interprofessional interaction (Reeves et al. 2010, p. 44). (Reproduced with permission from Wiley-Blackwell)

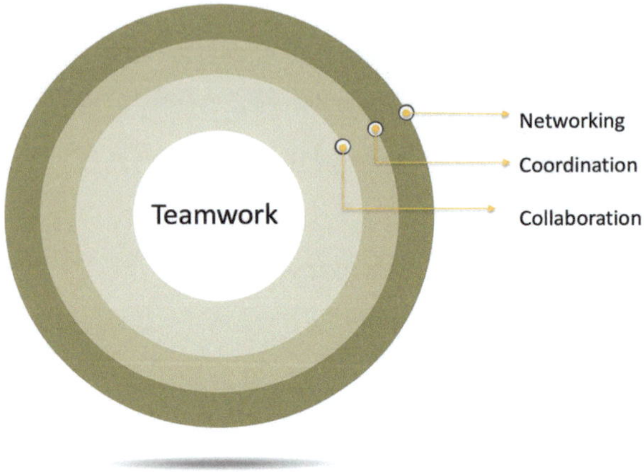

work systems that improve collaborative team performance by strengthening relationships and coordination among team members [15, 16].

The Institute of Medicine recognized effective teamwork as a means of coping with the increasing complexity in diagnosis and health care delivery [17]. The WHO defines interprofessional collaborative practice (ICP) as a situation in which "multiple health workers from different professional backgrounds work together with patients, families, carers, and communities to deliver the highest quality of care [18]. Collaborative practice is considered a priority by the WHO, which published a" Framework for Action on Interprofessional Action and Collaborative Practice" in 2010. The Canadian Interprofessional Health Collaboration (CIHC) [19] determines the elements of such practice to be respect, trust, shared decision making, and partnerships, Fig. 2.2.

> Definitions of Interprofessional Collaborative Practice: ICP happens when multiple health workers from different professions work together to care for patients, to deliver the highest quality of care. "Interprofessional collaboration is the process of developing and maintaining effective interprofessional working relationships with learners, practitioners, patients/clients/families, and communities to enable optimal health outcomes. Elements of collaboration include respect, trust, shared decision making, and partnerships." Canadian Interprofessional Health Collaborative (CIHC).

The Association of American Medical Colleges (AAMC) includes the ability to collaborate in an interprofessional team as a core professional activity [20]. Inadequate understanding of professional roles and processes of every member of the healthcare team are some of the knowledge gaps that interfere with ICP [21]. Behavioral practices that contribute to ICP include mutual support, between team members is one of the important practices.

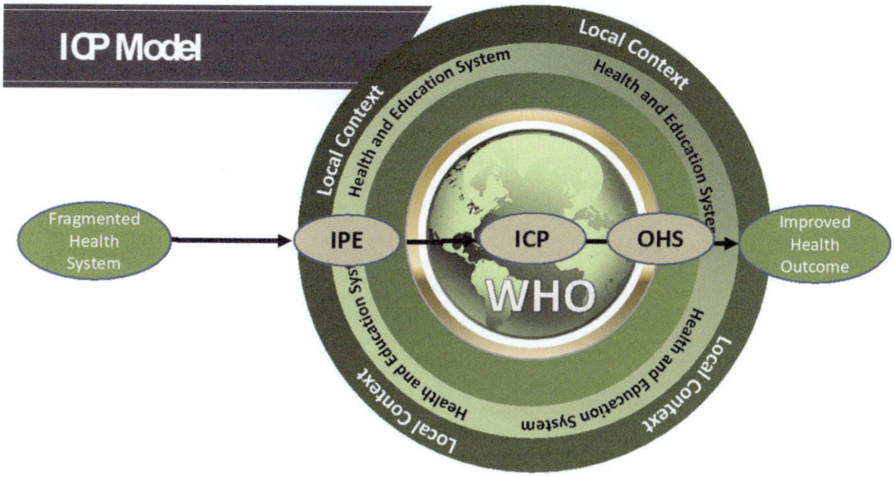

Fig. 2.2 The WHO Interprofessional Collaborative Practice Model. *IPE* Interprofessional education, *ICP* interprofessional collaborative practice, *OHS* Optimal Health Services. (World Health Organization: Framework for Action on Interprofessional Education and Collaborative Practice. Geneva, WHO, 2010. Available at: http://www.who.int/hrh/resources/framework_action/en/)

Traditionally, health care professionals are not grouped together in "official" teams before they start taking care of patients. Moreover, each member of the health care team works in a silo and follow strict boundaries set by their professional bodies. These boundaries limit their interaction and collaboration with other members of the healthcare team. Health care professions have hierarchical lines of authority and different degrees of autonomy. A nurse may be working in a health care team for one patient but follows and is managed by a leader who is outside that team, which is a nurse supervisor. These lines of authority and degrees of autonomy differ from one country to another. For example, the US system gives nurses a lot more autonomy and decision making power in relation to patient management than the European, Australian, Indian or Middle East system [22].

The roadmap to ICP is through various mechanisms that are summarized in the CIHC [19] and Sunnybrook ICP model [23], Fig. 2.3. The six core competencies and practices that are prerequisite to the establishment of ICP include "role clarification" which is awareness of each healthcare team member of the other team members' professional roles, scope of practice, and limits [18]. Interprofessional conflict resolution practice is achieved when the team can collaborate and define multiple solutions to deal with conflict within the healthcare team [24]. Collaborative leadership occurs when team members decide on actions together and share accountability for the selected decision. Then the team members put the plan for their action together and implement those decisions with consensus. Reflection is an integral component of an ICP team and should become one of the team norms. The team should debrief and take time to analyze the learning they gained from each case or project and define the successes and failures and the factors involved in each. Interprofessional

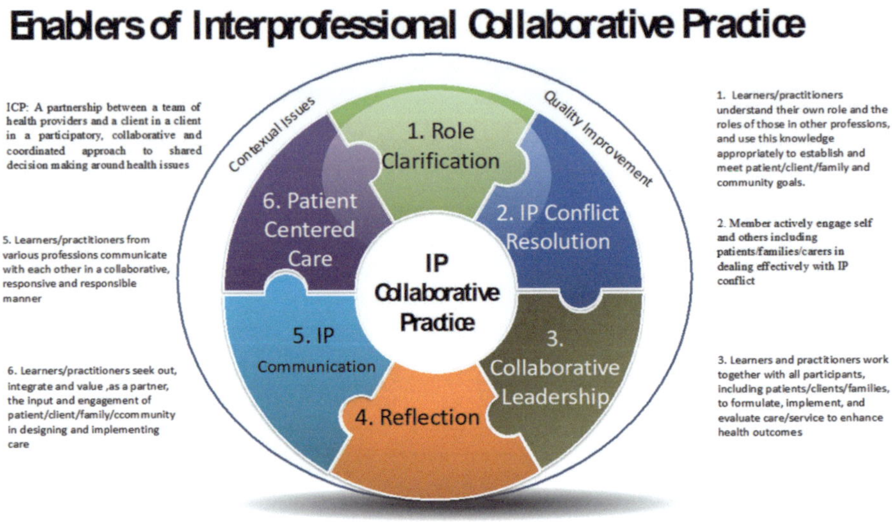
Enablers of Interprofessional Collaborative Practice
ICP: A partnership between a team of health providers and a client in a client in a participatory, collaborative and coordinated approach to shared decision making around health issues
5. Learners/practitioners from various professions communicate with each other in a collaborative, responsive and responsible manner
6. Learners/practitioners seek out, integrate and value ,as a partner, the input and engagement of patient/client/family/ccommunity in designing and implementing care
Contexual Issues
Quality Improvement
1. Role Clarification
2. IP Conflict Resolution
3. Collaborative Leadership
4. Reflection
5. IP Communication
6. Patient Centered Care
IP Collaborative Practice
1. Learners/practitioners understand their own role and the roles of those in other professions, and use this knowledge appropriately to establish and meet patient/client/family and community goals.
2. Member actively engage self and others including patients/families/carers in dealing effectively with IP conflict
3. Learners and practitioners work together with all participants, including patients/clients/families, to formulate, implement, and evaluate care/service to enhance health outcomes

Fig. 2.3 Enablers of ICP. (Modified from the Canadian Interprofessional Health Collaborative Framework and Sunnybrook Interprofessional Collaboration Framework)

collaborative practice is a great opportunity to practice reporting of medical errors and improve teamwork dynamics. Effective communication within the healthcare team ensures sharing of information and puts a common ground [25].

2.2 Impact of Interprofessional Education and Interprofessional Collaborative Practice on Health Outcome

Interprofessional education (IPE) was found to improve perceptions of collaboration and interprofessional practice and enhance collaborative knowledge and skills [26–29].

There is a systematic review evidence that ICP care pathways improve quality and effectiveness of organizational team collaboration [30], and that of a health care interprofessional team as measured by patient outcome in chronic obstructive pulmonary disease (COPD) and proximal femur fracture (PFF) [31]. The role of nurses in ICP is even more pronounced [32]. A recent systematic review found that ICP was associated with improvements in diabetic and hypertensive patient outcome in a primary care setting, as evidenced by reductions in cumulative blood glucose levels (HbA1c), systolic blood pressure (SBP), and diastolic blood pressure (DBP). There were statistically significant results of reduction of HbA1c values by 0.5%. Blood Pressure (BP) control rate improved to 66% during the first year of ICP and persisted, with 68% of patients reaching their goal BP by the end of the study [33]. There is evidence that ICP in the clinic led to significant improvements in adherence to supportive medications [34].

2.3 Tips

Tips for ICP

1. Leaders who are passionate about ICP and IPE
2. Administrative and institutional support
3. Teachers who have expertise with IPE
4. Shared vision and mission for collaboration
5. Flexible curricula that allow for IPE

2.4 Case Studies

The literature includes many case studies of ICP from all over the world [35]. The Brazilian case is an initiative of the ministry of health (MOH) and ministry of education (MOE) to enhance the relationship between academia, the community, and the primary health care (PHC) [36]. The Canadian Alberta initiative is about implementing interprofessional clinical training combining emergency care, rehabilitation, and primary care [37]. The interprofessional patient care team included nurses, speech therapists, social workers, occupational therapists, physical therapists, pharmacists, dieticians, physicians, administrators, and health educators. The Canadian Hamilton case was about providing ICP to geriatrics in the community including assessment and management of various geriatric conditions [38]. The Swedish Karolinska University Hospital emergency training for teams of medical, nursing, and physiotherapy students enhanced the professional identity and role identity among students and lead to provision of holistic patient care [39]. The team consisted of nurses, PHC physician, pharmacist, social worker, dietician, geriatric physician, and caregivers. In India the ICP is adopted by a non-governmental health association between hospitals, PHC centers, and social service [40]. The objective is to tackle HIV/AIDS cases at PHC centers in rural areas. In South Africa, the case is IPE of medical officers, nurses, pharmacists, social workers, medical technologists, community caregivers, midwives, and health educators. The objective was to combat HIV/AIDS, tuberculosis, and sexually transmitted disease. The USA case is collaboration between primary care physicians, specialists, pharmacists, nurses, physical therapist, nutritionist, religious leaders, and community associations to create a culturally sensitive community health care [41].

2.5 Health Issues That Requires ICP

Caring for patients with complex chronic diseases is a great burden on primary healthcare and very costly for governmental health sectors. Identification of individuals with complex and frequent needs for social and medical care, known as super-utilizers, is the cornerstone for the initiation of hot spotting programs that help students learn about social determinants of health and teamwork skills [42]. While actively participating in hot spotting programs, students engage in an interprofessional team and practice to manage patients who have complex health and social needs [43].

Patients who have chronic diseases such as: diabetes mellitus, bronchial asthma, chronic obstructive pulmonary disease (COPD), cardiovascular disease, and others need continuous care in a primary healthcare setting [44]. Multiple factors can impede the collaboration between different professionals in healthcare teams such as: prejudice, hierarchy, variations in work philosophy and ethics, different professional cultures, and unique occupational languages [45, 46]. One of the commonest chronic diseases that definitely needs collaboration of many professions is diabetes which requires coordination by the primary care physician with endocrinologist, podiatrist, diabetic educator, clinical nutritionist, dietician, nurse, exercise professional, and ophthalmologist. A Canadian study reported that despite the challenges of highly complex organization of health services, primary care physicians, and specialists succeeded to work together to care for patients with diabetes but needed to cope with challenges of sharing space, costs, and technology training [47].

Gonzalo et al. [48] analyzed 549 hospital rounds and showed that patients received an average of 8 min of team presence at the bedside with frequency exceeding 60%, and the independent predictors of increased BIR occurrence were in- experienced attending physician, senior resident, weekdays, and smaller team size. In hospital-based settings, the need for bedside interprofessional rounds (BIR), defined as "encounters that include the team of providers—at least two physicians plus a nurse or other care provider—discussing the case at the bedside with the patient" is important to improve the quality of healthcare provided to hospitalized patients. Some factors associated with increased incidence of BIR were intensive or moderate care units, long stay estimated as 5–7 or more days, using rounding script and perceived support from leadership. To attain patient satisfaction, we need an optimal interprofessional collaborative care model. The same authors suggested some strategies to support increasing BIR that includes billboard themes, reminders by email, nurse-physician gatherings, acknowledging providers who performed BIR, and the installment of touch pad buttons inside patient rooms that illuminate a colored light to alert the nursing staff to the initiation of BIR encounters [49].

> Definition: teamwork was described as "a collection of individuals who are interdependent in their tasks, who share responsibility for outcomes, who see themselves and who are seen by others as an intact social entity embedded in one or more larger social systems and who manage their relationships across organizational boundaries" [50].

2.6 Levels of Collaboration

The macro–meso–micro-individual model explains the contextual interrelated factors that can ensure effective collaboration in IPCs which includes global (policy or macro), local organizational (meso), within team (micro) and individual factors [51]. The input-output approach considers inputs as contextual variables within the policy environment, the organization or the team while the output is the team's overall collaborative performance. An interesting model called "gears model" was suggested to integrate the input-output approach, the macro-meso-micro-individual model, and the dynamic nature of health care teams which requires fast adjustment of relationship strategies between participants [52].

A systematic review showed that successful models of IPCP depend on multiple factors which can be summarized as "top down" organization, and "bottom up" intrinsic factors. The "top down" organizational factors such as available space and time, policies and structure can have a strong effect on "bottom up" intrinsic factors because it can enhance the informal communication that is considered as the most important component of interprofessional collaboration [53]. One of the key promoters of collaboration between different professions includes collocation which allows frequent interactions between members of healthcare team. Structuring intelligible policies such as regular meetings, written reports and synchronous/ asynchronous electronic communication will help clarify roles and responsibilities as well as sharing information to facilitate patient's care [54]. Patients with chronic conditions had a positive experience with IPCP if they were involved in the development of their care plan, received holistic care and were treated as a person rather than a patient [55].

Definition: "Collaboration is a process in which autonomous or semi-autonomous actors interact through formal and informal negotiation, jointly creating rules and structures governing their relationships and ways to act or decide on the issues that brought them together; it is a process involving shared norms and mutually beneficial interactions [56].

Definition: "Practice(s) are moments of human significance beyond self, by which people participate in and thus experience something greater than their own perceptions and perspectives of the world."

2.7 Enablers of ICP

Promoters of IPE and IPC between different health professionals

1. All involved professionals should be informed about each other's profession.
2. Explain the importance of IPE and IPC for all involved professionals.

3. Senior staff members should lead by role model.
4. Incorporate IPE activities within the working routine.
5. Explain individual's responsibilities for all members in the IPE activities.

2.8 Strategies

There is mismatch between what students learn in the formal curriculum about collaborative practice and the transmitted behaviors and values that they watch in clinical practice. There is no doubt that students and graduates need consistent team role models in practice instead of observing traditional hierarchical models of care [57]. The commitment to IPE/IPCP needs is required at all levels including "top down" governmental policies and accreditation standards that are aligned with the change in healthcare system. The new vision of integrated health and learning system require redesigning IPE needs in order to incorporate teams of students and residents into practice in a way that purposely adds value to patient care in community settings, transitional care, ambulatory and acute care [58, 59].

The world health organization designed a multipurpose classification called International Classification of Functioning, Disability and health known as ICF aiming to provide a consolidated standard language and framework of health and health-related status to facilitate communication between policymakers, healthcare workers, researchers, and the public [60]. The ICF conceptual framework is considered as a tool which can help in directing the attention of practitioners to identify enablers and hinders to participation which facilitate planning interventions to enhance functioning and well-being and assess modulations in health condition, interventions provided and adjustments in environmental factors [61]. A model known as MAGPIE was originally designed by an Australian health professional's team and stands for the following functions: Meet, Assess, Goal-Set, Plan, Implement and Evaluate, and has been adapted by health educators as a framework for interprofessional education [62].

2.8.1 Training Wards

Interprofessional training wards (IPTWs) are functioning hospital inpatient wards used to encourage students from different health professions to work together, over the last two decades IPTWs have been implemented in healthcare and medical training. The IPTWs were found to enhance supervised collaboration during which the students take full responsibility of medical treatment and rehabilitation of their patients [63]. In Australia a hospital collaborated with a university to establish an interprofessional training ward and the steering committee designed three rotations program which was conducted over 6 weeks for nursing, allied health, and medical students. Under supervision of a registered nurse the students perform all ward duties as an interprofessional team with profession specific tasks, facilitated group learning sessions, and reflective sessions. The impact of this innovative learning environment was found to improve students' attitude towards IPC and to increase the students' competencies required for interprofessional, patient centered health profession practice [64]. Another trial in Denmark, started by forming an interprofessional training unit (ITU), composed of nurses, occupational therapy, physiotherapy, and medical students, and making it in charge of running a ward of eight beds. The impact of engaging health profession students in a collaborative practice for an average of 5.5 days under supervision of experts helped them to gain interprofessional learning and practice skills. One important condition was that the training was highly authentic clinical practice in training wards with real patients and that all staff took an active role in the participants' learning by encouraging them to make decisions and implement the appropriate actions which established a culture of trust and respect with constructive feedback [65].

2.8.2 Students-Led Clinic

The student-Led Clinic (SLC), also known as Student-Run Clinic (SRC), was emerged from the needs of undeserved marginalized population for free primary healthcare services [66]. SLC is a tool that utilizes students to fill in the gaps in healthcare environment during which the students lead the care under supervision of licensed health care professionals [67]. SLC have been existing in the United States as early as 1960s, previously it has been estimated that 49 medical schools are managing 110 SLC at United States with numbers increasing dramatically during the last two decades [68]. In 1998 the first Canadian SLC was founded in Vancouver, British Columbia, however the clinical service was not started until 2000 after which several other SLC have been initiated across the country [69].

Student-Led Clinic usually incorporate a mixture of students from medicine, nursing, dentistry, pharmacy, social work, and other allied health disciplines who work together under supervision of preceptors from relevant professions [70]. Collaborative, interprofessional practice that relies on the effective communication and interaction between healthcare team members, including the patient, forms the cornerstone of safe patient care. Generally, encounters between students and patients in the clinical settings help to improve communication, establish trust rapport, and proper expressions of empathy [71]. When patients share the experience about their illness with students and staff their sense of empowerment and satisfaction may increase, additionally they feel that meeting others and sharing their stories with them increased their sense of community [71]. The clinical environment in SLC provides a chance for participating students to practice listening to patients' complaint and educating them about the management of their health problem which leads to the improvement of diagnostic accuracy, enhancement of patient compliance and satisfaction leading to fewer return visits [67].

In Saudi Arabia there are some charities that provide free healthcare services for uninsured patients by specialists who volunteer in their free time to serve the community. Until now the idea of SLC is not practiced in our community and needs to be addressed as a strategy to enhance the interaction of our future healthcare workers with the undeserved population in the community. Facilitating the involvement of our health sciences' students in an interprofessional collaborative practice to serve the community will have a dual favorable impact on the community and the students. Initiating SLC needs a huge support at macro, miso, and micro levels, therefore we need to study the community needs and prepare a detailed plan to convince higher authorities about its importance for medical education as well as community service.

2.8.3 Mobile Clinics

An innovative model for healthcare delivery to patients with chronic diseases and to those who are vulnerable is Mobile Health Clinics (MHCs) which could help alleviate health disparities by offering urgent healthcare, providing screenings for prevention, and initiating managements of chronic diseases [72]. Boston University School of Medicine initiated the Outreach Van Project aiming to provide both medical and non-medical services to improve the well-being of marginalized homeless individuals in the greater Boston area. The Outreach Van multidisciplinary approach provided their intended clients with a comprehensive and sustainable solution by offering basic medical care, such as blood pressure screenings and mental health services, in addition to offering connections to resources and homeless shelters, providing warm clothes, and supplying nutritious foods. Simultaneously, this outreach project create a chance for students to practice communication with clients and professionals and to develop important skills for their future career [73].

During the first half of 2019, as a part of the initiative of reforming and restructuring the primary healthcare, the Saudi Ministry of Health (MOH) estimated that its ten mobile clinics served over 85,000 patients. These clinics were launched to reach peripheral communities and provide essential healthcare services such as: screening and follow-up of non-communicable diseases, dental health, vaccinations and follow-up for healthy children, health education and support services including radiology (X-ray and ultrasound) and laboratory investigations. MOH receives all complaints and suggestions through the hotline (937) services center which help in following up projects' progress and evaluating the quality of performance with scientific methodology and performance indicators that are periodically evaluated by its senior officials [74].

2.9 Recommendation

Interprofessional mobile clinics were found to be efficient and reliable to provide safe patient centered care in rural and underprivileged areas [75]. The authors of this chapter take the opportunity to suggest interprofessional student mobile clinics (ISMC) as a medium for IPE and to establish and improve ICP knowledge and attitude among health profession students. This can be initiated by sponsoring multiprofessional mobile clinics in rural areas with students from all health professions as volunteers or as an elective course. Seasons like Haj (pilgrimage) and Umrah (visit to the holy mosque) can be targeted to have a concentrated exposure to a multitude of cases aiming to boost students' professional identity and ICP competencies.

2.10 Success Stories

Before COVID-19 pandemic the steering committee for IPEC in our institution was founded which involved the supervisor of the Deanship of skills development, faculty members and students from Pharmacy, Medicine, Nursing, and Emergency Medical Sciences colleges. Several meetings were conducted at the deanship of skills development to arrange for an IPE activity during 2019 academic year, however, it was difficult to find a suitable time for all the students and faculty members. After the lockdown took place due to the pandemic our committee continued meetings online and came up with an activity that aim to raise the awareness of our students about the crisis and how to deal with cases of COVID-19 infection. To construct a case study activity that attracts the interest of students from different disciplines we identified key aims, the framework was selected then case development and implementation of activity followed. To fulfill the primary aim of interprofessional collaboration, faculty from different professions worked together in designing a case scenario step by step using the toolkit for constructing IP simulation scenario by Health Sciences Education and research Commons', University of Alberta, Canada [76]. We used an online platform (Zoom) to monitor the performance of students during the activity while they worked collaboratively to solve the simulated scenario case step by step. Most of our students enjoyed the virtual IPE experience and have positive feedback, they reported an improvement of their communication and teamwork skills, and additionally they revealed that their roles and the roles of other professions was clarified during the activity [77].

In another occasion, King Saud University have launched a multidisciplinary event to raise patients' awareness about their rights and responsibilities in the health care system. The event was designed to simulate the hospital setting in the Kingdom of Saudi Arabia. During their visit, guests progress sequentially through the different departments such as the laboratory, radiology, and the pharmacy to simulate what might take place during a regular hospital visit. In each station/department, patient's rights and responsibilities are being delivered by role play and scenarios that mimic real-life situations. Although the event was primarily designed for public education it turned out to be a valuable opportunity for IPE for the student as well as the faculty members. Preparation for the event involved numerous meetings at the organizational level between students and staff representing different professions as well as parallel sub-meetings within each college. The preparation for the event required approximately 9 months during which students practiced brainstorming and conduct rehearsal of the educational scenarios under supervision of faculty members with varying backgrounds and specialties. Participating students appreciate the role play strategy as being very effective method that helped them to comprehend their roles and responsibilities towards their patients in addition to improving their communication and teamwork skills [78].

2.11 Summary

Interprofessional education was found to improve perceptions of collaboration and interprofessional practice and enhance collaborative knowledge and skills. ICP care pathways improve quality and effectiveness of organizational team collaboration, and that of a healthcare interprofessional team as measured by patient outcome in various diseases. To establish ICP we need leaders who are passionate about ICP and IPE, administrative and institutional support, teachers who have expertise with IPE, shared vision and mission for collaboration, and flexible curricula that allow for IPE. International and national success stories of IPE and ICP are discussed and analyzed.

References

1. Cutler S, Morecroft C, Carey P, Kennedy T. Are interprofessional healthcare teams meeting patient expectations? An exploration of the perceptions of patients and informal caregivers. J Interprof Care. 2019;33(1):66–75.
2. Classen DC, Resar R, Griffin F, Federico F, Frankel T, Kimmel N, et al. 'Global trigger tool' shows that adverse events in hospitals may be ten times greater than previously measured. Health Aff. 2011;30(4):581–9.
3. Aiken LH, Sermeus W, Van den Heede K, Sloane DM, Busse R, McKee M, et al. Patient safety, satisfaction, and quality of hospital care: cross sectional surveys of nurses and patients in 12 countries in Europe and the United States. BMJ. 2012;344(7851):20.
4. Deneckere S, Euwema M, Lodewijckx C, Panella M, Mutsvari T, Sermeus W, et al. Better interprofessional teamwork, higher level of organized care, and lower risk of burnout in acute health care teams using care pathways: a cluster randomized controlled trial. Med Care. 2013;51(1):99–107.
5. Nordang K, Hall-Lord ML, Farup PG. Burnout in health-care professionals during reorganizations and downsizing. A cohort study in nurses. BMC Nurs. 2010;9:8.
6. Nembhard IM, Edmondson AC. Making it safe: the effects of leader inclusiveness and professional status on psychological safety and improvement efforts in health care teams. J Organ Behav. 2006;27:941–66.
7. Buljac-Samardzic M, Dekker-van Doorn CM, van Wijngaarden JD, van Wijk KP. Interventions to improve team effectiveness: a systematic review. Health Policy. 2010;94(3):183–95.
8. Evans S, Shaw N, Ward C, Hayley A. "Refreshed…reinforced…reflective": a qualitative exploration of interprofessional education facilitators' own interprofessional learning and collaborative practice. J Interprof Care. 2016;30(6):702–9.
9. Thomas EJ. Improving teamwork in healthcare: current approaches and the path forward. BMJ Qual Saf. 2011;20:647–50.
10. Craig P, Dieppe P, Macintyre S, Michie S, Nazareth I, Petticrew M, et al. Developing and evaluating complex interventions: the new Medical Research Council guidance. BMJ. 2008;337(7676):979–83.
11. Salas E, King HB, Rosen MA. Improving teamwork and safety: toward a practical systems approach, a commentary on Deneckere et al. Soc Sci Med. 2012;75:986–9.
12. Lodewijckx C, Sermeus W, Panella M, Deneckere S, Leigheb F, Decramer M, Vanhaecht K. Impact of care pathways for in-hospital management of COPD exacerbation: a systematic review. Int J Nurs Stud. 2011;48(11):1445–56.
13. Kozlowski SWJ, Klein KJ. A multilevel approach to theory and research in organizations: contextual, temporal, and emergent processes. In: Klein KJ, Kozlowski SWJ, editors. Multilevel

theory, research, and methods in organizations: foundations, extensions, and new directions. San Francisco, CA: Jossey-Bass; 2000. p. 3–90.

14. Vanhaecht K, Panella M, van Zelm R, Sermeus W. An overview on the history and concept of care pathways as complex interventions. Int J Care Pathw. 2010;14(3):117–23.
15. Gittell JH. Coordinating mechanism in care provider groups: relational coordination as a mediator and input uncertainty as a moderator of performance effects. Manage Sci. 2002;48:1408–26.
16. Gittell JH, Seidner R, Wimbush JA. Relational model of how high performance work systems work. Organ Sci. 2010;21:490–506.
17. Tymitz K, Lidor A. The Institute of Medicine: crossing the quality chasm. In: The SAGES manual of quality, outcomes and patient safety. Boston, MA: Springer; 2011. p. 379–86.
18. World Health Organization. Framework for action on interprofessional education & collaborative practice. World Health Organization; 2010.
19. Canadian Interprofessional Health Collaborative (CIHC). A national interprofessional competency framework; 2010.
20. Loomis K, Amiel JM, Ryan MS, Esposito K, Green M, Stagnaro-Green A, et al. Implementing an entrustable professional activities framework in undergraduate medical education: early lessons from the AAMC core entrustable professional activities for entering residency pilot. Acad Med. 2017;92(6):765–70.
21. Garth M, Millet A, Shearer E, Stafford S, Bereknyei Merrell S, Bruce J, Schillinger E, Aaronson A, Svec D. Interprofessional collaboration: a qualitative study of non-physician perspectives on resident competency. J Gen Intern Med. 2018;33(4):487–92.
22. McLaney E, Morassaei S, Hughes L, Davies R, Campbell M, Di Prospero L. A framework for interprofessional team collaboration in a hospital setting: advancing team competencies and behaviours. Healthc Manage Forum. 2022;35(2):112–7.
23. Sunnybrook Interprofessional (IP) Working Group. Sunnybrook Interprofessional Collaboration (ICP) Framework; 2019. https://sunnybrook.ca/uploads/1/welcome/strategy/170630-icp-framework.pdf.
24. D'Alimonte L, McLaney E, Di Prospero L. Best practices on team communication: interprofessional practice in oncology. Curr Opin Support Palliat Care. 2019;13(1):69–74.
25. Bleich MR. Leadership responses to The future of nursing: leading change, advancing health IOM report. J Nurs Adm. 2012;42(4):183–4.
26. Paradis E, Reeves S. Key trends in interprofessional research: a macrosociological analysis from 1970 to 2010. J Interprof Care. 2013;27(2):113–22.
27. Reeves S, Goldman J, Burton A, Sawatzky-Girling B. Synthesis of systematic review evidence of interprofessional education. J Allied Health. 2010;39(Suppl 1):198–203.
28. Shrader S, Jernigan S, Nazir N, Zaudke J. Determining the impact of an interprofessional learning in practice model on learners and patients. J Interprof Care. 2023;37(1):S67–74.
29. Zook SS, Hulton LJ, Dudding CC, Stewart AL, Graham AC. Scaffolding interprofessional education: unfolding case studies, virtual world simulations, and patient-centered care. Nurse Educ. 2018;43(2):87–91.
30. Deneckere S, Euwema M, Van Herck P, Lodewijckx C, Panella M, Sermeus W, Vanhaecht K. Care pathways lead to better teamwork: results of a systematic review. Soc Sci Med. 2012;75(2):264–8.
31. Deneckere S, Euwema M, Lodewijckx C, Panella M, Sermeus W, Vanhaecht K. The European quality of care pathways (EQCP) study on the impact of care pathways on interprofessional teamwork in an acute hospital setting: study protocol: for a cluster randomized controlled trial and evaluation of implementation processes. Implement Sci. 2012;7:47.
32. Orchard CA. Persistent isolationist or collaborator? The nurse's role in interprofessional collaborative practice. J Nurs Manag. 2010;18(3):248–57.
33. Lee JK, McCutcheon LRM, Fazel MT, Cooley JH, Slack MK. Assessment of interprofessional collaborative practices and outcomes in adults with diabetes and hypertension in primary care: a systematic review and meta-analysis. JAMA Netw Open. 2021;4(2):e2036725.

34. Sisson EM, Dixon DL, Kildow DC, Van Tassell BW, Carl DE, Varghese D, et al. Effectiveness of a pharmacist-physician team-based collaboration to improve long-term blood pressure control at an inner-city safety-net clinic. Pharmacotherapy. 2016;36(3):342–7.
35. Johri M, Beland F, Bergman H. International experiments in integrated care for the elderly: a synthesis of the evidence. Int J Geriatr Psych. 2003;18:222–35.
36. Silva JA, Peduzzi M, Orchard C, Leonello VM. Interprofessional education and collaborative practice in primary health care. Rev Esc Enferm USP. 2015;49 Spec No:16–24.
37. Donovan ML, McCumber S. Interprofessional collaborative practice: dementia case studies engage nurse practitioner and occupational therapy students. J Nurs Educ. 2015;54(9):536.
38. Barr H. Editorial: Canada as a case study. J Interprof Care. 2005;19(1):5–7. https://doi.org/10.1080/13561820500081562.
39. Ericson A, Masiello I, Bolinder G. Interprofessional clinical training for undergraduate students in an emergency department setting. J Interprof Care. 2012;26(4):319–25.
40. Rajamani S, Westra BL, Monsen KA, LaVenture M, Gatewood LC. Partnership to promote interprofessional education and practice for population and public health informatics: a case study. J Interprof Care. 2015;29(6):555–61.
41. Yan J, Gilbert JH, Hoffman SJ. World Health Organization Study Group on interprofessional education and collaborative practice. J Interprof Care. 2007;21(6):588–9.
42. Cheng I, Powers K, Mange D, Palmer B, Chen F, Perkins B, et al. Interprofessional education through healthcare hotspotting: understanding social determinants of health and mastering complex care through teamwork. J Interprof Educ Pract. 2020;20:100340.
43. Camden Coalition of Healthcare Providers. The interprofessional student hotspotting learning collaborative: program overview 2020. https://camdenhealth.org/wp-content/uploads/2020/03/SH-Overview.pdf.
44. van der Gulden R, Haan ND, Greijn CM, Looman N, Tromp F, Dielissen PW. Interprofessional education and collaboration between general practitioner trainees and practice nurses in providing chronic care; a qualitative study. BMC Med Educ. 2020;20(1):1–9.
45. Johnson JM, Hermosura BJ, Price SL, Gougeon L. Factors influencing interprofessional team collaboration when delivering care to community-dwelling seniors: a metasynthesis of Canadian interventions. J Interprof Care. 2021;35(3):376–82.
46. Clark PG. The devil is in the details: the seven deadly sins of organizing and continuing interprofessional education in the US. J Interprof Care. 2011;25(5):321–7.
47. Gucciardi E, Espin S, Morganti A, Dorado L. Exploring interprofessional collaboration during the integration of diabetes teams into primary care. BMC Fam Pract. 2016;17(1):1–4.
48. Gonzalo JD, Wolpaw DR, Lehman E, Chuang CH. Patient-centered interprofessional collaborative care: factors associated with bedside interprofessional rounds. J Genl Int Med. 2014;29(7):1040–7.
49. Gonzalo JD, Himes J, McGillen B, Shifflet V, Lehman E. Interprofessional collaborative care characteristics and the occurrence of bedside interprofessional rounds: a cross-sectional analysis. BMC Health Serv Res. 2016;16(1):1–9.
50. Cohen SG, Bailey DE. What makes teams work: group effectiveness research from the shop floor to the executive suite. J Manag. 1997;23(3):239–90.
51. Mulvale G, Bourgeault IL. Finding the right mix: how do contextual factors affect collaborative mental health care in Ontario? Canad Pub Pol. 2007;33(1):S49–64.
52. Mulvale G, Embrett M, Razavi SD. 'Gearing Up' to improve interprofessional collaboration in primary care: a systematic review and conceptual framework. BMC Fam Pract. 2016;17(1):1–3.
53. Witt Sherman D, Flowers M, Alfano AR, Alfonso F, De Los Santos M, Evans H, et al. An integrative review of interprofessional collaboration in health care: building the case for university support and resources and faculty engagement. Healthcare (Basel). 2020;8(4):418.
54. Morgan S, Pullon S, McKinlay E. Observation of interprofessional collaborative practice in primary care teams: an integrative literature review. Int J Nurs Stud. 2015;52(7):1217–30.
55. Davidson AR, Kelly J, Ball L, Morgan M, Reidlinger DP. What do patients experience? Interprofessional collaborative practice for chronic conditions in primary care: an integrative review. BMC Prim Care. 2022;23(1):1–2.

56. Thomson AM, Perry JL, Miller TK. Conceptualizing and measuring collaboration. J Public Adm Res Theory. 2009;19(1):23–56.
57. Kemmis S, Trede F. Practice and developing future practice. 2010; p. 27–39.
58. Fraher E, Brandt B. Toward a system where workforce planning and interprofessional practice and education are designed around patients and populations not professions. J Interprof Care. 2019;33(4):389–97.
59. Earnest M, Brandt B. Aligning practice redesign and interprofessional education to advance triple aim outcomes. J Interprof Care. 2014;28(6):497–500.
60. World Health Organization. International classification of functioning, disability and health: ICF. Geneva: World Health Organization; 2001.
61. Kostanjsek N. Use of The International Classification of Functioning, Disability and Health (ICF) as a conceptual framework and common language for disability statistics and health information systems. BMC Public Health. 2011;11(4):S3.
62. Moran M, Bickford J, Barradell S, Scholten I. Embedding the international classification of functioning, disability and health in health professions curricula to enable interprofessional education and collaborative practice. J Med Educ Curric Dev. 2020;7:2382120520933855.
63. Falk AL, Hult H, Hammar M, Hopwood N, Dahlgren MA. One site fits all? A student ward as a learning practice for interprofessional development. J Interprof Care. 2013;27(6):476–81.
64. Brewer ML, Stewart-Wynne EG. An Australian hospital-based student training ward delivering safe, client-centred care while developing students' interprofessional practice capabilities. J Interprof Care. 2013;27(6):482–8.
65. Hansen TB, Jacobsen F, Larsen K. Cost effective interprofessional training: an evaluation of a training unit in Denmark. J Interprof Care. 2009;23(3):234–41.
66. Jakobsen F, Larsen K, Hansen TB. This is the closest I have come to being compared to a doctor: views of medical students on clinical clerkship in an Interprofessional Training Unit. Med Teach. 2010;32(9):e399–406.
67. Developing and sustaining student-led clinics: a toolkit. https://www.cfms.org/files/updates/SRC_ToolKit.pdf.
68. Simpson SA, Long JA. Medical student-run health clinics: important contributors to patient care and medical education. J Gen Intern Med. 2007;22(3):352–6.
69. Holmqvist M, Courtney C, Meili R, Dick A. Student-run clinics: opportunities for interprofessional education and increasing social accountability. JRIPE. 2012;2(3):264–77.
70. Warren S, Puryear E, Chapman M, Barnett TM, White LS. The role of social work in free healthcare clinics and student-run clinics. Soc Work Health Care. 2017;56(10):884–96.
71. Burgess A, Roberts C. Interprofessional student-led clinics: the volunteer patient experience. BMC Med Educ. 2022;22(1):1–6.
72. Yu SW, Hill C, Ricks ML, Bennet J, Oriol NE. The scope and impact of mobile health clinics in the United States: a literature review. Int J Equity Health. 2017;16(1):1–2.
73. Boston University School of Medicine Outreach Van Project: Project History. 2016. http://blogs.bu.edu/outreach/history/.
74. MOH: Over 85,000 patients served by mobile clinics. https://www.moh.gov.sa/en/Ministry/MediaCenter/News/Pages/news-2019-09-26-001.aspx.
75. Manusov EG, Diego VP, Smith J, Garza JR II, Lowdermilk J, Blangero J, et al. UniMóvil: a mobile health clinic providing primary care to the Colonias of the Rio Grande Valley, South Texas. Front Public Health. 2019;7:215.
76. Toolkit for constructing Interprofessional Simulation Scenarios, Health Sciences Education and Research Commons'. University of Alberta, Canada. https://sites.ualberta.ca/~hsercweb/viper/Toolkit_for_Interprofessional_Sims.pdf.
77. Alrasheed A, Altulahi N, Temsah MH, Almasri Z, Alghadeer S, Mubarak AM, et al. Interprofessional education competition during the COVID-19 pandemic at King Saud University: benefits and challenges. J Multidiscip Healthc. 2021;14:673–9.
78. Almalag HM, Saja M, Abouzaid HH, Aljuffali L, Alzamil H, Almater L, et al. Evaluation of a multidisciplinary extracurricular event using Kolb's experiential learning theory: a qualitative study. J Multidiscip Healthc. 2022;15:2957–67.

Theories of Team Working Relevant to Health and Social Systems

3

Farah Mansuri, Lubna Baig, Ganesh Kamath, and Mohammed Yahya Alnaami

3.1 Introduction

Interprofessional collaboration (IPC) is defined as a "partnership between a team of health providers and a client in a participatory collaborative and coordinated approach to shared decision making around health and social issues" [1]. It includes clarity of communication and precise decision making instigating out of a synergistic influence of grouped knowledge and skills that takes its roots from IPE. Originally, the educational strategy used in IPE is team-based learning (TBL), reflected later into effective collaborative team working or IPC. The TBL is a fairly new pedagogy in health professional education and designed to be learner-centered similar to problem-based learning (PBL). However, in TBL, one facilitator manages several groups in a large class room and guarantees a structured methodology in its conduct [2]. TBL is the mainstay in IPE and grounded in "constructivist learning theory" to engage the students actively and motivate them towards application of higher cognition, critical thinking, communication, and analytical or interpretation skills. The students are supposed to experience three phases of learning activities that include the preparation phase, readiness assurance phase, application phase, and concludes

F. Mansuri (✉)
Department of Family & Community Medicine, College of Medicine, Taibah University, Al Madina Al Munawwara, Kingdom of Saudi Arabia

L. Baig
APPNA Institute of Public Health, Jinnah Sindh Medical University, Karachi, Pakistan

G. Kamath
Manipal University College Malaysia, Melaka, Malaysia

M. Y. Alnaami
Department of Surgery, College of Medicine, King Saud University, Riyadh, Saudi Arabia

M. Y. Alnaami et al. (eds.), *Novel Health Interprofessional Education and Collaborative Practice Program: Strategy and Implementation*,
https://doi.org/10.1007/978-981-99-3420-1_3

with peer evaluations [2]. However, TBL steps are discussed in more details in "Chap. 9, *under initiative 1–4: To foster team-based learning and extracurricular team projects.*"

The following sections summarize the theories of TBL and IPC, interactions between IPE and IPC, enabling and disabling factors for IPC, evaluation of team and teamwork activities, and the challenges in developing and implementing the interprofessional team-based learning (IPTBL) program.

3.2 Theories of Team Working

Interprofessional teamwork is recognized as a core competency that all health care providers should acquire it with specific roles and professional identities and also in informal work-based interaction [3]. Teamwork is achieved by various interventions such as simulation-based training, role modeling, etc. Deriving through social-cognitive theory, it was found that team cohesiveness and collective efficacy are important predictors of collaboration outcomes that are measured as, teamwork satisfaction, overall satisfaction, and IPE goal attainment [4]. Each phase of interprofessional teamwork is explained by certain TBL theory to justify its application (Table 3.1) [5].

Based on these theoretical frameworks, activities of IPC are accordingly planned to meet the basic purpose of the enterprise and provide effective health care to individuals and groups. Therefore, the necessary approach to bridge a fragmented health care and to maximally utilize the available resources is to enhance collaboration and communication among related professionals and

Table 3.1 Social and learning theories applicable in TBL and team working

Theory	Use	Scope
Piaget and Vygotsky constructivist theory	Cognitive and social constructivism	Helps in understanding health problems in context to culture and social system
Kolb's experiential learning theory	To define sequence of activities	Active experimentation, concrete experience, reflective observation, abstract conceptualization
Dewey's theory	To reflect on thought process and action	Educational philosophy of pragmatism or hands-on approach
Schon's theory	Modified Kolb theory	Critical reflection at each stage of oneself, learning from other participants, facilitator
Bandura's theory	Self-efficacy	Social cultural context of teams
Turner's theory	Team members attributes	Social identity and conflict settlement
Goffman theory	Interactions	Team interaction
Engestőrm	Activity theory	Completion of team tasksand activities
Powell theory	Institutional influence	Effect of institutional policy on IPE
Friedson theory	Professionalization	Closure between professions
Foucalt theory	Disclosure and surveillance	Social power on IPE process

organizations through establishing quality interprofessional education and collaborative practice (IPECP) programs.

In IPC practice, more than one theoretical background can be used according to the scope of the program. Few models have been introduced by some universities to introduce IPC program including a didactic program for team development and IP clinical component, a community-based experience for training of teams to collaborate and interact in the environment, and a model of interprofessional-simulation experience to train students on clinical skills and leadership [6]. Other important considerations in IPC is that one can have multiple roles in the team and has to justify each one as per demand. Role adoption can be grounded in *Vygotsky theory* [7] of social constructivism in contrast to team building that requires cognitive constructivism.

3.3 Background of Health and Social Systems

Health is considered as one of the important social institutions, where not only the structure of the society and families do affect health situation, but importantly, many diseases and ill related health outcomes are directly determined by prevalent social factors. Hence, it is of utmost importance to understand the social system and its relevant cultures to prevent the health problems primarily and consequently provide the effective collaborative care.

Social science perspectives provide a firm pillar towards success of IPC, where social, psychological aspect of the patient or the community is targeted [8]. This interaction of environment is equally important for all spheres of ill health, communicable and non-communicable diseases, care of the elderly, women and child health, and emergency care.

Evidently, interprofessional collaborative practice (IPCP) in health care occurs when health workers from various specialties work together and provide high quality of comprehensive care by involving the patients, their families, and communities as a success to the IPCP program. In this context, a feasibility study was conducted in three districts of the Netherland to provide care of elderly through program participants (IPCP health professionals in primary care) and non-program participants (health care professionals for social networking). As a result, the interprofessional collaboration among professionals has increased by 42% after the IPCP program and also an increase in network diversity was reported [9].

In a training program, simulation-based education was used as a strategy to teach patient safety to medical interns and senior level nurses through workshops. They found it useful strategy to promote necessary skills to effectively reduce medical errors and provide hands-on training of patient safety to interns [10].

An integrated health and social care systems can lead to more patient satisfaction, patient acceptance of care and health outcomes, a more appropriate referral pattern, greater continuity and coordination of care, collaborative decision making, and reduced effects of negative workplace interactions [11].

3.4 Conceptual Framework of Team Organization

TBL and team working concept is based on personal attributes of team members, social values related to specific problem, organizational support, and the IPECP activity itself [5]. It is highly imperative to frame out the professional attributes of the team members and their willingness to participate in the activity. Besides, complexity of situation, conflicts, team stability, mutual trust or respect, and process of learning or problem solving altogether to be meticulously controlled.

Salas and colleagues [12] had analyzed 20 years of research on effectiveness of teamwork and identified the "big five competencies" as: (1) team leadership, (2) mutual performance monitoring, (3) backup behavior, (4) adaptability, and (5) team orientation. *Team leadership* is the ability to coordinate team members' activities, ensure appropriate task distribution, evaluate effectiveness, and inspire high-level performance. Whereas *mutual performance* helps to develop a shared understanding among team members regarding intentions, roles, and responsibilities. *Backup behavior* competency is the ability to anticipate the needs of other team members and cooperate during times of variable workload. In this particular regard, role of the IPC team's clinical supervisor is to bring these disparate team members together to form an integrated and equal team membership. Hence, the clinical supervisor requires additional information and training in order to effectively shape the skills and competencies of the team members. *Adaptability* is the ability of team members to adjust their strategy for completing tasks based on feedback from the work environment. Lastly, *team orientation* is focused on to prioritize team goals over individual goals and shows respect and regard for each team member [13].

3.5 Social Theories and Teamwork

Social or psychosocial theories are important to make us learn that how collaboration can be made more effective towards better care in the presence of fairly diverse health care provider team and the health care recipients. Professional socialization gears the team working in an effective manner [13]. Theories provide the ground to develop and train a team in order to carry out the desired activity accordingly (Table 3.2).

In this regard, *Piaget's theory* [14], also known as *"developmental stage theory,"* argued a century ago that operational (situational) intelligence is basic and it may translate into functional intelligence, and is applicable to all levels of learners. *Piaget* also mentioned that basic processes of assimilation and accommodation are to be understood well, in order to develop a culture of tolerance and respect. Similarly, the *"self-efficacy theory"* proposed by *Bandura* [15] addresses that how a person's belief in their own competence is useful in a group activity. Bandura had emphasized the importance of reflection on one's own experiences and exerting self-influence on the action or task done as a part of the group. *Kolb's theory* [16] identifies stages of effective learning as concrete learning, reflective observation,

Table 3.2 Theories applicable to various phases of IPECP

Phase of IPECP	Theory suited	Level of application	Benefit	Example
Training of team	Piaget's Vygotsky	Team building in educational programs; team building in health care organization	Well aware and well-developed teams to involve in learning or to get engaged in collaborative practice	Information exchange between the students allowed interprofessional learning to occur. Students from different disciplines collaborated in the development of strategies for planning, implementing, monitoring, and evaluating a health program through IPE
Activity/ task	Turner's theory	Interactions during team activity	Better communication and coordination; conflict resolutions if any	Contribution of the professional to interprofessional collaboration is achieved by *bridging* professional, social, physical, and task-related *gaps*, by *negotiating overlaps* in roles and tasks, and by *creating spaces* to be able to do so. Professionals from different professions seem to make different contributions
Evaluation of IPC	Self-efficacy theory	Reflection on roles in IPC program	Self-influence can be exercised of individuals as part of the whole	Simulation training enhanced participants' self-efficacy in clinical situations. It also led to increases in their perceived abilities relating to communication/teamwork and leadership

abstract conceptualization, and active experimentation. It also helps in recognizing learning styles as assimilating, accommodating, converging, and diverging. A team can be more effective if comprises of more than one type of learners. *Turner's theory* [17], also known as *"Social Identity Theory,"* is a very influential theory in various areas, like examining individual differences in task performance, leadership styles, and refining intergroup relations among its members [17].

Powell's theory [18], an "institutional theory," represents a macro-perspective and addresses concerns in the creative and prescriptive ways in which organizations and leaders inculcate and reflect their institutional pluralistic contexts. This theory would be useful in convincing the policy makers to have IPC policy at various levels of health care.

Recently, an evidence-driven *convergent care theory* [19] *(CCT)* has been introduced to be applied in a complex health care system with diverse needs of the stakeholders and that's how, able to achieve optimal health care outcomes. Caring culture is the basic principle in convergent care theory and in comparison, to other social theories, CCT not only based on concepts of organizational care, collaborative care, person/patient-centered care but also on health providers' or patients' self-care [19]. For more details on learning theories, see "Chap. 10".

3.6 Interprofessional Teamwork

Quality care, safety, and affordable cost are paramount in health care delivery. From the point of view of a health care professional, the main goal must be patient-centered care. In today's world, the delivery of care is complex and involves multiple professionals. These varied groups of health professionals with corresponding competencies and expertise in their profession intentionally cooperate to achieve specific goals for which they have collective responsibility. This is termed as interprofessional teamwork [13, 20, 21].

The history of health care interdisciplinary teams is said to have begun during World War II, when these interdisciplinary teams helped patients who were poor requiring treatment across the world [22]. IPE is typically described when various students or professionals learn *from with*, and *about* each other to develop collaboration and excellence in care [23–25]. Though the start of IPE was in the 1960s, educational paradigm shifts occurred towards IPE especially in the United Kingdom in the 1980s, and slowly progressed further on a larger scale during the next century [13, 26].

Interprofessional collaborative practice (IPCP) is termed as a collective exercise where the health care professionals work to collaborate with those inside their specific profession, other professionals, patients, and their relations [6, 27].

3.7 Why Interprofessional Teamwork Is Necessary?

Both IPE and IPCP require an amalgamation of varied professional beliefs, theoretical frameworks from various fields to work together towards one goal [28]. It requires active interprofessional teamwork for effective IPE or IPCP to transpire to address health care issues, resulting in quality patient care [28].

3.8 A Structural Framework for Interprofessional Teamwork

Reeves [21] and Reeves et al. [29] stated that there are four main pillars on which the structure of interprofessional teamwork is based upon, which are the Context, Organization, Relations, and Processual factors. Each of these factors, consisting of sub-factors, is significant and interlinked to complement each other and have a prominent effect on interprofessional teamwork. If one pillar factor is deficient, it affects the function and process of interprofessional teamwork. Let us examine each of these pillars.

Context Gender dynamics play a pivotal role in any team. Gender inequalities have existed over the centuries in various professions based on stereotypes and dominance. A similar situation prevails in the profession of health care. It is paramount that women should be part of the interprofessional team based on their expertise to achieve desired outcomes [31].

Culture and diversity of the team The culture of a team means how individual professionals perceive and understand the entire team and interprofessional cooperation [21]. Each interprofessional team may create their unique working culture based on each individual's belief, attitude, and professional outlook [31]. As a team culture, the diversity of the interprofessional team is significant since each professional would have the skill and experience to bring innovation to the forefront and help to achieve goals as an effective health care team. A diverse team produces enhanced outcomes as compared to those team members who think alike [21, 31].

Political intention for policies on interprofessional teamwork The willingness to initiate policies towards promoting interprofessional teamwork has been created by national governments of several countries (e.g., USA, UK, and Australia). These initiatives have helped in bringing quality care and enhanced patient safety.

Economics Interprofessional team-based care may play part in achieving better economics. However, there needs to be more evidence generated to say that interprofessional teamwork in health care is a profitable deal [21, 32].

Organization The support of the organization is crucial for the functioning and progress of the health care interprofessional team. The organization supports the interprofessional team for economic requirements and time, which are valuable and crucial for patient care. Less control may disrupt the functioning, whereas over control of the organization can result in less autonomy of the interprofessional team and may hinder the team goal of achieving the desired outcomes [21].

Fear of legal action Legal factors have effects on IPCP and how the interprofessional team works. Legal reforms in IPCP will bring about innovations and guidelines and will improve criteria for best practices and patient care [33]. Fears of legal action are likely to arise in an interprofessional team due to the overlapping of professional work and who in the team would be held responsible for the error on negligence. There must be changes in the laws and policies for IPCP per se [33, 34].

Relations The presence of a hierarchical system could disrupt the functioning of the interprofessional team, e.g., the senior professionals in the team may influence the junior professionals. An interprofessional hierarchy may also be present where one profession dominates the other. However, if the interprofessional team is aware, avoids dominance and traditional concepts of hierarchy, it could help the team towards an effective and positive outlook and outcomes [21].

Power of the profession Power imbalances within the interprofessional team have their effects on the decisions and the actions which follow. Thus, it is important that in an interprofessional collaboration power-sharing is balanced among the professionals through various interventions such as multifaceted interventions and shifting of roles within the interprofessional team [21].

Structure of the interprofessional team The number and those involved in the team are important, as research indicates that inappropriate composition and too high a number (e.g., >10) could result in the non-attendance of few professionals, the formation of subgroups, disrupting the work process [21, 35].

Role of the interprofessional team Clarity of the role for every member within the interprofessional team is vital for the relationships within the team and its functioning. Role clarification helps in avoiding encroachment or overlapping of the roles of every team member. Every member of the team is required to contribute to the task, process, and responsibility. The leader's role is crucial on how to take the team forward and steering the team positively towards the goal [21]. A leader of the interprofessional team may require to amalgamate various leadership styles (e.g., visionary, integrative, transactional, autocratic, authoritative, democratic, coaching, affiliative, transformational, etc.) and be a situational leader based on the circumstances, making sure that the decisions are patient-centered as per the local health care setting [36, 37].

Interprofessional team processes These include communication, emotions, trust, mutual respect, humor, conflicts within the team, stability of the team, inclination to collaborate, and activities for team building. Communication is paramount to the functioning of any team to overcome challenges, conflicts, and efficiently work towards the goal. Communication among the interprofessional team members may occur verbally or gestural. Inadequate communication among the interprofessional team can be disastrous in a clinical setting resulting in unfortunate events [21].

An emotional connection between the team member occurs when it is a gratifying experience to work with the individuals in the team. Acknowledging each other's work enriches the team effort resulting in better outcomes. Trusting other team members and having mutual respect are important components of healthier teamwork. Absence of trust and/or mutual respect in an interprofessional team will result in miscommunication leading to conflicts [21, 38].

Research indicates that use of humor eases the tension, reduces chances of conflict, and helps to build relationships among those in the interprofessional team [21, 39, 40]. Conflicts within the team members can result in fallout or disruption of the process and performance of the team. However, it is said that if conflicts can be controlled and resolved amicably, it can prove to be an effective method of moving forward towards the goal through training by a conflict management session [21, 41]. When the team is in a state of being stable, it augments the work process to achieve betterment. However, being stable may not be permanent as there may be a change in the members (professionals) upon a time [21]. The team would have to continuously construct relations with the new team member [21, 42]. Team building activities when conducted consistently and use of reflective practices conducted during fixed periods in time will enhance the team building processes and interpersonal relationships, resulting in instability of the interprofessional team [21].

Socialization Socialization is termed as the method of learning where the person behaves in a manner that is suitable to societal norms. Socialization in interprofessional teams occurs based on each individual's professional culture, upbringing, attitude, and principles. Each profession includes an attitude, hierarchy, or stereotypical belief that is generalized and imbibed by those in the profession from their professional learning years. This may result in hindering the interprofessional teamwork and process [21].

3.9 Processual Factors

Information Technology (IT) The plus point of IT is that effective communication between the interprofessional team members can occur at any time of the day or night, and on the go by reducing face-to-face interaction. The use of IT has been researched and used for the past two decades for interprofessional teamwork [43–45]. The use of IT has been promising for IPE and IPP by interprofessional teams, a recent example being the interprofessional teamwork during the COVID-19 pandemic in various parts of the world [44, 46, 47].

Unpredictability and Urgency Clinical work, for example, in the trauma/emergency or operation theater can be unpredictable for the interprofessional team. This kind of an unpredictable clinical setting can result in a stressful situation among the interprofessional team [21, 48]. Interprofessional team members must be aware that factors such as unpredictability could influence the team process and need to adapt to the situation [21]. Important clinical situations may require swift action (urgency) such as in the trauma/emergency or operation theater. These sorts of clinically urgent situations are challenging, so it is important that the interprofessional team members work together and work towards the intended outcome [21, 49].

Complexity Over the years, advances in organizations, technology, economics, and social development result in complex situations in health care delivery. For example, sub-specializations are on the rise, especially among physicians. When those with sub-specializations join an interprofessional team, they are required to adjust and rework the group dynamics to share and give space to other professionals [21].

Substitution Delegation (substitution) of work can occur when the professional hands over his or her role of the other professional in the team. This type of shifting the task to another professional within the team can help to ease the burden faced by one professional in the team [21].

Time and space factors Both time and space factors are interlinked socially and have their effects on the interprofessional team in a health care setting [21]. A general notion is that if the team spends more time, greater would be the teamwork and lesser the communication gaps [50]. When the team spends some informal time together, it can help build trust, understanding, and space between each individual in the interprofessional team during teamwork [21]. Health care workers and social care workers who are by tradition separated may separate the patient's illness and the patient, endorsing profession related tasks and resulting in disrupted interprofessional work [51].

Routine and rituals Standardized work processes or routines present in a health care setting are important as a map for the interprofessional health care team to reach the goal. Rituals are enactments that are established as a convention of traditionally assembled actions. Routines and rituals help in psychological and social aspects, identification of values, guidelines, and compromise of power of the interprofessional team and its members [21, 52, 53].

Other factors affecting Interprofessional teamwork Health care experts must be educated and possess skills to work together with other professionals to attain a successful, skilled, and socially sensitive health care delivery system [54]. To enhance interprofessional teamwork, students from varied professions must be provided with an interprofessional learning environment where they learn from, learn with, and socialize with each other. Pecukonis et al. [54] added that profession centric thinking should be avoided for actual interprofessional teamwork and collaboration to transpire. As previously stated, each profession has its own culture (principles, tradition, belief, attitude, and conduct), gender biases, and social status, therefore students must be trained to understand their work culture and evolve problem solving methods to sustain teamwork [31, 54].

Future scope of Interprofessional teamwork Recent times have shown that IPE and IPCP are gaining more attention. Langlois et al. [55] indicated that the COVID-19 pandemic has augmented teamwork and better collaborative practices among various health care professionals, which can be a reason for incorporation of IPE and IPCP practices in the future. Students from diverse health professions learn to function in teams early enough during their courses are likely to form effective interprofessional teams in the future. They create a culture and educational climate for collaborative practice that enhances the quality of patient care.

3.10 Summary of IPC Enabling and Disabling Factors and Values [56]

Factors and values that enhance effectiveness of IPC system may include:

- Proactive health policies.
- Organized health care system.
- Financial independence.
- Compassion.

- Competence.
- Accountability.
- Trust and respect.

The following factors may weaken interprofessional coordination and collaboration in general:

- Fragmented health care.
- Reactive health policies.
- Prolonged financial dependence.
- Donors' misalignment.
- Proliferation of donor and partners in health programs promotion.
- Longitudinal programs.
- Lack of sharing of responsibilities.

3.11 Summary of the Limitations of IPC Related Social/ Learning Theories

The followings are limitations of some social and learning theories applicable to TBL and team working [5]:

- Piagets' theory supports sharp stages rather than continuous development.
- Kolb's Experiential Learning theory criticized to be too simplistic in nature and only works in abstract isolation.
- Freidson's theory of professionalization can be criticized for its singular focus on the macro-level process of closure which overlooks individual resistance.
- Powells' theory also criticized for its macro-level process.
- Foucalt's theory may compromise the role of individual professionals.
- Turner's theory over emphasized the personal identity of team member while masking other sociodemographic profile.

3.12 Summary of Teams and Teamwork Evaluation

The following tools can be used in different situations for team and teamwork evaluation [57, 58]:

- Self-efficacy scales, which evaluate IPECP programs including all its components, the specific questions on teamwork and their roles, sharing problem solving, and accountability with other professions and taking informed decisions.
- Interprofessional socializing and valuing surveys.
- Student perception of interprofessional clinical education [SPICE-R].
- Performance assessment communication and teamwork.
- SF-36 health survey for patients' perception of their own health.

- Interdisciplinary team process and performance survey.
- Patient reported outcome measurement information survey.
- Assessment of interprofessional team collaboration scale.
- Team climate inventory.
- IPC scale.
- Oxford NO-TECHS Assessment.
- Program for assessment of care of elderly.

3.13 Evidence on Collaborative Practice

In a systematic review, Lavoie et al. [59] summarized that majority of the articles did not provide explicit theory and the ones reviewed commonly used Bandura's social-cognitive theory, Kolbs' experiential learning, Jeffries' simulation framework, and the self-efficacy theory.

Interprofessional and multiprofessional approaches have been used in different educational objectives without having any clear benefit of one approach to another. However, quality improvement can be assessed in both approaches by assurance of professional identity, hierarchies, and boundaries [60].

The health sector in Sierra Leone has been facing challenges of fragmentation of services, deficient emergency response capacities, and poor sustainable health system. This organizational disarray is accompanied with external threats like discontinuity of donors' funding and lack of coordination with international agencies to support horizontal programs. Fragmentation in policy and planning are repeatedly found in community health worker (CHW) programs, medical supply chains, and in-service level agreements (SLAs). Certain reactive rapid policies like Ebola policy have further shattered the development and health care funding was diverted to inadequately integrated vertical programs [61]. Therefore, CHW program could not be fully integrated in primary health care because of weak policies.

Another example is care of elderly program, that require special health and social services needs of older adults cannot be by single health expert and require a teamwork. The care needed by older adults is diverse, complex, and labor intensive. It encompasses different workforce from community health centers, hospitals, and nursing homes required to be well-skilled and highly committed to deliver quality, comprehensive, and effective geriatric care services [62].

Further details on evidence for IPE and IPC and their outcomes are outlined in "Chap. 7".

3.14 Team Strategies and Tools to Enhance Performance and Patient Safety (TeamSTEPPS)

Team STEPPS™ is an evidence-based framework to optimize team performance across the health care delivery system. It has five key principles. It is based on team structure and four teachable-learnable skills: Communication, Leadership, Situation

Monitoring, and Mutual Support. Situation monitoring is carried out by status of the patient, team members, environment, and the progress towards goal [63].

For implementing the curriculum of TeamSTEPPS, it is important to do needs assessment of the institution. Also, awareness and preparedness of all stakeholders is an important prerequisite, otherwise the process may not be successful. Furthermore, the evaluation of patient safety practices should be done before implementing TeamSTEPPS and during the training programs. After completion of training of health care teams, evaluation should be done frequently to see if TeamSTEPPS has been useful in enhancing performance and patient safety. In addition, the team working should also be evaluated using standard tools.

3.15 Challenges in Developing and Implementing IPECP Programs

Developing an effective health care team in either educational program or collaborative practices like in PHC or emergency hospital care, presents a significant challenge due to the complexities of curriculum requirements, professionals' behaviors, and interprofessional dynamics. In addition, greatly these professionals during their learning phase have never been trained for teamwork and for shared decision making and so take time to get accustomed to this novel philosophy of interprofessional care. Teams generally comprise of physicians, nurses, pharmacist, social or community workers, health managers, and psychologists, with diverse knowledge background and different roles. Nevertheless, team building and implementation of TBL in academic years would be the critical step to prepare future health care providers for their expected roles in collaborative practices and would deliver best standards.

Chan et al. [11] indicated that TBL is a viable pedagogy for IPE and can be implemented for undergraduate health and social care programs. However, the potential challenges like significant time involvement of the teachers, difficulty in matching students from different programs, difficulty in making summative assessment score from IPTBL, and inappropriateness of the venue are to be well thought off before its full implementation.

3.16 Summary

Team working is the central notion in collaborative health care practice with appropriate professional socialization of team members and their mutual harmony. It is evident that developing a committed team and helping them to understand their respective roles would ensure best outcome of IPC. In certain fields of health care practices such as emergency, natural disasters, and global health actions, which highly demand well-coordinated team with clarity of communication and informed timely decision making. Understanding the theories of social psychology and their proper use is of paramount importance to build a tangible IPECP program to maintain team dynamics and address team related problems. Social identity theory and self-efficacy theory provide worthy support in optimal team working and resultant quality health care. Students from diverse health professions who learn to function in teams early enough during their courses are likely to form effective interprofessional teams in the future, who create a culture and educational climate for collaborative practice that enhances the quality of patient care.

References

1. Canadian Interprofessional Health Collaborative. A national interprofessional competency framework. 2010. http://www.cihc.ca/files/CIHC_IPCompetencies_Feb1210.pdf.
2. Burgess A, van Diggele C, Roberts C, Mellis C. Team-based learning: design, facilitation and participation. BMC Med Educ. 2020;20(2):461.
3. Rees CE, Crampton P, Kent F, Brown T, Hood K, Leech M, et al. Understanding students' and clinicians' experiences of informal interprofessional workplace learning: an Australian qualitative study. BMJ. 2018;8:e021238.
4. Ganotice FA Jr, Chan L, Shen X, Ho Yan Lam A, Hoi Yan Wong G, Ka Wai Liu R, et al. Team cohesiveness and collective efficacy explain outcomes in interprofessional education. BMC Med Educ. 2022;22:820.
5. Reeves S, Lewin S, Espin S, Zwarenstein M. Interprofessional teamwork in health and social care. Hoboken: Wiley-Blackwell; 2010.
6. Bridges DR, Davidson RA, Odegard PS, Maki IV, Tomkowiak J. Interprofessional collaboration: three best practice models of interprofessional education. Med Educ Online. 2011;16:1.
7. Vygotsky LS. Mind in society: the development of higher psychological processes. Cambridge, MA: Harvard University Press; 1978.
8. Wagle K, Cottingham AH, Butler D, Grover J, Litzelman DK. Understanding social workers' hidden roles in medication safety for older adults: a qualitative study. Soc Work Health Care. 2021;60(4):369–86.
9. Smit LC, Dikken J, Moolenaar NM, Schuurmans MJ, de Wit NJ, Bleijenberg N. Implementation of an interprofessional collaboration in practice program: a feasibility study using social network analysis. Pilot Feasibility Stud. 2021;7:7.
10. Goolsarran N, Hamo CE, Lane S, Frawley S, Lu WH. Effectiveness of an interprofessional patient safety team-based learning simulation experience on healthcare professional trainees. BMC Med Educ. 2018;18:192.
11. Chan LK, Ganotice F Jr, Wong FKY, Lau CS, Bridges SM, Chan CHY, et al. Implementation of an interprofessional team-based learning program involving seven undergraduate health and social care programs from two universities, and students' evaluation of their readiness for interprofessional learning. BMC Med Educ. 2017;17(1):221.
12. Salas E, Sims DE, Burke CS. Is there a "big five" in teamwork? Small Group Res. 2005;36(5):555–99.
13. Leasure EL, Jones RR, Meade LB, Sanger MI, Thomas KG, Tilden VP, et al. There is no "i" in teamwork in the patient-centered medical home: defining teamwork competencies for academic practice. Acad Med. 2013;88(5):585–92.
14. Piaget J. The role of action in the development of thinking. In: Knowledge and development. New York: Springer US; 1977. p. 17–42.
15. Bandura A. Self-efficacy: toward a unifying theory of behavioral change. Psychol Rev. 1977;84:191–215.
16. Akella D. Learning together: Kolb's experiential theory and its application. J Manag Organ. 2010;16:100–12.
17. Freund R. Turner's theory of social evolution. Agric Hist. 1945;19(2):78–87.
18. DiMaggio PJ, Powell WW. The iron cage revisited: institutional isomorphism and collective rationality in organizational fields. Am Sociol Rev. 1983;48:147–60.

19. Wei H. The development of an evidence-informed convergent care theory: working together to achieve optimal health outcomes. Int J Nurs Sci. 2021;9(1):11–25.
20. Katzenbach JR, Smith DK. The wisdom of teams: creating the high-performance organization. Harvard Business Review; 2015.
21. Reeves S. Education in an interprofessional context. In: Dornan T, Mann K, Scherpbier A, Spencer J, editors. Medical education: theory and practice. London: Churchill Livingstone-Elsevier; 2011. p. 51–64.
22. Baldwin DW. Some historical notes on interdisciplinary and interprofessional education and practice in health care in the USA. J Interprof Care. 1996;10(2):173–87.
23. Barr H. Toward a theoretical framework for interprofessional education. J Interprof Care. 2013;27(1):4–9.
24. Centre for the Advancement of InterProfessional Education (CAIPE) on the definition and principles of interprofessional education. CAIPE Bulletin, 2006.
25. Gilbert JH. Interprofessional education for collaborative, patient-centred practice. Nurs Leadersh. 2005;18(2):32–8.
26. Fransworth TJ, Seikel JA, Hudock D, Holst J. History and development of interprofessional education. J Phon Audiol. 2015;1(1):1–5.
27. Canadian Interprofessional Health Collaborative. 2009. www.cihc.ca/resources-files/CIHC_Factsheets_CP_Feb09.pdf.
28. Lateef F. Inter-professional education, inter-professional practice and team science: learning together; working together. Educ Med J. 2018;10(4):81–91.
29. Reeves S, Xyrichis A, Zwarenstein M. Teamwork, collaboration, coordination, and networking: why we need to distinguish between different types of interprofessional practice. J Interprof Care. 2018;32(1):1–3.
30. Bell AV, Michalec B, Arenson C. The (stalled) progress of interprofessional collaboration: the role of gender. J Interprof Care. 2014;28(2):98–102.
31. Kochan T, Bezrukova K, Ely R, Jackson S, Joshi A, Jehn K, et al. The effects of diversity on business performance: report of the diversity research network. Human Resource Management: published in cooperation with the School of Business Administration, the University of Michigan and in alliance with the Society of Human Resources Management. Hum Resour Manag. 2003;42(1):3–21.
32. Oxman AD, Bjørndal A, Flottorp SA, Lewin S, Lindhal AK. Integrated health care for people with chronic conditions. A policy brief. Open Arch Initiative. 2008;6(13):106–8.
33. Ries NM. Law matters: how the legal context in Canada influences interprofessional collaboration. J Interprof Care. 2017;31:417–9.
34. Bentley M, Freeman T, Baum F, Javanparast S. Interprofessional teamwork in comprehensive primary healthcare services: findings from a mixed methods study. J Interprof Care. 2018;32(3):274–83.
35. Williams G, Laungani P. Analysis of teamwork in an NHS community trust: an empirical study. J Interprof Care. 1999;13(1):19–28.
36. Hersey PW, Blanchard KH. Management of organizational behaviour: utilizing human resources. ILR Rev. 1971;24(3):491–2.
37. Chatalalsingh C, Reeves S. Leading team learning: what makes interprofessional teams learn to work well? J Interprof Care. 2014;28(6):513–8.
38. Walby ST, Greenwell J, Mackay L, Soothill K. Medicine and nursing: professions in a changing health service. New York: SAGE Publications; 1994. p. 206.
39. Brewer ML, Flavell H. High and low functioning team-based pre-licensure interprofessional learning: an observational evaluation. J Interprof Care. 2021;35(4):538–45.
40. Dobai A, Hopkins N. Humour is serious: minority group members' use of humour in their encounters with majority group members. Eur J Soc Psychol. 2020;50(2):448–62.
41. Bajwa NM, Bochatay N, Muller-Juge V, Cullati S, Blondon KS, Perron N, et al. Intra versus interprofessional conflicts: implications for conflict management training. J Interprof Care. 2020;34(2):259–68.
42. Ong YH, Koh MY, Lim WS. Shared leadership in interprofessional teams: beyond team characteristics to team conditions. J Interprof Care. 2020;34(4):444–52.

43. Patel VL, Kaufman DR, Allen VG, Shortliffe EH, Cimino JJ, Greenes RA. Toward a framework for computer-mediated collaborative design in medical informatics. Methods Inf Med. 1999;38(3):158–76.
44. Natale JE, Boehmer J, Blumberg DA, Dimitriades C, Hirose S, Kair LR, et al. Interprofessional/interdisciplinary teamwork during the early COVID-19 pandemic: experience from a children's hospital within an academic health center. J Interprof Care. 2020;17:1–5.
45. Wada RK. Leadership, behavioral science, and interprofessional teamwork. Transl Behav Med. 2020;10(4):905–8.
46. Bautista CA, Huang I, Stebbins M, Floren LC, Wamsley M, Youmans SL, et al. Development of an interprofessional rotation for pharmacy and medical students to perform telehealth outreach to vulnerable patients in the COVID-19 pandemic. J Interprof Care. 2020;12:1–4.
47. Chen YY, Zhuang J. Roles of medical social workers in interprofessional teams: a case study of a Shanghai COVID-19 quarantine center for medical observation. Asia Pac J Soc Work. 2020;3:1–9.
48. Annandale E, Clark J, Allen E. Interprofessional working: an ethnographic case study of emergency health care. J Interprof Care. 1999;13(2):139–50.
49. Skjørshammer M. Co-operation and conflict in a hospital: interprofessional differences in perception and management of conflicts. J Interprof Care. 2001;15(1):7–18.
50. Jaques D, Salmon G. Learning in groups: a handbook for face-to-face and online environments. 4th ed. Oxford: Routledge; 2007.
51. Pryor J. A nursing perspective on the relationship between nursing and allied health in inpatient rehabilitation. Disabil Rehabil. 2008;30(4):314–22.
52. Helman CG, editor. Culture, health and illness. 5th ed. Boca Raton: CRC Press; 2007.
53. Strange F. Handover: an ethnographic study of ritual in nursing practice. Intensive Crit Care Nurs. 1996;12(2):106–12.
54. Pecukonis E, Doyle O, Bliss DL. Reducing barriers to interprofessional training: promoting interprofessional cultural competence. J Interprof Care. 2008;22(4):417–28.
55. Langlois S, Xyrichis A, Daulton BJ, Gilbert J, Lackie K, Lising D, et al. The COVID-19 crisis silver lining: interprofessional education to guide future innovation. J Interprof Care. 2020;34(5):587–92.
56. Reeves S, Fletcher S, Barr H, Birch I, Boet S, Davies N. A BEME systematic review of the effects of interprofessional education: BEME Guide No. 39. Med Teach. 2016;38(7):656–68.
57. Kottorp A, Keehn M, Hasnain M, Gruss V, Peterson E. Instrument refinement for measuring self-efficacy for competence in interprofessional collaborative practice: development and psychometric analysis of IPECC-SET 27 and IPECC-SET 9. J Interprof Care. 2019;33(1):47–56.
58. National Centre for International practice and Education. https://nexusipe.org/advancing/assessment-evaluation/.
59. Lavoie P, Michaud C, Bélisle M, Boyer L, Gosselin É, Grondin M, et al. Learning theories and tools for the assessment of core nursing competencies in simulation: a theoretical review. J Adv Nurs. 2018;74(2):239–50.
60. Goldman J, Kuper A, Whitehead C, Baker G, Bulmer B, Coffey M, et al. Interprofessional and multiprofessional approaches in quality improvement education. Adv Health Sci Educ. 2021;26:615–36.
61. Barr A, Garrett L, Marten R, Kadandale S. Health sector fragmentation: three examples from Sierra Leone. Glob Health. 2019;15(8):1–8.
62. Moncatar TRT, Nakamura K, Siongco K, Seino K, Carlson R, Canila CC, et al. Interprofessional collaboration and barriers among health and social workers caring for older adults: a Philippine case study. Hum Resour Health. 2021;19:52.
63. Guimond ME, Sole ML, Salas E. TeamsSTEPPS. Am J Nurs. 2009;109(11):66–8.

Learning In and About Interprofessional Teams and Wider Collaborations

4

Jill Thistlethwaite and Nichola McLarnon

4.1 Introduction

Interprofessional education (IPE) aims to improve collaboration between health and social care professionals and the quality of care for patients and clients. In this chapter we mainly focus on teamwork and explore 'learning together to work together' [1] through IPE. However, collaborative practice encompasses more than co-located teamworking and IPE should also aim to introduce learners to the complexities of modern health care delivery with its diverse models of 'working together'.

Collaboration is a complex concept with one definition being 'a process in which autonomous or semi-autonomous actors interact through formal and informal negotiation, jointly creating rules and structures governing their relationships and ways to act or decide on the issues that brought them together; it is a process involving shared norms and mutually beneficial interactions' [2]. The widely used definition of interprofessional collaborative practice specifies the actors and the purpose: 'the process of developing and maintaining effective interprofessional working relationships with learners, practitioners, patients/clients/ families and communities to enable optimal health outcomes' [3].

J. Thistlethwaite (✉)
University of Technology Sydney, Sydney, Australia

N. McLarnon
Glasgow Caledonian University, Glasgow, UK

M. Y. Alnaami et al. (eds.), *Novel Health Interprofessional Education and Collaborative Practice Program: Strategy and Implementation*, https://doi.org/10.1007/978-981-99-3420-1_4

4.1.1 Types of Interprofessional Practice

Reeves et al. have identified six common elements that affect interprofessional working: shared team identity; clear roles/goals; interdependence; integration; shared responsibility; and team tasks—'the predictability, urgency and complexity of a team's actual work' [4]. These six elements occur along a continuum and taken together help describe four types of interprofessional work with collaboration considered as a looser form than teamwork, the latter being the 'most focused of activities with high levels of interdependence, integration and shared responsibility' [5]. An ideal team is typically a small number of people, with optimal membership ranging from 4 to 12 members depending on its objectives [6]. Collaboration, coordination, and networking are conceptualised as increasingly broader activities with correspondingly reduced levels of interdependence, integration, and shared responsibility as the number of people involved increases. Later work to refine the typology of interprofessional work activities has added two sub-categories to collaboration—consultative collaboration and collaborative partnership, and three to coordination—coordinated collaboration, delegative coordination, and consultative coordination [7].

Entry-level pre-qualification students need to learn about teamwork. The nuances of other types of interprofessional practice should be discussed once learners are in clinical settings. Subsequently, IPE for licensed health professionals helps them develop a comprehensive insight into the range of interprofessional work activities. The principles of teamwork apply across many contexts, whereas the performance of other forms of interprofessional work may differ depending on a jurisdiction's health system. It is important for all health professional students and practising professionals to have a good understanding of their own context: the governance and working of their health system and the hierarchies within it, as well as patients'/clients' perspectives including access to and costs of health care.

There are challenges in providing students and novice health professionals (HPs) with authentic experiences of teamwork and wider collaboration in healthcare settings. At the pre-qualification level students tend to work in small groups for teamwork activities and observe bounded teams in clinical settings as they are easier for faculty to identify. After qualification, HPs begin to experience a wider range of collaboration as 'teams in healthcare span the full spectrum of team taxonomies' [8]. 'Teams' tend to be fluid in many settings with frequent membership changes depending on the context; yet students may see them as stable rather than complex. Adaptive expertise is required but may cause tensions in relation to role definitions and scopes of practice [9]. Engeström introduced the term 'negotiated knotworking' described as 'rapidly pulsating, distributed, and partially improvised orchestration of collaborative performance between otherwise loosely connected actors and activity systems' [10]. Bleakley considers how teams work in both space and time with their knotworking grounded in complexity and uncertainty. Teams that knotwork effectively produce new knowledge and innovative practice strategies *because* they tolerate high levels of ambiguity and work at maximum complexity without falling into chaos and are adaptive [11].

Such teams require reflective capacity: discussion amongst members using practice-based discourse. In routine teamwork, things simply get done without the need for dialogue. In more complex work, the need for communication exchange increases [11]. Students and less-experienced HPs learning 'teamwork' need to become familiar with both stable and adaptable knotworking practices. Adaptable knotworking requires education about tolerance of uncertainty and ambiguity, key attributes of health professionals who collaborate well both intra- and interprofessionally [12].

4.2 Interprofessional Learning Outcomes and Competencies for Interprofessional Practice

A curriculum designed for HP education students (i.e., pre-qualification) to learn about and participate in teamwork and collaborative practice needs to define what students are expected to achieve: the endpoint of learning at that stage of education. There are several ways in which this may be framed [13], of which the most common in IPE are as follows:

- Learning objectives: the specific knowledge, skills, and attitudes the learner will have acquired by the end of the curriculum.
- Intended outcomes: stated in clear and specific terms that allow for assessment.
- Competencies: what graduates should be able to do in practice [14].
- Capabilities: what learners need to be able to achieve to become effective (capable) interprofessional workers [15].

The interprofessional outcomes should be written in similar words to the overarching curriculum as an integral component of learning. However, health professional curricula are also informed by a health profession's specific national accreditation body. Typically, interprofessional outcomes/competencies are written in diverse ways for each profession even if the underlying aim of interprofessional learning (IPL) is similar. Therefore, IP educators and curriculum designers need to ensure that IPL outcomes/competencies meet the needs of accreditation bodies at the same time as being equitable for all learners. It can be difficult to reach consensus on the same set of outcomes for all professions. Some countries, such as Canada and the USA, are in the process of agreeing on interprofessional competencies for all health professions that will inform national accreditation standards.

There are interprofessional competency frameworks, including national examples such as those of the Canadian Interprofessional Health Collaborative (CIHC) of 2010 (currently under review) [3], the Interprofessional Education Collaborative of the United States (IPEC) published in 2011 [16] and updated in 2016 [17], an Australian set of common IPL competencies [18], and the Qatar Competency Framework [19], as well as single institutions such as Curtin University, Western Australia [20]. In addition, interprofessional competencies are listed in broader frameworks such as the World Health Organization's *Global Competency and*

Outcomes Framework for Universal Health Coverage [21]. As would be expected, there are commonalities across these frameworks that have remained constant in the last 15 years. Variations on teamwork and team functioning are prominent as well as items referring to roles and responsibilities, communication, collaborative practice, and patient/client-centred care [22]. However, not all the frameworks have been widely adopted, the two most frequently cited being those of the CIHC and IPEC. Examples of frameworks and items are listed in Table 4.1.

More recently, particularly in medical education, competencies have been reframed and amalgamated as entrustable professional activities (EPAs) that aim to bridge the gap between the approach of competency-based education and clinical practice. EPAs are framed as real-life tasks that learners/trainees need to perform well in their professional role at designated stages of training. They define the level of supervision required at each stage of training, based on the level of trust (entrustment) the supervisor has in the supervisee [23]. However, the problem with team-based EPAs is that they are in danger of being too broad and without an endpoint that is required for an entrustment decision. For example, the Association of American Medical Colleges has set 13 EPAs for medical students one of which is 'collaborate as a member of an interprofessional team' [24]. This EPA has been critiqued by the founders of the EPA movement as not representing a discrete task. Rather, working interprofessionally should be a feature of many EPAs as much clinical practice relies on collaboration [25]. A better example is an EPA for patient handovers, a specific task that requires communication with other professionals.

Table 4.1 Examples of interprofessional frameworks

Framework/list	Description	Themes/domains	Examples more specific to teamwork itself
Australia common set of IPL competencies (2017) [18]	Eight competency statements for students; 'team' not mentioned explicitly	Not applicable	Plan patient/client care goals and priorities with involvement of other health professionals
Canadian Interprofessional Health Collaborative (2010) [3]	Six domains	Interprofessional communication Patient/client/family / community-centred care Role clarification Team functioning Collaborative leadership Interprofessional conflict resolution	Learners/practitioners understand the principles of teamwork dynamics and group/team processes to enable effective interprofessional teamwork

Table 4.1 (continued)

Framework/list	Description	Themes/domains	Examples more specific to teamwork itself
Curtin University, Western Australia. Interprofessional capability framework (2011) [20]	Three core elements: client-centred service; client safety and quality; collaborative practice	5 collaborative practice capabilities: Communication Team function Role clarification Conflict resolution Reflection	The collaborative worker analyses the process of team development; engages in shared decision making to establish and achieve commonly agreed goals
Interprofessional Education Collaborative (2016), USA [17]	Four core competencies	Interprofessional communication practices Roles and responsibilities for collaborative practice Values/ethics for interprofessional practice Interprofessional teamwork and team-based practice	Describe the process of team development and the roles and practices of effective teams Use available evidence to inform effective teamwork and team-based practices
Qatar Competency Framework (2019) [19]	Four domains	Role clarification Interprofessional communication Patient-centred care Shared decision-making	Demonstrate through application an understanding of the principles of teamwork communication Include patients and their family members as part of the health care team

4.3 The Patient as a Member of the Team

Patient centredness is an important learning outcome for team education. The phrase 'the patient at the centre of the team' is a similar but not identical aspiration. There is no consensus definition of patient centredness in health care delivery, but terms frequently used in describing the concept are understanding the patient's perspective, recognising the patient's needs, patient as partner, shared decision making, and from the patient: 'nothing about me, without me'. It is the patient involvement that transforms generic teamwork learned in classrooms and non-patient facing activities into patient-centred healthcare focused collaborative practice. This is more than case-based learning in which the script is already written and patients cannot be actively involved.

Organised encounters with patients in clinical settings enable interprofessional teams of students to explore and recognise patients' health issues and perspectives, however, they may not lead to the integration of the patient into the team [26]. There may be tension between the students' learning imperatives and the care offered to patients depending on the task the students have been given.

4.4 Topics for Learning About Teamwork

As indicated in Table 4.1, IPL outcomes include understanding team development and functioning as well as the roles and responsibilities of team members. Theories of teamwork may be learned in classroom settings and then applied in team exercises and on clinical placements. Alternatively, team-based learning can be introduced experientially with guided reflection on team processes and subsequent underpinning with theory.

Common content of IPL includes definitions of a team and generic requirements for effective teams, such as clear team goals, shared team commitment, role clarity, interdependence, and integration between team members [5]. Types of healthcare teams should also be discussed, including co-located teams, for example, multidisciplinary teams in a primary care health centre and specialties such as mental health or palliative care, as well as teams that come together for specific tasks such as the cardiac arrest team.

Real-world experiences show that teams may become dysfunctional. There are five frequently described characteristics of dysfunctional teams: absence of trust; fear of conflict; lack of commitment; avoidance of accountability; inattention to results [27]. Conflict may be productive as successful conflict management enhances team cohesion [28]. It should be addressed rather than ignored, making sure that discussions have ground rules, and every voice and profession is heard. IPL should include discussion and reflection on dysfunction and conflict, and triggers such as professional stereotyping and differences in personal and professional values [29]. In addition, more experienced learners should be able to identify situations that commonly lead to conflict in practice-based settings, how professional identities may impact on collaborative practice and how to establish a safe environment incorporating psychological safety for addressing concerns [30].

4.5 Learning From and Learning in Teams

The World Health Organization has identified four principles for developing an interprofessional curriculum at any level of training: relevance to learners' current or future practice; the incorporation of typical and priority health issues that are solved through interprofessional approaches; IPL based on clinical practice; and interactive learning methods such as small group and case-based learning [31]. In addition, curriculum alignment is important at the pre-qualification level, with learning activities and experiences designed and offered to meet defined learning outcomes or competencies followed by appropriate and relevant assessment [32].

When planning learning activities, it is important to consider the learning space(s) and the learning and teaching approaches, which are informed by the level of training, logistics, feasibility, cost, availability of facilitators and supervisors, and relevant learning theories.

4.5.1 Pre-Qualification Students

A helpful model for situating learning within an undergraduate curriculum is that of the University of British Columbia (UBC) with its three levels of exposure, immersion, and mastery [33]. Students in their first 1 or 2 years are exposed to IPL with other professions while beginning to understand their own health profession. They learn mainly in the classroom and simulation spaces, though there may be opportunities for early patient contact in the community and hospitals. Immersion in clinical placements allows for learning in teams with practice-based collaborative education helping the development of an interprofessional world view and identity. The third level that incorporates the final year of university and postgraduate training focuses on mastering interprofessional concepts, incorporating them into daily practice while fostering critical reflection [33].

A major challenge for many institutions is the large number of students from different schools and faculties to involve in IPL. Timetabling and space require logistical solutions. An institution-wide leader and a dedicated centre or staff for IPE help with planning and evaluation. E-learning is one way to include all health (and perhaps social) care students in IPL. The use of online learning has increased during the pandemic [34] though it has been a feature of IPE for many years prior to this [35]. Virtual teams for IPL can highlight the advantages and disadvantages of telehealth for care delivery.

4.5.1.1 Learning Activities in the Classroom

Students should be in mixed professional groups; learning is interactive. Guided discussion should focus on the process of group or team learning as well as the content. Well-established pedagogics include problem-based learning (PBL) and case-based learning (CBL), which involve learning in and about teams. PBL and CBL focus on clinically related problems or patient case histories to provide triggers for learning and for IPL should include examples of interprofessional approaches to teamwork. Team-based learning (TBL) is a type of blended learning that involves one facilitator working with several groups of students in one classroom, each group having between 5 and 7 members. The groups self-manage and work as teams to solve problems that should foster complex reasoning and ensure constructive debate [36]. Case triggers within an interprofessional team reasoning framework together with video examples of interprofessional interactions have been shown to improve students' team skills and case presentations [37].

4.5.1.2 Simulation-Enhanced Interprofessional Education (Sim-IPE)

Simulation-based learning activities are defined as 'structured activities that represent actual or potential situations in education and practice' [38]. They are recognised as a highly effective and powerful way for students to develop clinical competence and reasoning skills, knowledge, self-efficacy, and self-confidence, in an authentic but most importantly 'safe' and controlled environment [39]. In addition to bridging theory to practice, students can make and learn from mistakes, without risk of harm to patients or service users [40].

Simulation-enhanced IPE (Sim-IPE) is at the intersection of the pedagogy of simulation and IPE. It 'prepares students to function as part of an interprofessional team and carry learned knowledge, skills, and values into future collaborative practice' [41]. The use of Sim-IPE, which emerged in the 1950s, has increased exponentially over the past three decades, allowing students from different professions to participate in simulation-based exercises to achieve defined and higher order learning outcomes [40, 42]. Within an IPE context, simulation activities facilitate the additional development of interprofessional competencies, such as team functioning, collaboration and communication, roles and responsibilities, values, and conflict resolution [41, 43]. A number of Sim-IPE initiatives also reinforce simulated activities with the didactic TeamSTEPPs® (team strategies and tools to enhance performance and patient safety) approach [44]. Examples of Sim-IPE activities cited within the literature relate to paediatrics [45], death notification [46], obstetrics [47], perinatal care [42], anaphylaxis [48], medication safety [49], and care of the older adult [41]. Sim-IPE activities are highly valued by students and have been shown to have a positive impact on their learning, motivation, and preparedness for practice [39, 43, 46, 49–51]. The use of Sim-IPE may also help address some of the logistical challenges associated with sourcing of interprofessional placement experiences, such as capacity or student numbers [50].

Although inherently valuable, the development and delivery of effective Sim-IPE activities can be challenging for educators [52]. The degree of complexity and fidelity, 'the degree to which the simulator replicates reality' [53], should therefore be carefully considered against available resource and expertise [54]. Additionally, it is important to ensure that tasks remain focused on interprofessional competencies and not practice skills and knowledge [48]. High-fidelity simulations are frequently cited in relation to Sim-IPE activities, with the employment of standardised or simulated patients a common feature [55]. Trained to act as a patient, or other individual, such as a carer or family member, standardised or simulated patients are considered to substantially enhance the fidelity of simulation activities, bringing the patient voice into learning. Sim-IPE and virtual adaptations with case studies, standardised patients, and small and large group discussions were adopted during the COVD-19 pandemic when placement challenges were particularly acute [51, 56]. However, Velásquez et al. highlight, that higher-level learning outcomes can in fact be achieved through lower fidelity approaches and diversification of pedagogical approach [55].

4.5.1.3 Team Learning in Clinical Practice

Students' observation through, for example, shadowing of clinical teams in their workplaces requires facilitated reflection to be actively processed [57]. This type of activity contributes to an understanding of health professional roles, responsibilities, constraints, expertise, hierarchies, and models of practice [58]. Active learning in teams is important as a follow-on to the more passive observation role. Students may be placed in existing clinical teams or may form interprofessional teams of students for specific tasks such as formulating a care plan for an allocated patient.

Interprofessional training wards (IPTW) and student-run clinics (SRC) are two examples where students provide patient care in service delivery settings under expert supervision. There are logistical and legal considerations for these activities within the context of the local jurisdiction.

Sweden introduced the first IPTWs in 1996 [59] with other examples in Germany [60], Australia [61], and the United Kingdom [62]. An IPTW is a functioning hospital inpatient ward where a diversity of health professional students has full responsibility for the management of patients. A review of 37 articles from 14 examples of IPTWs found that students rate IPL opportunities on IPTWs highly and value their team-activities. However, evaluations showing that students meet the learning outcomes have been short term only; longer term follow-up is required to show their impact on teamwork competencies [63].

SRCs in the USA provide free access to health care for uninsured and underserved populations. In countries with universal health care access, they are called student-led or student-assisted clinics. In such clinics, students from a wide range of health professions work under appropriate supervision. One systematic review has indicated that SRCs give students 'the optimal and most realistic form of learning by doing' [64], while a rapid review indicated that a benefit of such clinics is increasing students' understanding of working in interprofessional teams [65].

4.5.2 Training Qualified Health Professionals in Teamwork

Newly qualified healthcare professionals are likely to become members of healthcare teams at some level unless they work in solo practice, though even in this case they will collaborate with other health professionals regularly through referral processes. Novice health professionals typically join established teams as new members and require orientation to the team and how it functions. If they have received some teamwork training through IPE, these fledgling practitioners will have some understanding of the roles and responsibilities of their colleagues, the context of healthcare delivery and team dynamics.

Team training may be provided to improve team performance and may form part of quality improvement in certain healthcare settings. Such training may also contribute to professional reaccreditation as continuing professional development (CPD) reimagined as continuing interprofessional development (CIPD) [66]. Interventions include crew (also referred to as crisis) resource management (CRM) derived from the aviation industry [67], TeamSTEPPs® [68], simulation training and debriefing, and specific location/specialty training such as for the operating theatre or primary care. A systematic review of team training restricted to publications between 2008 and 2018 included 297 articles [69]. Simulation-based training was the most frequent intervention mentioned, while outcomes mainly focused on non-technical skills such as team working, communication, situational awareness, leadership, decision making, and team management. Most studies took place in hospitals and in acute care. Similar to other healthcare education interventions, most evaluations are restricted to short-term changes with low quality of evidence. The authors do, however, conclude that training is likely to be effective.

IPL may and should also occur in the workplace: informal learning in the teams of which health professional are members during day-to-day practice [70]. For example, interprofessional team meetings are opportunities to learn together, with sharing of tacit knowledge gained through experience and context, as well as the sharing of information about patient care [71]. For collective learning, IPL needs to be introduced as an integral part of the meeting with time for reflection on team processes [72].

4.6 Assessment of Teams and Team Members

Assessment is necessary 'to meet the needs and expectations of patients, clients and communities, as well as carers and families, for effective cooperation and interprofessional communication between health and social care workers' [73].

The tension when assessing teamwork is between the role of an individual member and the performance of the team as a whole unit, particularly as professional licensure is based on individual competency [74]. Who and what is being or should be assessed? Lingard has argued for consideration of the concept of collective competence [75]. She notes three regularly observed occurrences in team research: 'competent individuals can come together to form an incompetent team; individuals who perform competently in one team may not in another team; one incompetent member functionally impairs some teams but not others'. These phenomena emphasise the importance of context that is rarely considered in non-workplace assessment such as objective structured clinical examinations (OSCEs) and simulations, particularly where a team is formed specifically for the assessment itself.

4.6.1 Pre-Qualification and Undergraduate

Assessment of IPL outcomes/competencies at the pre-qualification level is the important endpoint of curriculum alignment. The purpose of such assessment is to check whether learning outcomes have been achieved and to contribute to the evaluation of whether a program is effective in promoting learning. Assessment at this level of education is typically of an individual student's learning based on marks or grades, though team-based assessment may also take place. The 2016 international consensus statement on the assessment of interprofessional learning outcomes, based on contributions from 75 respondents from 15 countries advocated for situated and contextualised assessment [73]. For registration with the relevant professional accreditation body, a student needs to meet individual profession-specific standards. Professional registration bodies usually mandate that staff from the same profession assess students for summative decisions. Considerations for assessment include:

- Timing of assessments.
- Format of assessments.
- IPL outcomes/competencies to be assessed.
- Whether formative, summative or programmatic.
- Weighting such as grading or pass/fail only.
- Individual and/or team-based assessment.
- Moderation processes.
- Professions to be assessed.
- Professions to assess and recruitment.
- Which professions may assess which professions.
- Faculty development required to assess.
- Impact of assessment on learning.

Interprofessional teamwork assessment for prequalification students is challenging. Written knowledge tests may focus on the theory of teamwork and HPs' roles and responsibilities, with case-based scenarios that promote application of knowledge to clinical practice. Observation and assessment of teamwork in action is more difficult, raising the question of what a team consists of at this level. Students may work in teams for course work and projects; they may be in interprofessional student groups for clinical placements, but not necessarily for sufficient time to form a team and then be observed; a student may be placed in an existing clinical team as an observer or participant, or be treated as a member of a clinical team during a longitudinal clinical placement lasting several months to a year [76]. Teams may be newly formed for specific learning experiences and/or assessments, such as simulations (for example, dealing with a cardiac arrest or deteriorating patient) or T-OSCEs (team objective structured clinical examinations) [77]. Assessment for such episodes will differ from that of a team that has been working together for some time. A group of students constituted for an assessment of collaboration is unlikely to function well compared to a team that has already been working together [78].

Programmatic assessment aims to reduce the reliance on single point summative decisions. It consists of combining a range of methods, including less than perfect instruments, for ongoing assessment throughout a program, where the combination is more important than the quality of the components administered individually. The validity of non-standardised assessment resides in the users and not so much in the instruments, and expert judgment is imperative [79]. Therefore, interprofessional competencies are not judged by a one-off observation or written test but rather over a longer time frame, with the collection of structured evidence of learning. This allows for high-stakes decisions at the end of phases of education based on multiple sources of information [80]. One approach is via an interprofessional passport or portfolio. Students are given the list of interprofessional competencies or learning outcomes they need to achieve during their program of study. The institution provides suitable opportunities for students to learn, many of which have a grade or narrative mark. Students provide evidence of learning in the portfolio such as work-based assessments (WBA), for example, multisource feedback and team observation tools, peer assessment, rotation grades, and reflections on how they know they have learned and what they have learned [81].

4.6.2 Postgraduate

Following qualification and licensure, the approach to assessment depends on its purpose. Again, there may be individual forms of assessment such as written and practical examinations, and work-based assessment for postgraduate qualifications.

4.6.3 Assessment of Clinical Teams

There are many teamwork tools to choose from that measure in diverse ways team functioning, processes, and outcomes. Teamwork assessment is also used to evaluate training, such as comparing teamwork before and after a learning activity. As well as 'tools' there are indices, instruments, measures, questionnaires, scales, and surveys. Some of these are to be completed by individuals in relation to their perception of some aspect of their team's functioning (i.e., self-report of behaviour or performance). There are attitudinal measures for individuals and tools to be used by observers of teams in action. Some tools are validated for generic team performances and some for teams working in specific areas/specialties such as emergency departments or operating theatres. Decisions on what tool to use are based on the following considerations:

- What is being measured (e.g., attitudes, confidence, competency, behaviour, clinical performance).
- Who is being measured (e.g., individual team members, the whole team, students, health professionals).
- Who is measuring (e.g., external observer, team members, tutor/trainer, peers, self).
- Location (e.g., generic settings or specific hospital departments, primary care, community-settings).
- Timing of assessment (before, during, after a task or learning activity).
- How data will be used.
- Psychometrics of the tool from previous usage.

Descriptions of teamwork assessment instruments are available from the National Center for Interprofessional Practice and Education at https://nexusipe.org/advancing/assessment-evaluation. Examples and descriptions of some tools are given in Table 4.2.

Table 4.2 Examples of team/teamwork assessment tools

Authors/date	Tool/instrument	Description	Metrics	Comments	Examples of items
Andreoli et al. (2010) [82]	Team orientation scale	Used before and after training to look at team orientation in rehabilitation settings 10 items	States shown to be valid and reliable, but no data given	Assessment of whole team	Team has agreed methods of communication; all team members' perspectives are important
Chiu et al. (2014) [83]	PACT: performance assessment communication and teamwork tools set	Toolbox of two self-report instruments and three observational rating tools	Validity study: acceptable to very good inter-rater reliability for the observational tools	Derived from the 5 domains of Team STEPPS	Team members refer to established protocols and checklists for the procedure/intervention
Curran et al. (2011) [84]	ICAR: interprofessional collaborator assessment rubric	Observation of teamwork with 6 domains Can be used for individual team members or the whole team		Developed through literature review and Delphi process for validity	Establishes collaborative relationships with other in planning and providing patient/client care
Earnest et al. (2022) [85]	CATME: comprehensive assessment of team member effectiveness	Web-based, peer and self-assessment tools; five items behaviourally anchored rating scale with five domains	Validity evidence provided	Originally developed for use in engineering; for use in classroom team-based learning	Contributing to the team's work Keeping the team on track
Hall et al. (2011) [86] Solomon et al. (2011) [87]	T-OSCE: Team OSCE	Observation of students in teams in scenario-based stations	Data given for inter-rater reliability; face and content validity		Wording depends on the station but covers communication, collaboration and team functioning

(continued)

Table 4.2 (continued)

Authors/date	Tool/instrument	Description	Metrics	Comments	Examples of items
Orchard et al. (2012) [88]	AITCS: assessment of interprofessional team collaboration scale	37 items with four subscales Measures collaboration within teams Individual self-report of team performance	Overall reliability = 0.98 Extensive testing with factor analysis	Can be used to compare before and after training scores	
Simmons et al. (2011) [77]	iOSCE: interprofessional OSCE	Behavioural indicators Specific skills for each station		Stations need to be developed for context and metrics calculated for each station and overall iOSCE	Demonstrates ability to work well with different members of the team
Thistlethwaite et al. (2016) [89]	iTOFT: individual teamwork observation and feedback tool	Two versions: 1. Basic for novice learners (11 observable behaviours); 2. Advanced for senior students and juniors HPs	Field tested pilot tool—Reliability 0.89	Developed through literature review and Delphi process for validity	Demonstrates respect for others in and outside the team (novice) Works with other team members to manage conflict (advanced)

4.7 Faculty Development

Faculty development for health care professionals, with responsibilities for facilitating teamwork and collaborative practice, occurs within a constantly evolving and complex environment and must, therefore, be agile and responsive to changes in healthcare delivery, professional roles, and educational practices [90]. For the purposes of this chapter, the term 'faculty' refers to all individuals involved in the delivery of IPE to learners from all levels, disciplines and settings. Anderson et al. outline the importance of faculty development in the delivery of a successful interprofessional curriculum and define the key faculty roles as:

- **the local IPE champion**, a leader who acts as an 'ambassador' for both the strategic and operational aspects of the IPE curriculum,
- **the IPE professional lead**, with in-depth understanding about their profession-specific curriculum, working in tandem with the IPE champion,
- **the IPE facilitator**—the educator who assists the student in their learning and are usually university academics or practice educators (or potentially service users) [91].

4.7.1 The Importance of Interprofessional Faculty Development

Faculty confidence, knowledge, skills, attitudes, and behaviours are perceived to be integral to interprofessional practice and fundamental to the successful implementation of IPE initiatives. Carefully designed faculty development is, therefore, intended to improve the knowledge, skills, and attitudes and preparedness of the IPE facilitator, ultimately resulting in successful implementation of IPE curricula and initiatives and a quality student experience [92–97]. Barr noted that IPE is only as effective as those who deliver it [98]. It is essential, therefore, that faculty tasked with the development and implementation of IPE curricula and initiatives receive the appropriate support and guidance to undertake these tasks effectively [91, 97, 99, 100]. Virant-Young et al. highlight that for IPE faculty development to be successful, however, it must be strategic in design, include an experienced leadership team with a shared vision and be adequately supported, both financially and administratively [101].

Rubeck and Witzke define faculty development as the 'enhancement of faculty members' educational knowledge and skills so that they can make educational contributions that advance the educational program rather than only teaching within it' [102]. 'Those who need faculty development the most attend the least' [103], therefore authenticity is crucial for the engagement of faculty in any proposed development initiative [96, 104]. The knowledge and skills developed should align with both the individual's role and the institution in which they teach [99], and should prepare faculty to design and facilitate IPL activities in both the classroom and the practice environment [90]. The use of 'IPE champions' and engaged faculty has also been identified by a number of authors as critical to successful IPE faculty development [96, 101, 104].

4.7.2 The Effective IPE Facilitator

Anderson et al. highlight five challenges to the development and delivery of IPE and advocate faculty development as essential in addressing these: the crossing of professional boundaries, the integration of IPE into existing curricula; maintaining focus on theoretical rigour and evidence; IPE's changeable and unpredictable nature; and the recognition that it is both complex and different [91]. For students to engage with and value IPE, the skill of the facilitator is therefore paramount. However, it is frequently assumed that experienced educators are inherently skilled at facilitating within an interprofessional context. Facilitators may feel they have the appropriate experience and expertise to teach within their own discipline, but research has demonstrated that faculty frequently feel unprepared or even challenged by the additional demands of interprofessional teaching [105, 106]. In IPE, the concept of the 'expert teacher' is superseded with a more facilitative approach, whereby facilitators 'work with' learners [107]. For many educators, this requires a conscious shift from a more didactic role towards an interactive, facilitative role. Facilitators, therefore, need to be familiar with these differences and the techniques and principles of facilitation across a range of disciplines and diverse student cohorts with differing learning requirements [108].

Furthermore, IPE facilitators should endeavour to foster their own interprofessional skills and bring experience of interprofessional working [109]. Faculty with little or no exposure to IPE may harbour negative attitudes towards colleagues from other professions, interprofessional working or IPE in general [100, 106, 110, 111], whereas faculty *with* exposure to IPE have been shown to exhibit more positive attitudes towards interprofessionalism [112, 113]. From a student perspective, faculty act as role models and learners are more likely to perceive IPE activities favourably when these are authentic and faculty have 'personal and professional' IPE experience [105]. Conversely, the perceived importance of interprofessional initiatives may be adversely affected if poorly executed, or if faculty are not able to 'walk the talk' [106]. Novice educators may also require more teaching experience in addition to the specific skills necessary for the delivery of IPE [92, 94, 100, 114].

Either IPE facilitators must present with positive attitudes towards IPE or this must be cultivated through faculty development [93]. IPE facilitators should hold an active interest and belief in the value of IPE, as well as collaborative practice, and possess an understanding of the challenges and processes involved [113]. Ideally, they should be volunteers, not conscripts. Fostering learning environments, where diversity among professions is appreciated and respected, commands attributes such as compassion, empathy, humour, and flexibility of approach [108, 115]. In addition, facilitators require an understanding of group dynamics and process, conflict resolution, the ability to encourage participation from all students, and the ability to reflect upon their own learning and teaching practices [99, 100, 107, 110, 113, 116, 117].

In terms of facilitator effectiveness, and ultimately student satisfaction with IPE, the quality of faculty is considered one of the most important contributors [105] and a key factor in developing sustained interprofessional practice attitudes in students [118]. Skilled, confident, enthusiastic, and knowledgeable educators, who keep abreast of current evidence, are essential to ensure a positive outcome for students [90, 94, 96, 108, 119].

4.7.3 Strategies for Successful IPE Faculty Development

Just as IPE faculty serve as role models for students in relation to interprofessional practice and behaviour, the objectives of faculty development initiatives should reflect core interprofessional principles [110]. The literature provides a valuable insight into the different approaches to IPE faculty development over recent years [120–122]; however, concern still remains as to the most effective [96, 123, 124]. Whichever the adopted approach, Silver and Leslie [110] advocate use of an outcomes-based approach, where faculty are encouraged to develop interprofessional initiatives that are competency-driven [96].

A recent 'Train the Trainer' model for IPE faculty development, a team-based development approach, has been advocated in helping drive the development and implementation of IPE initiatives [125]. Other successful documented approaches within the literature have included didactic, experiential, face-to-face, online and hybrid methods—including shadowing, observation, co- or team teaching, peer coaching and mentorship, away days, workshops, seminars, and longitudinal programmes [90, 104, 109]. Steinert [99] suggests such strategies should include the showcasing of best practice and the use of case studies and examples from a range of professions, with experiential learning a valuable approach. It is also important to ensure that any faculty training initiatives are strongly aligned to practice and that there are inbuilt opportunities for reflective practice [96].

4.7.3.1 Shadowing/Observation/Co or Team Teaching/Peer Coaching and Mentorship

Co-teaching, peer coaching, observation, and mentorship have been discussed extensively within the literature in relation to faculty development and advocated in the support of novice or inexperienced faculty [94, 96, 101, 113, 126]. In particular, team or co-teaching can serve to role model the collaborative behaviours integral to IPE [117]. Woltenberg et al., also highlight the importance of peer networks and learning communities in supporting IPE faculty [127].

4.7.3.2 Away Days/Time Out

Anderson et al. propose protected time for faculty development activities, through 'away days' or 'time-out' to encourage buy in and ownership. It is important that these events are interactive and discursive, and a series of faculty development events may be necessary [91].

4.7.3.3 Workshops

Faculty development workshops for IPE facilitators have been employed by Chappell et al. [109]. The workshop design included both theoretical and educational concepts, including cognitive dissonance, reflection, role play and feedback, clinical relevance, and intergroup contact theory [128]. The results from seven faculty development workshops (in USA, Europe, Asia, and the Middle East) were mixed, demonstrating significantly improved faculty knowledge and skills, but not significant changes to faculty attitudes or practices.

4.7.3.4 Debriefing Sessions

In addition, Lindqvist and Reeves highlight the importance of regular debriefing sessions [108], which are perceived by IPE faculty to be useful in terms of ongoing peer support, reflection on, and sharing of experiences. Shrader et al. similarly advocate regular debriefing sessions, 'pearls', and celebratory events to facilitate continued collegiality and camaraderie among IPE faculty [129].

4.7.4 Online Facilitation

One further consideration is online facilitation of IPE, which is increasing in prevalence, partly due to the pivot to online delivery and assessment during the COVID-19 pandemic, where innovation of approach has been fundamental to continuity of student learning [130, 131]. The evidence as to the advantages or disadvantages of such approaches in relation to teamwork is conflicting. Online instruction can be used to facilitate IPE where logistics of delivery prove challenging, for example in relation to geography [132], or where there is a need for greater flexibility of delivery or learning. However, online delivery of teamwork related experiences must be carefully deployed as this medium can prove challenging for students and faculty alike. Both may struggle with digital literacy; students may also struggle with motivation, engagement, and the social and communicative aspects of remote groupwork, for example, through the absence of non-verbal cues [133, 134]. For facilitators, online IPE requires enhanced digital knowledge and skills and the ability to support learners to overcome the 'transactional distance' of online learning' [135].

With regard to faculty development in preparation for delivery within an online environment, consideration should be given to hosting any development initiatives on the platform on which the students will learn. This should help promote familiarity with and development of the necessary digital skills and knowledge for delivery [136].

4.8 Evaluation

An important component of interprofessional interventions for learning in and about teams is evaluation. Formal episodic IPE is typically evaluated with participant surveys straight after an intervention, which is useful for learner reaction but says little about its effectiveness in the longer term [137]. Changes in team performance may be evaluated with a team assessment, while faculty development can be evaluated through self-assessment measures, such as the interprofessional facilitation scale (IPFS) [138]. A frequently used framework for outcomes-based evaluation is the modified Kirkpatrick model that was adapted for IPE by the Joint Evaluation Team (JET) under the auspices of CAIPE (Centre for the Advancement of Interprofessional Education) [139]. Process evaluation looks at factors affecting learning with one approach being that of realist evaluation [140], which acknowledges that education and health involve complexity rather than linear causation [141].

4.9 Conclusion

This chapter has focused primarily on teamwork and 'learning together to work together' through IPE for the benefit of patients and clients. It has explored various types of interprofessional practice, in relation to contemporary frameworks, learning outcomes and competencies. Consideration has been given to the transformative role of the patent, within IPL and patient centred care; in addition to the approaches and considerations for learning, teaching and assessment of teams and team members. Engaged faculty and associated faculty development has been shown to be pivotal in the successful implementation of IPE and a high-quality learner experience.

References

1. World Health Organization. Learning together to work together for health. Geneva: WHO; 1988.
2. Thomson AM, Perry JL, Miller TK. Conceptualising and measuring collaboration. J Publ Admin Theory. 2009;19(1):23–56.
3. Canadian Interprofessional Health Collaborative (CIHC). A national interprofessional competency framework. 2010. https://drive.google.com/file/d/1Des_mznc7Rr8stsEhHxl8XMjgiYWzRIn/view.
4. Reeves S, Xyrichis A, Zwarenstein M. Teamwork, collaboration, coordination, and networking: why we need to distinguish between different types of interprofessional practice. J Interprof Care. 2018;32(1):1–3. https://doi.org/10.1080/13561820.2017.1400150.
5. Reeves S, Lewin S, Espin S, Zwarenstein M. Interprofessional teamwork for health and social care. London: Blackwells; 2010.
6. Knowledge at Wharton. Is your team too big? Too small? What's the right number? Wharton School of the University of Pennsylvania; 2006. https://knowledge.wharton.upenn.edu/article/is-your-team-too-big-too-small-whats-the-right-number-2/.
7. Xyrichis A, Reeves S, Zwarenstein M. Examining the nature of interprofessional practice: an initial framework validation and creation of the InterProfessional activity classification tool (InterPACT). J Interprof Care. 2018;32(4):416–25. https://doi.org/10.1080/13561820.2017.1408576.
8. Rosen MA, Diaz Granados D, Dietz AS, Benishek LE, Thompson D, Pronovost PJ, Weaver SJ. Teamwork in healthcare: key discoveries enabling safer, high-quality care. Am Psychol. 2018;73(4):433–50. https://doi.org/10.1037/amp0000298.

9. Cristancho S, Field E, Lingard L, et al. Ecological interchangeability: supporting team adaptive expertise in moments of disruption. Adv Health Sci Educ. 2022;27:1361. https://doi.org/10.1007/s10459-022-10160-4.
10. Engeström Y. From teams to knots: activity-theoretical studies of collaboration and learning at work. Cambridge: Cambridge University Press; 2008.
11. Bleakley A. Working in 'teams' in an era of 'liquid healthcare': what is the use of theory? J Interprof Care. 2013;27(1):18–26. https://doi.org/10.3109/13561820.2012.699479.
12. Bleakley A, Bligh J, Browne J. Medical education for the future: identity, power and location. Dordrecht: Springer; 2011.
13. Grant J. Principles of curriculum design. In: Swanwick T, Forrest K, O'Brien B, editors. Understanding medical education. Evidence, theory and practice. 3rd ed. Oxford: ASME/Wiley Blackwell; 2019. p. 71–88.
14. Gruppen LD, Mangrulkar RS, Kolars JC. The promise of competency-based education in the health professions for improving global health. Hum Resour Health. 2012;10:43.
15. Walsh CL, Gordon FM, Marshall M, Wilson F, Hunt T. Interprofessional capability: a developing framework for interprofessional education. Nurse Educ Pract. 2005;5(4):230–7. https://doi.org/10.1016/j.nepr.2004.12.004.
16. Interprofessional Education Collaborative. Core competencies for interprofessional collaborative practice: 2011 original. https://ipec.memberclicks.net/assets/2011-Original.pdf.
17. Interprofessional Education Collaborative. Core competencies for interprofessional collaborative practice: 2016 update. https://ipec.memberclicks.net/assets/2016-Update.pdf.
18. O'Keefe M, Henderson A, Chick R. Defining a set of common interprofessional learning competencies for health profession students. Med Teach. 2017;39(5):463–8. https://doi.org/10.1080/0142159X.2017.1300246.
19. Smilski A, Parrott M. Interprofessional competency frameworks in education. MedEdPublish. 2019;8:56. https://doi.org/10.15694/mep.2019.000056.1.
20. Curtin University. Interprofessional capability framework. 2013. https://s30991.pcdn.co/about/wp-content/uploads/sites/5/2021/03/interprofessional_A5_broch_1-29072015.pdf.
21. WHO. Global competency and outcomes framework for universal health coverage. Geneva: World Health Organization; 2022. Licence: CC BY-NC-SA 3.0 IGO.
22. Thistlethwaite JE, Moran M. Learning outcomes for interprofessional education (IPE): literature review and synthesis. J Interprof Care. 2011;24:503–13. https://doi.org/10.3109/13561820.2010.483366.
23. ten Cate O, Scheele F. Competency-based postgraduate training: can we bridge the gap between theory and clinical practice? Acad Med. 2007;82:542–7.
24. Englander R, Flynn T, Call S, Carraccio C, Cleary L, et al. Core entrustable professional activities for entering residency—curriculum developers guide. Washington, DC: Association of American Medical Colleges; 2014.
25. ten Cate O, Pool IA. The viability of interprofessional entrustable professional activities. Adv Health Sci Educ. 2020;25:1255–62. https://doi.org/10.1007/s10459-019-09950-0.
26. Jensen CB, Norbye B, Dahlgren MA, et al. Getting real in interprofessional clinical placements: patient-centeredness in student teams' collaborative learning. Adv Health Sci Educ Theory Pract. 2022:1–17. https://doi.org/10.1007/s10459-022-10182-y.
27. Lencioni P. The five dysfunctions of a team. Lafayette, CA: The Table Group; 2002.
28. Tekleab AG, Quigley NR, Tesluk PE. A longitudinal study of team conflict, conflict management, cohesion and team effectiveness. Group Org Manag. 2009;34:170–205.
29. Thistlethwaite JE. Values-based interprofessional collaborative practice. Cambridge: Cambridge University Press; 2012.
30. Thistlethwaite JE, Jackson A. Conflict in practice-based settings: nature, conflict and resolution. Int J Pract Based Learn Health Social Care. 2014;2(2):2–13. https://doi.org/10.11120/pblh.2014.00036.
31. World Health Organization. Transforming and scaling up health professionals' education and training. In: WHO Education guidelines 2013. Geneva: WHO; 2013.

32. Biggs JB, Tang C. Teaching for quality learning at university: What the student does. 4th ed. Maidenhead: McGraw-Hill, Open University Press; 2011.
33. Grant C, Bainbridge L, Gilbert J. The University of British Columbia model of interprofessional education. J Interprof Care. 2010;24(1):9–18. https://doi.org/10.3109/13561820903294549.
34. Khalili H. Online interprofessional education during and post the Covid-19 pandemic: a commentary. J Interprof Care. 2020;34(5):687–90. https://doi.org/10.1080/13561820.2020.1792424.
35. Bluteau P, Jackson A. An e-learning model of interprofessional education. In: Bluteau P, Jackson A, editors. Interprofessional education. Making it happen. Basingstoke: Palgrave Macmillan; 2009. p. 107–24.
36. Haidet P, Levine RWE, Parmelee DX, Crow S, Kennedy F, Kelly PA, et al. Perspective: guidelines for reporting team-based learning activities in the medical and health sciences education literature. Acad Med. 2012;87:292–9.
37. Packard K, Chelal H, Maio A, et al. Interprofessional team reasoning framework as a tool for case study analysis with health professions students: a randomized study. J Res Interprofession Pract Educ. 2012;2(3):250–63. https://doi.org/10.22230/jripe.2012v2n3a96.
38. Lioce L, Lopreiato J, Downing D, Chang TP, Robertson JM, Anderson M, Diaz DA, Spain AE, editors. Healthcare simulation dictionary. 2nd ed. Rockville, MD: Agency for Healthcare Research and Quality; 2020. https://doi.org/10.23970/simulationv2.
39. Zhang C, Thompson S, Miller C. A review of simulation-based interprofessional education. Clin Simul Nurs. 2011;7(4):e117–26. https://doi.org/10.1016/j.ecns.2010.02.008.
40. Palaganas JC, Epps C, Raemer DB. A history of simulation-enhanced interprofessional education. J Interprof Care. 2014;28(2):110–5. https://doi.org/10.3109/13561820.2013.869198.
41. Tilley CP, Roitman J, Zafra KP, Brennan M. Real-time, simulation-enhanced interprofessional education in the care of older adults with multiple chronic comorbidities: a utilization-focused evaluation. MHealth. 2021;7(3):3.
42. Tullmann D, Shilling A, Goeke L, Wright E, Littlewood K. Recreating simulation scenarios for interprofessional education: an example of educational interprofessional practice. J Interprof Care. 2014;27(5):426–8. https://doi.org/10.3109/13561820.2013.790880.
43. Trotter K, Blazar M, Muckler VC, Kuszajewski M, Molloy MA. Perinatal IPE simulation can improve collaborative competencies. J Interprofessional Educ Pract. 2019;15:30–3. https://doi.org/10.1016/j.xjep.2019.01.011.
44. Welsch LA, Hoch J, Poston RD, Parodi VA, Akpinar-Elci M. Interprofessional Education involving didactic TeamSTEPPS® and interactive healthcare simulation: a systematic review. J Interprof Care. 2018;32(6):657–65. https://doi.org/10.1080/13561820.2018.1472069.
45. Sanders M, Richards D, Panahi L. Interprofessional education (IPE) in a pediatric simulation: case of an infant with fever. MedEdPORTAL. 2013;9:9515. https://doi.org/10.15766/mep_2374-8265.9515.
46. Galbraith A, Harder N, Macomber CA, Roe E, Roethlisberger KS. Design and implementation of an interprofessional death notification simulation. Clin Simul Nurs. 2014;10(2):E95–E102. https://doi.org/10.1016/j.ecns.2013.08.003.
47. Shaw-Battista J, Belew C, Anderson D, van Schaik S. Successes and challenges of interprofessional physiologic birth and obstetric emergency simulations in a nurse-midwifery Education program. J Midwif Womens Health. 2015;60(6):735–43. https://doi.org/10.1111/jmwh.12393.
48. Hodgkins SR, Marian KM, Shrader S, Averett E, Crowl A, Kalender-Rich JL, Laverentz DM, Shaw P, Schell K, Johnston K. A case of anaphylaxis: IPE simulation as a tool to enhance communication and collaboration. J Interprofessional Educ Pract. 2020;18:18. https://doi.org/10.1016/j.xjep.2019.100303.
49. Ellis DM, Hickey S, Prieto P, McLaughlin C, Felgoise SH, Becker M, O'Connor M, Puleo M, Reddy T, Kim L, Markey D, Bernhardt PW. Interprofessional mock code simulation promotes collaboration and competency in Parkinson's medication safety during transition in care. J Interprofessional Educ Pract. 2021;25:100468. https://doi.org/10.1016/j.xjep.2021.100468.

50. Buckley S, Hensman M, Thomas S, Dudley R, Nevin G, Coleman J. Developing Interprofessional simulation in the undergraduate setting: experience with five different professional groups. J Interprof Care. 2012;26(5):362–9. https://doi.org/10.3109/13561820.2012.685993.
51. Saldanha K, Myler L, Seurynck K. Building interpersonal care teamwork skills in a virtual IPE simulation event. Social Work Groups. 2022;45(1):39–45. https://doi.org/10.1080/01609513.2020.1859073.
52. INACSL Standards of Best Practice. Simulation simulation-enhanced Interprofessional Education (Sim-IPE). Clin Simul Nurs. 2016;12(Suppl):S34–8. https://doi.org/10.1016/j.ecns.2016.09.011.
53. Cant RP, Cooper SJ. Simulation-based learning in nurse education: systematic review. J Adv Nurs. 2010;66(1):3–15. https://doi.org/10.1111/j.1365-2648.2009.05240.x.
54. Reese CE, Jeffries PR, Engum SA. Learning together: using simulations to develop nursing and medical student collaboration. Nurs Educ Perspect. 2010;31(1):33–7.
55. Velásquez ST, Ferguson D, Lemke KC, Bland L, Ajtai R, Amezaga B, Cleveland J, Ford LA, Lopez E, Richardson W, Saenz D, Zorek JA. Interprofessional communication in medical simulation: findings from a scoping review and implications for academic medicine. BMC Med Educ. 2022;22:204. https://doi.org/10.1186/s12909-022-03226-9.
56. Hutchings M, McLarnon N, McDermott J, Watson A, Power A, Anderson ES, Owens M. Practice-based learning and the impacts of COVID-19: doing it for real? Br J Midwifery. 2022;30(6):333–44. https://doi.org/10.12968/bjom.2022.30.6.333.
57. Kent F, Glass S, Courtney J, Thorpe J, Nisbet G. Sustainable interprofessional learning in clinical placements: the value of observing others at work. J Interprof Care. 2020;34(6):812–8. https://doi.org/10.1080/13561820.2019.1702932.
58. Freeth D, Savin-Baden M, Thistlethwaite JE. Interprofessional education. In: Swanwick T, O'Brien B, Forrest K, editors. Understanding medical education. 3rd ed. Oxford: Wiley; 2018. p. 191–206.
59. Fallsberg M, Hammar M. Strategies and focus at an integrated interprofessional training ward. J Interprof Care. 2000;14:337–50.
60. Mink J, Mitzkat A, Krug K, Mihaljevic A, Trierweiler-Hauke B, Götsch B, Wensing M, Mahler C. Impact of an interprofessional training ward on interprofessional competencies—a quantitative longitudinal study. J Interprof Care. 2021;35(5):751–9. https://doi.org/10.1080/13561820.2020.1802240.
61. Brewer ML, Stewart-Wynne EG. An Australian hospital-based student training ward delivering safe, client-centred care while developing students' interprofessional practice capabilities. J Interprof Care. 2013;27(6):482–8. https://doi.org/10.3109/13561820.2013.811639.
62. Reeves S, Freeth D. The London training ward: an innovative interprofessional learning initiative. J Interprof Care. 2002;16(1):41–52. https://doi.org/10.1080/13561820220104159.
63. Oosterom N, Floren LC, ten Cate HE, Westerveld HE. A review of interprofessional training wards: enhancing student learning and patient outcomes. Med Teach. 2019;41(5):547–54. https://doi.org/10.1080/0142159X.2018.1503410.
64. Haines TP, Kent F, Keating JL. Interprofessional student clinics: an economic evaluation of collaborative clinical placement education. J Interprof Care. 2014;28(4):292–8.
65. Hopkins S, Bacon R, Flynn A. Student outcomes for interprofessional education in student led clinics: a rapid review. J Interprof Care. 2022;36(2):234–44. https://doi.org/10.1080/13561820.2020.1858767.
66. Thistlethwaite JE. Engaging health professionals in continuing interprofessional development. In: Orchard C, Bainbridge L, editors. Interprofessional client-centred collaborative practice. New York: Nova; 2015. p. 83–94.
67. Helmreich RL, Merritt AC, Wilhelm JA. The evolution of crew resource management training in commercial aviation. Int J Aviat Psychol. 1999;9(1):19–32. https://doi.org/10.1207/s15327108ijap0901_2.
68. Agency for Healthcare Resource and Quality. Pocket guide: TeamSTEPPS. 2013. https://www.ahrq.gov/teamstepps/instructor/essentials/pocketguide.html.

69. Buljac-Samardzic M, Doekhie KD, van Wijngaarden JDH. Interventions to improve team effectiveness within health care: a systematic review of the past decade. Hum Resour Health. 2020;18:2. https://doi.org/10.1186/s12960-019-0411-3.
70. Billett S. Constituting the workplace curriculum. J Curric Stud. 2006;38:31–48.
71. Nisbet G, Dunn S, Lincoln M. Interprofessional team meetings: opportunities for informal interprofessional learning. J Interprof Care. 2015;29(5):426–32. https://doi.org/10.3109/13561820.2015.1016602.
72. Nisbet G, Lincoln M, Dunn S. Informal interprofessional learning: an untapped opportunity for learning and change within the workplace. J Interprof Care. 2023;27(6):469–75. https://doi.org/10.3109/13561820.2013.805735.
73. Rogers GD, Thistlethwaite JE, Anderson ES, et al. International consensus statement on the assessment of interprofessional learning outcomes. Med Teach. 2017;39:347–59. https://doi.org/10.1080/0142159X.2017.1270441.
74. Smeets HWH, Sluijsmans DMA, Moser A, et al. Design guidelines for assessing students' interprofessional competencies in healthcare education: a consensus study. Perspect Med Educ. 2022;11:316. https://doi.org/10.1007/s40037-022-00728-6.
75. Lingard L. Rethinking competence in the context of teamwork. In: Hodges BD, Lingard L, editors. The question of competence. reconsidering medical education in the twenty-first century. Ithaca, NY: Cornell University Press; 2012. p. 42–69.
76. Thistlethwaite JE, Bartle E, Chong AL, et al. A review of longitudinal community and hospital placements in medical education: BEME Guide No. 26. Med Teach. 2013;35(8):e1340–64.
77. Simmons B, Egan-Lee E, Wagner SJ, Esdaile M, Baker L, Reeves S. Assessment of interprofessional learning: the design of an interprofessional objective structured clinical examination (iOSCE). J Interprof Care. 2011;25(1):73–4.
78. Oakley B, Felder RM, Brent R, Elhajj I. Turning student groups into effective teams. J Student Center Learn. 2004;2:9–34.
79. Van Der Vleuten CPM, Schuwirth L, Driessen EW, Dijkstra J, Tigelaar D, Baatman LKJ, van Tartwijk J. A model for programmatic assessment fit for purpose. Med Teach. 2012;34:205–14. https://doi.org/10.3109/0142159x.2012.652239.
80. Schuwirth L, van der Vleuten C, Durning SJ. What programmatic assessment in medical education can learn from healthcare. Perspect Med Educ. 2017;6(4):211–5. https://doi.org/10.1007/s40037-017-0345-1.
81. Domac S, Anderson E, O'Reilly M, Smith R. Assessing interprofessional competence using a prospective Reflective portfolio. J Interprof Care. 2015;29(3):179–87.
82. Andreoli A, Fancott C, Velji K, et al. Using SBAR to communicate falls risk and management in interprofessional teams. Healthc Q. 2010;13:94–101.
83. Chiu CJ. Development and validation of performance assessment tools for Interprofessional communication and teamwork (PACT) (doctoral dissertation, University of Washington), 2014. https://nexusipe.org/advancing/assessment-evaluation/performance-assessment-communication-and-teamwork-tools-set-pact.
84. Curran V, Hollett A, Casimiro LM, et al. Development and validation of the interprofessonal collaborator assessment rubric (ICAR). J Interprof Care. 2011;25(5):299–344.
85. Earnest M, Madigosky WS, Yamashita T, Hanson JL. Validity evidence for using an online peer-assessment tool (CATME) to assess individual contributions to interprofessional student teamwork in a longitudinal team-based learning course. J Interprof Care. 2022;36:923. https://doi.org/10.1080/13561820.2022.2040962.
86. Hall P, Marshall D, Weaver L, et al. A method to enhance students teams in palliative care: piloting the McMaster Ottawa team observed structured clinical encounter. J Palliat Med. 2011;14(6):744–50.
87. Solomon P, Marshall D, Boyle A, et al. Establishing face and content validity of the McMaster-Ottawa team observed structured clinical encounter (TOSCE). J Interprof Care. 2011;25(4):302–4.
88. Orchard CA, King GA, Khalili H, Bezzina MB. Assessment of interprofessional team collaboration scale (AITCS). J Contin Educ Health Prof. 2012;32(1):58–67.

89. Thistlethwaite JE, Dallest K, Moran M, Dunston R, Roberts C, Eley D, et al. Introducing the individual teamwork observation and feedback tool (iTOFT): development and description of a new interprofessional teamwork measure. J Interprof Care. 2016;30(4):526–8.
90. Steinert Y. Faculty development in the health professions: a focus on research and Practice. Dordrecht: Springer; 2014.
91. Anderson L, Hean S, O'Halloran C, Pitt R, Hammick M. Faculty development for interprofessional education and practice. In: Steinert Y, editor. Faculty development in the health professions. Innovation and change in professional education. Dordrecht: Springer; 2014. https://doi.org/10.1007/978-94-007-7612-8_14.
92. Kwan D, Barker KK, Austin Z, Chatalsingh C, Grdisa V, Langlois S, Meuser J, Moaveni A, Power R, Rennie S, Richardson D, Sinclair L, Wagner SJ, Oandasan I. Effectiveness of a faculty development program on interprofessional education: a randomized control trial. J Interprof Care. 2006;20(3):314–6. https://doi.org/10.1080/13561820500518712.
93. Buring SM, Bhushan A, Brazeau G, Conway S, Hansen L, Westberg S. Keys to successful implementation of interprofessional education: learning location, faculty development, and curricular themes. Am J Pharm Educ. 2009;73(4):60. https://doi.org/10.5688/aj730460.
94. Anderson ES, Thorpe LN, Hammick M. Interprofessional staff development: changing attitudes and winning hearts and minds. J Interprof Care. 2011;25(1):11–7. https://doi.org/10.3109/13561821003721311.
95. Simmons B, Oandasan I, Soklaradis S, Esdaile M, Barker K, Kwan D, Leszcz M, Lowe M, Moaveni A, Richardson D, Silver I, Sinclair L, Tassone M, Wagner S. Evaluating the effectiveness of an interprofessional education faculty development course: the transfer of interprofessional learning to the academic and clinical practice setting. J Interprof Care. 2011;25(2):156–7. https://doi.org/10.3109/13561820.2010.515044.
96. Hall LW, Zierler BK. Interprofessional Education and Practice Guide No. 1: developing faculty to effectively facilitate interprofessional education. J Interprof Care. 2015;29(1):3–7. https://doi.org/10.3109/13561820.2014.937483.
97. Watkins KD. Faculty development to support interprofessional education in healthcare professions: a realist synthesis. J Interprof Care. 2016;30(6):695–701. https://doi.org/10.1080/13561820.2016.1209466.
98. Barr H. In: Howkins E, Bray J, editors. Preparing for interprofessional teaching, theory and practice. Oxford: Radcliffe Publishing; 2008.
99. Steinert Y. Learning together to teach together: interprofessional education and faculty development. J Interprof Care. 2005;19(Suppl 1):60–75. https://doi.org/10.1080/13561820500081778.
100. Anderson ES, Cox D, Thorpe LN. Preparation of educators involved in Interprofessional Education. J Interprof Care. 2009;23(1):81–94. https://doi.org/10.1080/13561820802565106.
101. Virant-Young D, Forrest K, McCaskey S, Smith C, Saadeh C, Gudakunst J, Sefcik D. Faculty development in interprofessional education: designing and implementing a successful program. Med Sci Educ. 2014;24:401–7. https://doi.org/10.1007/s40670-014-0071-9.
102. Rubeck RF, Witzke DB. Faculty development: a field of dreams. Acad Med. 1998;73(Suppl):S32–7.
103. Steinert Y, McLeod PJ, Boillat M, Meterissian S, Elizov M, Macdonald ME. Faculty development: a 'Field of Dreams'? Med Educ. 2009;43(1):42–9. https://doi.org/10.1111/j.1365-2923.2008.03246.x.
104. Doll J, Maio A, Potthoff M. Epic failure: lessons learned from Interprofessional faculty development. Perspect Med Educ. 2018;7(6):408–11. https://doi.org/10.1007/s40037-018-0488-8.
105. Hammick M, Freeth D, Koppel I, Reeves S, Barr H. A best evidence systematic review of Interprofessional Education: BEME Guide No. 9. Med Teach. 2007;29(8):735–51. https://doi.org/10.1080/01421590701682576.
106. Howkins E, Bray J, editors. Preparing for interprofessional teaching, theory and practice. Oxford: Radcliffe Publishing; 2008.
107. Oandasan I, Reeves S. Key elements for interprofessional education. Part 1: the learner, the educator and the learning context. J Interprof Care. 2005;19(Suppl 1):21–38. https://doi.org/10.1080/13561820500083550.

108. Lindqvist SM, Reeves S. Facilitators' perceptions of delivering interprofessional education: a qualitative study. Med Teach. 2007;29(4):403–5. https://doi.org/10.1080/01421590701509662.
109. Chappell KB, Sherman L, Barnett SD. An interactive faculty development workshop designed to improve knowledge, skills (competence), attitudes, and practice in interprofessional continuing education. Med Teach. 2018;40(9):896–903. https://doi.org/10.1080/0142159X.2018.1481286.
110. Silver I, Leslie K. Faculty development for continuing interprofessional education and collaborative practice. J Contin Educ Health Prof. 2017;37(4):262–7. https://doi.org/10.1097/CEH.0000000000000178.
111. Freeman S, Wright A, Lindqvist S. Facilitator training for educators involved in interprofessional learning. J Interprof Care. 2010;24(4):375–85. https://doi.org/10.3109/13561820903373202.
112. Curran VR, Sharpe D, Forristall J. Attitudes of health sciences faculty members towards interprofessional teamwork and education. Med Educ. 2007;41(9):892–6. https://doi.org/10.1111/j.1365-2923.2007.02823.x.
113. Christianson TM, Bainbridge L, Halupa C. A pilot study on interprofessional education: how prepared are faculty to teach? Prof Dev Educ. 2019;45(4):659–69. https://doi.org/10.1080/19415257.2018.1474490.
114. Freeth D, Hammick M, Reeves S, Koppel I, Barr H. Effective interprofessional education: development, delivery and evaluation. Oxford; England: Blackwell Publishing; 2005.
115. Nicol P, Forman D. Attributes of effective interprofessional placement facilitation. J Res Interprofession Pract Educ. 2014; 4(2). https://doi.org/10.22230/jripe.2014v4n2a155
116. Hammick M. Interprofessional education: concept, theory and application. J Interprof Care. 1998;12(3):323–32. https://doi.org/10.3109/13561829809014123.
117. Crow J, Smith L. Using co-teaching as a means of facilitating interprofessional collaboration in health and social care. J Interprof Care. 2003;17(1):45–55. https://doi.org/10.1080/1356182021000044139.
118. Reeves S, Goldman J, Oandasan I. Key factors in planning and implementing interprofessional education in health care settings. J Allied Health. 2007;36(4):231–5. PMID: 18293805.
119. Shrader S, Mauldin M, Hammad S, Mitcham M, Blue A. Developing a comprehensive faculty development program to promote interprofessional education, practice and research at a freestanding academic health science center. J Interprof Care. 2015;29(2):165–7. https://doi.org/10.3109/13561820.2014.940417.
120. Steinert Y, Mann K, Centeno A, Dolmans D, Spencer J, Gelula M, Prideaux D. A systematic review of faculty development initiatives designed to improve teaching effectiveness in medical education: BEME Guide No. 8. Med Teach. 2006;28(6):497–526. https://doi.org/10.1080/01421590600902976.
121. cLean M, Cilliers F, Van Wyk J. Faculty development: yesterday, today and tomorrow. Med Teach. 2008;30(6):555–84. https://doi.org/10.1080/01421590802109834.
122. Steinert Y, Naismith L, Mann K. Faculty development initiatives designed to promote leadership in medical Education. A BEME systematic review: BEME Guide 19. Med Teach. 2012;34(6):483–503. https://doi.org/10.3109/0142159X.2012.680937.
123. Ratka A, Zorek JA, Meyer SM. Overview of faculty development programs for interprofessional education. Am J Pharm Educ. 2017;81(5):96. https://doi.org/10.5688/ajpe81596.
124. da Silva JAM, da Costa MV, Mininel VA, Rossit RAS, Xyrichis A. The effectiveness of faculty development activities for interprofessional education: a systematic review protocol. J Interprof Care. 2022;36(4):630–3. https://doi.org/10.1080/13561820.2021.1929105.
125. Blakeney EA, Owen JA, Ottis E, Brashers V, Summerside N, Haizlip J, Dyer C, Hall L, Zierler BK. Measuring the impact of the National Train-the-Trainer Interprofessional Team Development Program (T3-ITDP) on the implementation of interprofessional education and interprofessional collaborative practice. J Interprofessional Educ Pract. 2021;24:100442. https://doi.org/10.1016/j.xjep.2021.100442.
126. Reeves S, Tassone M, Parker K, Wagner SJ, Simmons B. Interprofessional education: an overview of key developments in the past three decades. Work. 2012;41(3):233–45. https://doi.org/10.3233/WOR-2012-1298.

127. Woltenberg LN, Aulisio MC, Taylor SA. Fostering an interprofessional learning community of scholars: a model for contemporary faculty development. J Interprofessional Educ Pract. 2021;23:100390. https://doi.org/10.1016/j.xjep.2020.100390.
128. Allport GW. The nature of prejudice. Cambridge, MA: Addison-Wesley; 1954.
129. Shrader S, Hodgkins R, Laverentz D, Zaudke J, Waxman M, Johnston K, Jernigan S. Interprofessional Education and Practice Guide No. 7: development, implementation and evaluation of a large-scale required Interprofessional Education Foundational Programme. J Interprof Care. 2016;30(5):615–9.
130. Power A, Sy MP, Hutchings M, Coleman T, El-Awaisi A, Kitema GF, Gallagher J, Herath C, McLarnon N, Nagraj S, O'Carroll V, Owens M, Park V, Pope E, Wetzlmair LC, Greaves PJ, Anderson ES. Learning in lockdown: exploring the impact of COVID-19 on interprofessional education. Br J Midwifery. 2021;29(11):648–52. https://doi.org/10.12968/bjom.2021.29.11.648.
131. McLarnon N, Hutchings M, O'Carroll V, Wetzlmair LC, Blumenthal S, Boyle L, El-Awaisi A, Greaves PJ, Park V, Power A. Rethinking assessment for Interprofessional learning during COVID-19: steering a middle course. Br J Midwifery. 2022;30(10):572–81. https://doi.org/10.12968/bjom.2022.30.10.572.
132. Hayward K, Brown M, Pendergast N, Nicholson M, Newell J, Fancy T, Cameron H. IPE via online Education: pedagogical pathways spanning the distance. J Interprofessional Educ Pract. 2021;24:100447. https://doi.org/10.1016/j.xjep.2021.100447.
133. Saghafian M, O'Neill DK. A phenomenological study of teamwork in online and face-to face student teams. High Educ. 2018;75:57–73. https://doi.org/10.1007/s10734-017-0122-4.
134. Khalili H. Online Interprofessional Education during and post the COVID-19 pandemic: a commentary. J Interprof Care. 2020;34(5):687–90. https://doi.org/10.1080/13561820.2020.1792424.
135. Sargeant J, Curran V, Allen M, Jarvis-Selinger S, Ho KJ. Facilitating interpersonal interaction and learning online: linking theory and practice. J Contin Educ Health Prof. 2006;26(2):128–36. https://doi.org/10.1002/chp.61.
136. Evans S, Ward C, Shaw N, Walker A, Knight T, Sutherland-Smith W. Interprofessional education and practice guide No. 10: developing, supporting and sustaining a team of facilitators in online interprofessional education. J Interprof Care. 2020;34(1):4–10. https://doi.org/10.1080/13561820.2019.1632817.
137. Thistlethwaite JE. Research and evaluation: the present and the future. In: Forman D, Jones M, Thistlethwaite JE, editors. Leading research and evaluation in interprofessional education. Basingstoke: Palgrave; 2016. p. 355–68.
138. Sargeant J, Hill T, Breau L. Development and testing of a scale to assess interprofessional education (IPE) facilitation skills. J Contin Educ Health Prof. 2010;30(2):126–31. https://doi.org/10.1002/chp.20069.
139. Barr H, Freeth D, Hammick M, Koppel I, Reeves S. Evaluations for interprofessional education. A United Kingdom review for health and social care. London: CAIPE/BERA; 2000.
140. Pawson R, Tilley N. Realistic evaluation. London: Sage; 1997.
141. Wong G, Greenhalgh T, Westhorp G, Pawson R. Realist methods in medical education research: what are they and what can they contribute? Med Educ. 2012;46:89–96.

Part II

Formulation and Implementation of Strategies for Effective Interprofessional Education and Collaborative Practice

Developing a Novel Health Interprofessional Education Curriculum: Strategies and Implementation

5

Alla El-Awaisi and Susan Waller

5.1 Introduction

Evidence continues to emerge globally in favor of interprofessional education as the critical first step in developing the interprofessional collaborative competencies to graduate a collaborative practice-ready workforce [1, 2]. Today, the value placed on interprofessional practice permeates all facets of worldwide policy and practices in the delivery of health profession education and services [3]. Despite widespread acceptance, it has been challenging integrating IPE into curriculum for health profession education [3]. The mostly used definition for IPE is the one defined by the Centre for Advancement of Interprofessional Education (CAIPE) as "occasions when two or more professions learn with, from and about each other to improve collaboration and the quality of care" [4]. This chapter will apply Biggs' 3P model of learning and teaching in terms of presage, process, and product which provides a useful approach when considering developing and evaluating an interprofessional curriculum [5–8].

A. El-Awaisi (✉)
Department of Clinical Pharmacy and Practice, College of Pharmacy, QU Health, Qatar University, Doha, Qatar

S. Waller
Department of Medical Education, College of Medicine and Health Sciences, UAE University, Al Ain, United Arab Emirates

M. Y. Alnaami et al. (eds.), *Novel Health Interprofessional Education and Collaborative Practice Program: Strategy and Implementation*, https://doi.org/10.1007/978-981-99-3420-1_5

5.2 PRESAGE: The Learning Context

Interprofessional education (IPE), alongside competency-based education and the integration of information technology facilitated education are among the transformative developments to health profession education in the last decade [9]. IPE is a necessary curricular component at the pre-licensure level to prepare a "collaborative practice-ready" future health workforce who are better able to address local health needs [1]. Needs assessments are required to understand the status of IPE in the institution, identify the drivers necessitating the inclusion of IPE in the curriculum, and to explore facilitators and barriers to be the basis for moving forward. Presage factors define the context in which the learning experience takes place and will have an impact on IPE design, delivery, and outcomes [10]. Freeth et al. in their self-help guidebook evaluating IPE suggested asking questions focused on presage concerning the drivers for IPE within a particular institution, learner and champion characteristics, facilitators and challenges affecting IPE planning and delivery that might have an impact on the learners [11]. These questions include:

- Why was IPE initiated in this particular organization?
- What learner characteristics allow them to benefit from this approach to learning?
- Who, if anyone, championed the IPE and how did this affect the planning and delivery of the education?
- What are the pressures that could/do inhibit effective delivery of the education?
- Where are the challenges to establishing IPE as an accepted part of mainstream provision in this organization and for these particular groups of learners?
- What tensions, if any, exist within the planning and delivery teams.

A "one size fits all" approach does not work for IPE and hence it is important to learn from others' experiences. It is important to appraise existing models of IPE to identify which model would work within respective programs and adapt it to the local context [1, 12]. The barriers to IPE implementations are widely documented in the literature, and have been categorized into three different levels: government and professional, institution, and individual [13]. The institutional barriers can be further categorized into structural, cultural, financial, and curricular issues [9]. The needs assessment must also identify future healthcare practice needs and demands taking into consideration the local context, global health, advancement in health technology, and educational reforms [14].

In a recent scoping review exploring models of IPE for health profession students, a popular starting point for integrating IPE within health profession curricula included:

- A benchmarking exercise to map competencies of the health profession curricula to international IPE competency frameworks and identify areas of strengths and weakness within their curricula [12].

- The establishment of IPE steering committee that includes various stakeholders that are IPE champions to advocate for IPE and guide the curriculum development of IPE [12, 14]. Advocates need to include representatives of the different health professions. Institutional support with dedicated structure, shared institutional vision, and funding are of crucial importance to ensure sustainability [14].

The IPE program must ensure learning outcomes and expectations are clearly defined and understood by learners. A number of interprofessional competency/capabilities frameworks exist that could serve as the basis for developing an IPE curriculum. In a recent scoping review, the most frequently used frameworks were the Canadian National Interprofessional Competency Framework followed by the Core Competencies for Interprofessional Collaborative Practice.

- The National Interprofessional Competency Framework developed in Canada in 2010 by the Canadian Interprofessional Health Collaborative required for effective interprofessional collaboration which is defined as: "A partnership between a team of health providers and a client in a participatory, collaborative and coordinated approach to shared decision-making around health and social issues" [15]. It includes six competency domains which are as follows:
  - Role clarification.
  - Team functioning.
  - Collaborative leadership.
  - Interprofessional conflict resolution.
  - Interprofessional communication.
  - Patient/client/family/community-centered care.

  Each domain contains a competency statement, descriptors, and explanation/rationale. The knowledge, skills, attitudes, and values that collectively shape the judgements necessary for interprofessional collaborative practice are highlighted by six competence domains [15]. Three factors can influence how the framework applied and these include the learning or practice context, the complexity of the situation and the need for quality improvement.
- The core competencies for interprofessional collaborative practice were developed originally in 2011 and updated in 2016 in the USA. Four competencies listed needed for effective collaborative practice:
  - Values/Ethics for Interprofessional Practice.
  - Roles/Responsibilities for Collaborative Practice.
  - Interprofessional Communication Practices.
  - Interprofessional Teamwork and Team-Based Practice.

  Each domain has a general competency statements and related sub-competencies. Competencies are intended to be patient and family centered, community and population oriented, integrated across the learning continuum from education to practice settings, and applicable to all health professions [16].

IPE tends to be integrated into health profession curriculum either as [12]:

- Extra-curricular or partially integrated curriculum designs that do not require major restructure of profession-specific curricula including elective Interprofessional Enrichment Activities, elective IPE courses, and IPE clinical placements.
- Integrated curriculum designs throughout the whole program based on a phased curriculum model that is continued beyond graduation in the form of continuing professional development.

However, it is important to ensure IPE is an integral and well-developed component of the health professions curricula and not optional.

5.3 PRESAGE: Teacher and Program Developer Characteristics

Two critical features of this presage element are essential for the success of IPE activities and these are: the quality of IPE facilitation experience and faculty development for facilitators [17]. IPE facilitators and champions are of great importance to the success of effective and high-quality IPE activities [18]. To ensure the effectiveness of IPE sessions, several attributes are needed including commitment to IPE concepts and values, preparedness and readiness for IPE facilitation, experiences in IPE facilitation, understanding of team functioning and group dynamics, ability to handle conflict resolution [18–21]. Furthermore, for IPE to be effective, educators must engage in, create, and ensure positive role modeling for interprofessional collaboration for students [9].

Regular faculty development sessions focused on the importance of IPE in teamwork and collaboration, IPE core principles, development of core facilitation skills for interprofessional teams, ensuring a balance between uniprofessional and interprofessional identity are all crucial faculty development topics to ensure facilitators are equipped with the needed skills to facilitate effectively [9, 18, 22].

5.4 PRESAGE: Learner Characteristics

The delivery of IPE may be impacted by a variety of learner characteristic-related factors, including attitudes towards IPE, desire to engage in IPE, perceived professional hierarchies and stereotypes, and health profession background [17]. Furthermore, gender, age, previous IPE experiences are considered as influential student characteristics impacting students' attitudes and perceptions of IPE [17]. Student-led IPE initiatives can also have an impact on students' willingness to participate in IPE activities and become IPE advocates [23].

Application of the 12 steps and strategies for introducing IPE into pre-registration health profession education from Qatar are as demonstrated in Case Study 5.1 [24]. An additional step was added at the end related to sustainability.

Case Study 5.1 Application of Steps for Introducing Interprofessional Education into Health Profession Education: Case Study from Qatar [24–31]

Step 1: get started	• Driver: Accreditation was a key driver for integrating IPE with health profession curricula at Qatar University. It started at the College of Pharmacy where its Bachelor of Pharmacy degree program is fully accredited by the Canadian Council for Accreditation of Pharmacy Programs (CCAPP). As part of CCAPP accreditation standards, there was a need to demonstrate evidence for creating IPE opportunities within the pharmacy curriculum • Establishing a committee: An interprofessional education committee was established in 2014 at the College of Pharmacy and then moved to QU Health level in 2017. The committee included representatives from all the health professions programs in Qatar University and Qatar. Currently, representatives include members from QU Health which includes five health colleges: College of Pharmacy, College of Medicine, College of Dental Medicine, College of Nursing and College of Health sciences with its four programs: Biomedical Science, Public Health, Human Nutrition and physiotherapy. In addition to representatives from Weill Cornell Medicine in Qatar, University of Calgary—Qatar and University of Doha for Science and Technology • Needs assessment: Readiness and the perspectives of key stakeholders towards IPE and collaborative practice was assessed. These included: faculty members, students, and practicing health professionals. Findings from these studies were used as the basis for developing IPE initiatives • Faculty development: In 2015, IPEC hosted the First Interprofessional Education Symposium in Qatar for faculty members to equip them with the knowledge and skills needed to design and deliver IPE within the different curricula. This was followed by hosting the first Middle Eastern conference on Interprofessional Education
Step 2: Adopt a definition, values and principles	• Definition: IPEC adopted the Center for Advancement of Interprofessional Education (CAIPE) definition and core values and principles
Step 3: Formulate outcomes	• Learning outcomes: These were based on the IPE shared competency domains and statements adapted to the Qatar context. These included interprofessional communication; role clarification; patient-centered care; and shared decision-making
Step 4: Decide who is going to participate and select the students and faculty	• Initially, IPE was mandatory for pharmacy students and optional for all the other health professions. However, with the move of IPEC to QU Health level, gradually IPE became an integral and well-developed component of the health professions curricula at Qatar University
Step 5: Select themes	• IPE topics: In consultation with IPEC members, themes chosen based on overlapping curricular topics appropriate for the: Intended level, IPE event and professions involved

Step 7: Determine levels and stages	• IPE levels: These were based on the University of British Columbia model which takes into consideration the learning needs across their professional years. The model is based on three main categories: Exposure, Immersion, and Mastery • IPE program: – First professional year (exposure level): introducing IPE with first topic focused on roles and responsibilities for the fall semester and on mental Health and wellbeing for second semester – Second professional year (exposure level): smoking cessation and being an effective team player in the second semester – Third professional year (immersion level): case-based discussion on diabetes in the fall semester and case-based discussion on pneumonia and antibiotic stewardship for the spring semester – Fourth professional year (immersion/mastery level): vaccination and COVID-19 vaccine hesitancy in the spring semester and part of clinical placement across the year • IPE passport program: in 2020, IPEC established the IPE passport program. Benefits of the IPE Passport: – To motivate students to attend, participate and engage in the IPE activities as part of a structured program – To enables students to participate in IPE activities as part of their courses in a progressive level tailored to their professional year – To meet the IPE shared competencies and enhance learners understanding of IPE concepts and principles – To demonstrate that learners have met the IPE requirement
Step 6: Be collaborative in case and activity design and mix up learning methods	• IPE activity development: the content of each of the IPE activity is developed collaboratively. There is a lead for each activity that work with other representatives to ensures the activity is appropriate to the participating professions. Various learning methods are employed including case-based discussion, simulation and experiential learning
Step 8: Facilitate the learning Step 9: Strive to ensure a positive student experience and raise students' expectations	• IPE facilitation: Each IPE activity has a lead facilitator that oversees the planning and delivery for the IPE session. For each IPE session, students are divided into small groups of interprofessional teams (7–10 students) and each group is assigned a facilitator. Facilitators are usually faculty members, alumni and in some cases senior students. Prior to each IPE activity, an orientation takes place with all participating facilitator with tips to follow on best practices in facilitating an IPE session including the inclusion of an ice breaker and opportunity for interprofessional interactive learning

Step 10: Assess and utilize feedback	• Assessment: Though IPE was integrated in the different health profession curricula at Qatar University, the methods to assess the learning outcomes varied across the colleges such as reflective accounts in College of Pharmacy and College of Health Science, portfolio in College of Medicine and Dental Medicine and MCQs and short answers in midterm and final exams in College of Pharmacy for introductory IPE activities. Reflective accounts and portfolio were usually post reflection of the IPE activity they participated in or related to an IPE task within their clinical placement. The variation and absence of assessment of IPE learning outcomes across the different profession had an influence on student engagement for some of the participating profession affecting students' ability to write reflective account post the event. Therefore, discussion with IPE members took place to reflect on our assessment strategies and work towards unifying assessment across the different health colleges to ensure: – Similar IPE exposure to all QU Health students ensuring equal opportunities to all – Structured integration/ assessment of IPE – Graduating capable and competent collaborative practice ready workforce who are equipped with the skills to work interprofessionally • For the IPE passport program, we designed and implemented a comprehensive assessment plan that targets the goals and educational competencies of IPE in discussion with all the participating professions. All health profession students must now complete a minimum of four IPE activities with at least one at each level of exposure, immersion, and mastery. For each IPE activity, students must submit a reflective assignment as per their assigned course/ module to add the event to their passport. These assignments were graded by the respective colleges with a score assigned to the course/ module. The assessment was mapped to the University of British Columbia IPE model which is based on three key concepts: Exposure, Immersion, and Mastery. A rubric for each level was developed
Step 11: Evaluate the intervention	• A pre-post intervention quantitative research design including the use of validated instruments, qualitative studies and mixed method studies have been used to evaluate IPE initiatives. Currently, we are working on a plan to evaluate the IPE passport program and the comprehensive assessment plan introduced. In addition to assessing the impact of IPE program on learners and graduates
Step 12: Share your experience	• Since 2014, there has been significant scholarly output with peer-reviewed articles published, by IPEC members, regarding IPE in Qatar and the Middle East. In addition to presentations at national and international conferences

Sustainability	• Dedicated IPE unit: In 2017, Qatar University established a health cluster, referred to as QU Health which is an umbrella of the five health colleges at Qatar University. Colleges work together to maximize efficiencies prepare 'competent graduates capable of shaping the future of health care in Qatar' [32]. IPE is now part of QU Health strategy and in 2022 a dedicated office for IPE has been established. The office is led by a section head and two academic specialists (one for pre-clinical phase and the other to focus on IPE clinical placements). In addition to an administrative specialist • IPE passport program: Compulsory for all health profession students at Qatar University • Leading the establishment of Interprofessional collaborative Arab Network which is an emerging network part of the global Confederation for Interprofessional Education and Collaborative Practice • Will be hosting the 11th International Conference on Interprofessional Education and Collaborative Practice (IPECP), All Together Better Health (ATBH) XI in November 2023

5.5 PROCESS: Teaching and Learning Methodologies

Constructive alignment is required between defined learning outcomes, teaching and learning activities, and assessment methods [33]. Constructive alignment ensures that learning outcomes are directly matched with the activity and to pertinent assessment tasks when creating interprofessional activities. Designing teaching and learning activities aligned to learning outcomes for interprofessional learning, student interaction, and a mix of disciplines, begin with the adoption or development of a competency framework (Case Study 5.2).

Case Study 5.2 Development of the Collaborative Competency Curriculum Framework at Monash University

The Faculty of Medicine Nursing and Health Sciences at Monash University is large, with around 13,000 students across five campuses in Victoria, Australia, a campus in Malaysia, and numerous international partnerships and co-operative ventures. The health professions represented in the Faculty are Medicine, Midwifery, Nursing, Nutrition and Dietetics, Occupational Therapy, Paramedicine, Pharmacy, Physiotherapy, Psychology, Radiography, Radiation therapy, Sonography and Social Work. Despite multiple successful IPE initiatives, the Faculty did not have a structured IPE framework that afforded integration of these activities in the curriculum. In 2016 the process to develop a framework was initiated with the appointment of a faculty lead and formation of a Collaborative Care Curriculum Committee [34].

Appointment of a committed and knowledgeable interprofessional leader, with protected time, clear agendas and outcome-focused deliverables, facilitated the project—(Maddock et al. 2019 [35])

A six-stage process was undertaken (Maddock et al. [35]).

1. **Group formation**-nominated representatives from all programs, a patient advocate and student representatives.
2. **Review of existing literature.**
3. **Synthesis of accreditation documents**-multiple themes were inducted, and consensus reached on 4 themes through group discussion.
4. **Final themes and student learning outcomes**- additional outcomes added from student and consumer feedback.
5. **Working with multimedia**-design representation of framework, produce documents and facilitate communication across faculty.
6. **The Monash University FMHS Collaborative Competency Curriculum Framework**- academic overview briefing paper and an explanatory document for students and the wider community were approved for dissemination.

The objectives of the Collaborative Care Curriculum [34] are to:

- Establish an overarching education framework for collaborative practice, learning outcomes at novice, intermediate and entry to practice levels.
- Support the development and promotion of interprofessional learning opportunities within profession specific curricula.
- Support the pursuit of educational research in the design, delivery and evaluation of the Collaborative Care Curriculum.
- Advise on the development of educational resources to support the Collaborative Care Curriculum learning outcomes.

The curriculum is structured as a continuum rather than aligned to years of study. This enables the development of targeted learning programs, where the curriculum is used to plan in relation to learning needs, rather than assumed knowledge, skills or behaviors. Collaborative learning outcomes from accreditation documents for each profession formed the starting point for this curriculum framework. Existing interprofessional curriculum frameworks were sourced; the Canadian CIHC National Interprofessional Competency Framework and Curtin University Interprofessional Capability Framework were key references [34].

Student learning outcomes were devised in four themes: Person-centered care; role understanding; interprofessional communication; and collaboration with and across teams

Consumer representatives were not in agreement in their preference for the word 'client', 'patient' or 'person'. Ultimately, 'person' was agreed upon by the group because of the tendency to align the word 'patient' with illness and 'client' with consumer, rather than active participant—[35]

The achievement standards for the student learning outcomes are presented in three levels reflecting the emphasis in each theme within the stage of learning:

- Novice (first year of an undergraduate degree).
- Intermediate (second or third year of an undergraduate degree, or first year of a graduate entry).
- Entry to practice (final year).

Students felt that any new framework should replicate the structure of existing curriculum documents, and be uncomplicated for students to grasp the main concepts and skills required for graduation—[35]

Keys to the successful development of the framework included:

- reference to profession specific accreditation requirements,
- incorporating patient and student perspectives, and,
- working with multimedia to produce clear professional documents.

The outcome of the six-stage structured process was the establishment of an agreed framework for use across professions when planning an interprofessional curriculum. Shared language, vision and priorities were developed in this process [35]

Replicating the proposed framework development process at other universities, or in countries outside of Australia, would require additional consideration of the range of professions represented at the university, and the variations in professional groups and accreditation documents—[35]

IPE curricular frameworks support the development of appropriate teaching and learning (T&L) activities and assessment strategies to facilitate alignment with outcomes. They are often devised with three levels: beginning, intermediate, and the advanced. These levels are labeled according to the stage of the student program and the depth of the IPE teaching and learning process and expected outcomes.

1. Early/Exposure – an IPE learning activity that meets the minimum education requirements related to interprofessional education and collaborative practice concepts and is case-based or problem-based but does not need to involve patients/clients either simulated or actual. The exposure level provides students with an introduction to the principles of interprofessional collaborative practice.

2. Intermediate/ Engagement - an IPE learning activity that builds on previous learning about the concepts of interprofessional education and collaborative practice and involves patients/clients either simulated or actual, affording development of teamwork, collaboration, and communication skills. Activities may involve simulation, and this may be combined with early clinical exposure in community settings.
3. Later/ Immersion - an IPE learning activity that builds on previous learning about collaborative practice and is based in a clinical workplace where students participate in usual care; the term 'complex immersion activity' has been used to denote an extended clinically based module [36]. This level is also referred to other frameworks as Competency or Transition to Practice and students are supported to develop interprofessional communication and teamwork skills while working in clinical settings with patients and other health professionals.

To ensure that IPE competencies linked to communication, teams, and collaboration are attained, it is important to choose appropriate T&L methodology.

All IPE learning activities must have as a minimum prerequisite:

- Full involvement of students from two or more professions; and of facilitators from two or more professions wherever possible.
- At least one IP learning outcome must be explicit to students and staff at the outset.
- The learning must be predominantly interactive or experiential.
- There must be explicit assessment of at least one IP competency domain.

These requirements for T&L methods in IPE reflect the definition of IPE mentioned earlier [1].

In a systematic review investigating the T&L approaches for pre-registration programs, the most often reported teaching and learning strategies for IPE were simulation-based education (SBE), e-learning, and PBL [37]. There are multiple other T&L methods cited in the literature but in the following section, a sample of these will be included to illustrate the diversity of options for various levels of the curriculum. Although T&L methods are presented at different levels, none are bound to that level and educators are best placed in their own context to decide where a particular activity works best and is aligned to outcomes and assessment methods. It does seem that to prepare novice students or more experienced students with less clinical exposure to patients and other health professionals' practice, there is a need for didactic content to be delivered about person-centered care, drivers of collaborative practice, and roles and responsibilities of various health professions with a system focus. Case-based learning appears to be constructive at any level as is the opportunity for practice-based learning where there are explicit opportunities for reflection on interprofessional competencies.

5.5.1 Beginning/Exposure

At this stage of an interprofessional curriculum, the concepts, and drivers of interprofessional education and collaborative practice are introduced.

In this early phase, multiple programs are included which often cater to large cohorts of students. Technology assisted T&L methods may be useful at this stage. E-Learning IPE activities might include virtual games, discussion boards, live web-based seminars, web-based discussion forums, and virtual environment interactive exercises. At the University of Queensland in Australia, the blended format of a flipped classroom approach is used to deliver a core first year course in all programs. In the flipped classroom approach, there is directed self-learning assigned before the class comes together for discussion and interactive exploration. The multidisciplinary approach to the course's delivery seeks to provide students with a basic understanding of the variety of health professions' responsibilities within Australia's health system and how they contribute to individuals' and the community's health and well-being. By using a flipped format, the course is delivered to students in a way that allows them to independently engage with online learning resources while also meeting face-to-face with peers and teaching staff once a week in tutorials [38].

At the Université Laval in Canada, the first portion of each of the three courses in the curriculum is structured as self-study online learning, while the second portion adopts an action learning strategy where students work in small groups. This design is also inspired by the flipped classroom paradigm. As a result, students have the chance to collaborate while addressing real-world problems and considering their actions. Students are coached in the classroom by experienced clinicians from multiple participating disciplines who have participated in facilitator training to promote interprofessional learning [39]. The advantage of these online methodologies is their ability to be scaled up and to be used during situations, such as experienced during the pandemic, when face to face teaching may be suspended.

As students are introduced to various professions during IPE activities in the preclinical curriculum, they learn that there is a group of healthcare experts they will eventually collaborate with, each with their own set of skills. While gaining exposure to their distinctive skill sets, unique perspectives, it becomes clear to students, with facilitator and peer guidance, that there are numerous shared bodies of knowledge, abilities, and ideals throughout the various health professions. Various IPE exposure actions are possible even in the early stages of an IPE curriculum. For instance, one occupation (and related students) may consent to early career learners from other disciplines shadowing them in a community setting. Supporting medical students to work as a pharmacist's assistant alongside pharmacy students is one instance. As each profession's students learn side by side while participating in typical clinical activities, they can learn to collaborate with others.

5.5.2 Intermediate/Engagement

In the intermediate phase of an interprofessional curriculum, concepts of IPE and collaborative practice are further developed and the competencies of interprofessional communication and teamwork applied in practice.

SBE has been frequently employed as a transitional phase between basic learning components and clinical workplace learning. At Griffith University in Australia, SBE activities are designed to give students a realistic taste of working in an interprofessional team in a supervised and safer setting. Interprofessional student teams are formed, and these teams collaborate on the assessment and management of simulated patients. Student teams should ideally be able to collaborate for long enough to experience a variety of team dynamics and interactions. This is accomplished either through a single lengthy simulation or a string of shorter-duration regular simulations [40].

Simulation scenarios are designed to afford students the opportunity to demonstrate to their peers the knowledge and skills unique to their field of study. An interprofessional workgroup of faculty from Thomas Jefferson University in the USA with experience in geriatrics and collaboration dynamics devised a clinical skills scenario [41]. This learning exercise was designed to give students the chance to work in interprofessional teams and to highlight the crucial roles that all healthcare providers play in providing for a patient and family. The development of the clinical case scenario and the definition of the learning objectives were the first steps in constructing the activity. The activity's specific learning goals required students to show that they could communicate and work collaboratively with patients, family members, and co-workers, construct a care plan with others, and reflect on the experience. A patient chart and a film were made by the faculty workgroup to demonstrate the case of the fictitious patient. The case of a 76-year-old patient admitted with left-sided hemiparesis because of an acute stroke was recorded in the clinical scenario's simulated chart. A doctor, nurse, occupational therapist, physical therapist, pharmacist, and social worker were each seen evaluating the patient in the acute care setting in the 30-minute interprofessional movie [41]. Such an activity that is case-cased, person-centered with a need for multidisciplinary teamwork affords for students to learn with, from and about each other and for that learning to result in a collaborative plan.

Several universities also use structured IPE, which includes patient-centered case studies for student debate [42]. To maximize the learning opportunities for the students from these interactions, small groups were formed that included a representative from a real work environment. Discussions about various patient care strategies not only emphasized the value of interprofessional collaboration (IPC) but also improved the educational process. The idea of patient and caregiver partnership in care is one distinctive aspect of this IPE curriculum at the University of Montreal in Canada [42]. Patients were trained to co-facilitate interprofessional discussion workshops and patients' representatives were included in the course preparation process. They provided students with input on how to use and integrate the patient partnership idea from the perspective of the patient.

Case-based learning interventions can be used to develop interprofessional collaboration competencies across multiple domains and at all levels [43]. Case-based learning teaches students how to deal with the dynamics of interprofessional teams and to cultivate shared values and is also considered an effective teaching strategy to promote role identification, team communication, and team functioning. Problem-based learning (PBL) is the perfect vehicle for IPE case-based learning where a case that would be managed by a multidisciplinary team can enable discovery and discussion of roles and responsibilities with the patient at the center of the care team. The utilization of scenarios, or actual cases, as learning prompts and as facilitators of student interaction, significantly contributes to improving IPE program effectiveness.

A constructive way to ensure centrality of the patient or service user and prevent discipline division is to use a common framework to present a case such as the World Health Organization's International Classification of Functioning, Disability and Health (ICF) [44, 45]. The shared language and conceptual framework based on functional aspects of a case enhances a collaborative approach to a case presentation which transcends disciplinary boundaries. Students at the University of Stellenbosch in South Africa used the ICF in their approach and management of patients on clinical placements [46]. Students, preceptors, and patient have found that this framework has enabled patient-centered care. Moran et al. [45] proposed that the ICF framework can be introduced at any of the stages of an interprofessional curriculum and affords opportunities for educators to embed principles and values of collaborative practice in T&L activities to facilitate interprofessional learning. The MAGPIE model, informed by the ICF is also recommended for use as a process to support students to design and reflect on collaborative care and can be used in work-based learning activities. This model can guide case-based teaching as students follow the steps to **m**eet, **a**ssess, **g**oal-set, **p**lan, **i**mplement, and **e**valuate a person's presentation [45].

Team-based learning (TBL) has been used to support interprofessional learning, used to build collaborative capability in students [47]. During the process of TBL, health professions educators from different disciplines, clinicians, and scientists can role model interprofessional teamwork. The small group and task-focused characteristics of TBL provide an opportunity to develop collegiality and collaboration among health professional students at an early stage in healthcare curricula. Early years medical and physiotherapy students at the University of Sydney in Australia participated in a musculoskeletal system focused TBL activity. Students appreciated the opportunity to learn about the curriculum of another healthcare discipline, and their scope of practice; gain multiple perspectives on a patient case from different disciplines; and recognized the importance of multidisciplinary teams in patient care. The important elements of across discipline interactive problem solving, and relevance to patient-centered care for participant groups, along with skilled content design and interprofessional facilitation, are demonstrated in appropriate choice of T&L activities for interprofessional learning.

Existing curriculum materials can be accessed to supplement locally developed IPE curricula. TeamSTEPPS is an evidenced based initiative developed by the Agency for Healthcare Research and Quality (AHRQ) in the USA. Based on teamwork principles, the materials can be accessed freely and support understanding of team roles, effective interprofessional communication, and conflict management. Three educational institutions in the USA used TeamSTEPPS alongside the IPEC Competency framework to inform IPE curricula and to support faculty development [48]. Although the materials are implemented at each institution in slightly different ways, T&L methods of active small group learning with debriefing and reflection, facilitating constructive discussion across disciplines, are commonly used. Students participate in these activities using scenarios related to interprofessional relations with a patient-centered focus based on developing collaborative practice-ready health professionals [48].

5.5.3 Later/Transition to Practice/Competency

At this stage of the interprofessional curriculum, students will be expected to demonstrate developing competencies in IPE and collaborative practice.

5.5.3.1 Practice Placements

Practice placements offer work-integrated learning and support the application of theory learned to practice. A placement is any period where a student is in a practice setting. Students must be active members of the clinical team to experience team processes and to develop an understanding of how the needs of the patient are met collaboratively. It is possible that students may be placed in multidisciplinary teams and further develop disciplinary competencies without developing collaborative competencies. It is essential to the effectiveness of a placement which includes an interprofessional learning objective that there is explicit reflection on team roles and processes so that collaborative competence is recognized and participated in.

A team-based interprofessional learning practice placement (TIPP) has been defined as "a dedicated and prearranged opportunity for several students from health, social care and related professions to learn together for a period of time in the same setting as they perform typical activities of their profession as a team focused on a client-centered approach" [49]. Students from different disciplines and programs who are present at the same time and site can collaborate on various activities including ward rounds, patient admission and assessment, management planning, and case conferences. Students who are co-located in the health service may conduct service improvement projects and review and revise placement resources while learning and working together. Elements to consider when planning a TIPP are the learning and collaboration culture of the placement site partner, support for the placement from all stakeholders, ways that students will consolidate their learning and inclusion of a quality improvement process [49]. Essential to success of interprofessional learning on practice placements are opportunities for students to learn and work together that reflect authentic practice. Affording specific activities to ensure reflection on interprofessional practice experiences is also essential to building the student's identity as a health professional team member as well as their uniprofessional identity.

5.5.4 Interprofessional Training Wards and Student-Led Clinics

Whole wards and clinics may be serviced by a multidisciplinary group of students supervised by health professionals. Managing patients in these settings affords students from multiple disciplines the opportunity to learn and work together but also in many cases to offer healthcare to those who may not have service access otherwise. The details of the teaching and learning methodologies in these settings has not been clear in the published studies ([50]. In a systematic review of student-led clinics, studies reported on the students' experiences and perceptions of interprofessional learning. It was found that students gained better understanding of their own role and of others, positively perceiving the opportunity to work together [50].

Interprofessional training wards (ITWs) have been established in Sweden, United Kingdom, Australia, and Canada. The composition of ITWs was found in most countries to be informed by the original Swedish model and including medical and nursing students with various combinations of allied health disciplines [51]. There was again, positive reception of interprofessional education and practice reported in evaluations of ITWs but issues have been raised about the limited length of time and unclear goals being constraints that require consideration [51].

5.5.5 Managing Challenges: Intense and Distributed Methods

For interprofessional T&L to be included regularly and sustainably in multiple programs, it is necessary for approaches to curricula inclusion to be varied and nimble. One solution is to have a regular intense program. At the University of Maryland Baltimore (UMB) in the USA, IPE Day is hosted annually by the UMB Center for Interprofessional Education. The IPE Day brings together students from Health, Law, and Social Services to learn and work together on a complex case. The case is presented by a community member with lived experience or a simulated patient (an actor). In 2022, students attended a panel of faculty and students who presented on their experience of working in an interprofessional clinic sharing components of collaborative care. The case is then presented, and students are divided into smaller multidisciplinary groups. They interact with the simulated patient and consider not just the health of the person but how that impacts on all aspects of life. Learning and working together across disciplines and professions improves their understanding of collaborative person-centered problem solving [52].

In larger institutions, campuses may be distributed. Regional and rural campuses offer excellent opportunities for facilitators and students to develop interprofessional rapport, particularly if they are collocated in a smaller health service [53]. This does pose challenges with participating in IPE T&L activities organized and delivered on the main campus. Technology assisted solutions are possible [54] but there are also multiple practice and project-based activities that can be done locally [55, 56].

Table 5.1 Constructive alignment examples in an interprofessional curriculum

Learning objective	Teaching and learning approach	Assessment task
Describe role, responsibilities, and practices of own and other professions	Flipped classroom introductory lecture followed by small group learning	Reflection and short answer
Recognize own limitations and seek interprofessional involvement as indicated	Interprofessional case-based simulation scenario (e.g., Family meeting with Multidisciplinary Team)	Mock referral requests to appropriate health professionals
Synthesize the input of other professionals and devise a shared care plan	Joint patient assessment on practice placement	Collaborative case management plan

5.5.6 Opportunistic or Informal Learning on Practice Placement

When a discipline specific placement is taking place in a multidisciplinary team, there is value in the placement manual containing suggestions and templates for interprofessional learning activities. For example at the University of Toronto, "flexible" IPE activity guidelines can be accessed by students from their website [57]. Students from different professions may work together to jointly assess a patient and to collaboratively devise a management plan. With the supervisor facilitating reflection on this activity, the collaboration experience can be unpacked and interprofessional learning reinforced.

The structure of such an interprofessional activity can be taken from a template in the university's IPE resource pack or practice placement guideline. Sharing knowledge about each profession, aspects of person-centered care, negotiating, and commenting on what was learned about collaborating with other professions are constructive aspects of such a template. Essential to the success of IPE activities on placement is the explicit linking of the performance of the student with their competency assessment document [58].

At each stage of an IPE curriculum, alignment of learning objectives, T&L methods, and assessment tasks is essential to support effective development of the collaborative practice-ready health professional (see Table 5.1).

5.6 Process: Assessment

Best practice in assessing interprofessional learning requires constructive alignment between desired learning outcomes, learning activities, and how they are assessed [30, 33]. Both formative assessment, assessment *for* learning and summative assessment, assessment *of* learning are important processes in an interprofessional curriculum. A call to "raise the bar for innovative IPE assessment approaches" [59] followed several major initiatives to strengthen summative assessment of interprofessional learning [60–62]. Most published studies describe formative assessment procedures (feedback) without reference to measurement or grading of knowledge, skills, or performance [59]. In an IPE curriculum there is a need for a combination of various types of assessments to capture the complex competencies that represent interprofessional learning for future effective collaborative practice [30]. Evidence informed assessment techniques, standardized usage of common tools, and longitudinal assessment from a variety of data streams are required for inclusion in an IPE curriculum for the field to advance and to be in line with the requirements of evolving clinical care systems [60–62].

Assessment drives learning and historically summative assessment of IPE has not always been regularly included or well aligned to learning outcomes and T&L activities. An international group of expert IPE educators reached consensus that role understanding, interprofessional communication and values and coordination and collaborative decision-making, reflexivity, and teamwork require assessment in an interprofessional curriculum [61]. It is also recommended that the assessment must be matched to the environment in which the student experiences the IPE activity and measures what is planned; that it is constructively aligned. [61].

5.6.1 Formative Assessment for Learning

Programs for health professional education must include the accurate and prompt feedback of learners on their progress towards achieving IPE outcomes. Feedback should be viewed as a proactive process that highlights the learner's agency as a proactive seeker of feedback so they can enhance their performance. Peer feedback exchanges in an interprofessional setting can be quite effective to build insight in understanding of one's own role and that of others. One's ability to reflect on oneself is frequently enhanced by constructive feedback of healthcare professionals from different specialties and from patients; actual or simulated. Effective interprofessional facilitation includes constructive feedback and a tool such as the Individual Teamwork Observation and Feedback Tool (iTOFT) offers excellent criteria to inform feedback on an individual's performance in a team [63]. At the University of Kansas in the Doctor of Pharmacy program, iTOFT was used to assess the student's ability to work effectively in an interprofessional team and preceptors reported that use of the tool led to improved feedback [64].

Constructive multidisciplinary feedback encourages reflection on communication styles and terminology use. Utilizing an interprofessional competency framework or the interprofessional practice standards of a health professional body can support educators and students with assessment for learning. By comparing performance in written assessments, oral presentations, team projects or clinical placement performance, to these resources, learning or skills gaps can be identified, and remediation plans made.

5.6.2 Summative Assessment of Learning

Students are generally assessed as individuals although many programs, even in courses which include group projects and assignments. These collaborative activities require rubrics which include assessment of the individual's ability to work with others but may also include criteria describing expected levels of group performance which are judged collectively. Assessments geared towards assessing competence may not address that important outcome of collective competence. A holistic, person-centered approach to healthcare management necessitates collective competency which is dependent on the complex interaction between practitioners, the patients/community and the health service [65]. This need to summatively assess for both individual and team-based competence requires a different view of assessment.

Interprofessional learning may be assessed using multiple tools including multiple choice questions or short answer questions on professional roles and responsibilities, team projects rubrics of a quality improvement activities, review of a service information document, community visits or direct observation in interprofessional simulations and practice settings. Reflective journaling with appropriate rubrics may be used to demonstrate the development of collaborative competencies. ePortfolios are a portal for the recording and assessment of interprofessional learning including reflection. The challenge with reflection that is summative is that students may chose not to share openly and explore areas of doubt and therefore negate the value of looking back on experiences to reinforce learning.

Design guidelines have been published that were developed by a qualitative consensus study using nominal group technique [62]. IP assessment development requires balance across a curriculum, with different IP assessment tasks focusing on distinct but overlapping clusters of IP competencies and ensuring that IPE assessment is focused on the individual but also on the IPE team performance. Equally necessary is consideration of the experience and expertise if the assessors as IPE assessment is more complex and requires clear guidelines as to how a student's performance is graded [62].

To describe that elusive readiness to collaborate, The American Association of Medical Colleges (AAMC) has included in a set of 13 core entrustable professional activities (EPAs) which pre-registration medical students must demonstrate in learning and assessment, EPA 9, to "Collaborate as a member of an interprofessional team." Educators and researchers from three US medical schools worked together to devise a tool to deconstruct the EPA and align it with collaborative competencies for education and assessment [66]. It was found that this EPA could be best assessed in the practice setting, however, funding and supervision regulation must be considered when assessing entrustment to collaborate which basically equates to unsupervised practice. A review of tools to assess teamworking as an indicator of the competency of interprofessional collaboration was undertaken. It was noted that the AAMC expects students "to demonstrate collaboration in interprofessional teams so as to provide patient and population-centered care" [67]. The reviewers found that a deficit existed in tools that would assess change is behavior and improved patient outcomes as expected by the AAMC.

Finding a tool to assess both individual and team performance is challenging, and it is more feasible that a combination of tools is necessary. Examples of such assessments might be MCQs to assess role and responsibilities of health professionals, presentation of a project which demonstrates collaborative practice, direct observation in simulation and practice, and reflective journaling with clear rubrics for performance aligned to learning outcomes.

The Individual Teamwork Observation and Feedback Tool (iTOFT), devised by a consortium of seven universities, is a validated tool designed to assess an individual's performance on a team rather than the performance of the entire team; it employs a consistent evaluation scale; and it is relatively brief (11 items) [63]. Pharmacy students at University of Wisconsin-Madison School of Pharmacy in the USA were assessed using the iTOFT during advanced pharmacy practice experiences to assess and give feedback on performance in the interprofessional team. Although not used summatively, preceptors were encouraged to use the iTOFT score to inform an IPE item on the student's final placement performance assessment [68].

When selecting or creating an assessment tool, Crowl et al. [64] recommend that the following should be considered:

1. Alignment with interprofessional competencies,
2. Clear descriptors or examples and ease of utilization.
3. Applicable to all health professions.
4. Training of assessors is imperative on how to complete the assessment tool as recommended by the IPE experts.
5. Consider expanding the assessor pool to include non-discipline specific supervisors/ preceptors in the assessment of team-ready behaviors to provide a 360-degree evaluation to students [64]. The behaviors needed for collaborative practice by health professionals must be learnt and demonstrated in the context of tasks practiced in the healthcare system. A practice-based, authentic, integrated assessment that can evaluate many different aspects of emerging abilities compared to criterion referenced standards is required [30].

Recommendations to both formatively and summatively assess IPE particularly in the later stages of a curriculum are that there is regular and continuous direct observation and assessment of collaborative behavior linked to improved patient experience and healthcare outcomes, that there are multiple data points and multiple raters, over time and multiple contexts, a programmatic approach to IPE assessment.

5.7 PRODUCT: Evaluation

In contrast to evaluations of complete interprofessional curricula, published IPE evaluations typically focus on specific initiatives that are a part of a curriculum. This incomplete approach disregards the entirety of the program, which would provide a better grasp of how to constructively align IPE inside core profession-specific curricula [69, 70]. Students may positively experience multiple IPE activities but without constructive alignment, it will be challenging to understand a clear pathway to the collaborative practice ready graduate. Curricular evaluation affords an understanding of the staged development required to build collaborative competency and meet IPE outcomes and should support identification of gaps and areas of strength in that educational pathway.

Although often written as the last step in any model of curricular development, evaluation must be considered from the beginning of curriculum development. Certainly, most curricular development models begin with a needs assessment such as that referred to earlier in the section on presage. To make sure that the curriculum or course is operating as intended and to pinpoint areas for improvement, it must be continuously monitored and evaluated with the results used to guide further development.

Observation, feedback surveys, focus groups, interviews, student assessment results, and reports that the institution is required to produce for internal use (such as absence data) or external organizations such as accreditation bodies, are some of the monitoring and evaluation approaches that can be used to evaluate an interprofessional curriculum.

Why evaluate interprofessional education curricula? There are several important uses for it:

- To determine which elements of a curriculum, need to be changed and which are effective.
- To evaluate the success of the modifications that have previously been made.
- To show that the current program is effective.
- To fulfill regular program review obligations.
- To fulfill professional accreditation requirements.

The Kirkpatrick Model has been the most widely used and referenced approach for evaluating learning and change because of an IPE intervention and in fact, is its use is increasing in all educational evaluations [71]. Originally designed to evaluate business activities, it is now frequently used as an evaluation model in higher education or health professional learning activities. The Kirkpatrick model is a 4-step outcome-based approach that is widely used to evaluate training programs. Often used to evaluate pilot and one-time IPE activities, the model has been adapted for IPE outcome evaluation to 6 levels, Reaction, Modification of perceptions and outcomes, Acquisition of knowledge and skills, Behavioral change, Change in organizational practice and Benefits to Patients or Clients [72, 73].

To understand how and why outcomes occur from an interprofessional curriculum, it is necessary to use a more comprehensive program evaluation rather than an exclusively outcomes focused model [71]. If evaluation of a complex intervention is focused only on outcomes, evaluators may overlook unintended positive or negative consequences of curricular implementation [70, 71]. It is necessary to consider evaluation methods that investigate the environment, the context into which the interprofessional curriculum is implemented (presage) and the processes that operationalize the curriculum.

The Indiana University Interprofessional Practice and Education Center in the US devised an interprofessional curriculum, Team Education Advancing Collaboration in Health (TEACH) for 8,000 students in 20 health professions programs at multiple institutions. Following 5 years of this curriculum and regular collection of student and faculty data for continuous quality improvement, a recent review was conducted utilizing the Modified Kirkpatrick Model to represent educational outcomes. Following completion of the external evaluation, interviews and focus groups were conducted with evaluators and stakeholders from the multiple institutions and programs to discuss evaluation outcomes and development improvement strategies [74]. Resembling an action research approach, all stakeholders were engaged in regular meetings to review recommendations and development improvement strategies. Changes to the curriculum included efficiencies of delivery, additional use of online learning, new content to support flexibility, and fidelity and establishment of new committees to increase student and faculty engagement. The challenging issue of assessment was also addressed with measures to approve new approaches. A further recommendation was also made to evaluate the costs of IPE [74]. Although an outcome focus framed the beginning of this evaluation, a comprehensive review and investigation with all stakeholders followed and produced data that informed the quality improvement strategies developed for the interprofessional education curriculum.

An interprofessional curriculum's quality is best continuously monitored by structured feedback processes that are ongoing and geared at acquiring timely data. It is crucial to incorporate evaluation activities to determine the curriculum's successes and failures with a view to addressing deficiencies, to gauge whether stated goals have been met, to determine whether the curriculum is meeting the needs of students and the community, and to assess the cost effectiveness of the curriculum.

One method that have been used effectively is a realist approach. A realist approach enables evaluation which investigates what works for whom in what context and why and is appropriate for complex interventions such as an interprofessional curriculum. Mechanisms are identified that impact on the intervention and lead to various outcomes so that evaluation with this approach can identify the "why" and the "how," affording greater guidance for improvement. Researchers used this approach to evaluate interprofessional practice placements and discovered that interaction and reflection helped students better comprehend the roles and responsibilities of the healthcare team. Patients were integral to interprofessional learning on placement and helped students understand their experience as service users. This study further underlined the value of strong interprofessional facilitation [75]. Such findings may have been hidden in a solely outcomes-based evaluation and would therefore not be available for informing improvement in these areas.

Three institutions in the USA participated in an interprofessional initiative where a multidisciplinary group of students were assigned a community member as a mentor to better understand their experience of a chronic health condition. The Dalhousie Health Mentors Program (DHMP) aimed to evaluate the students intended and unintended learning experiences [76]. Using a mixed methods approach to program evaluation, researchers found three curriculum issues that limited learning, team composition, DHMP integration into discipline programs, and variability in team effectiveness. These findings will afford process improvement which could not result from an outcome only evaluation model. Educational benefits in the areas of patient centeredness, interprofessional skills, and collaborative attitudes were reported by students and can potentially be strengthened with attention to the context and process issues uncovered in the evaluation [76].

Longitudinal follow-up across the university and the health service offers rich data to evaluate collaborative ready practitioners. Researchers in New Zealand conducted a longitudinal evaluation of students who participated in an interprofessional practice placement using validated tools and free text comments [77]. Learner attitudes and self-perceived teamwork skills were assessed over their first 3 years as health professions. Students who had participated in an interprofessional practice placement had higher positive attitudes to healthcare teams than those who had not according to the quantitative and qualitative data collected [77]. They reported a readiness to work in teams and this evaluation enables an understanding of the sustained potential of interprofessional learning to positively influence collaborative practice.

As in the preceding study, the focus of evaluation needs to be expanded from short-term pre- and post-single activity measurement points to longer term measurement points. There is also a need to use tools and methods which evaluate the whole system of an interprofessional education curriculum.

A meta-analysis of an IPE curriculum for ten programs in the UK combined the Biggs' 3P Framework and the Kirkpatrick model [7]. An external evaluator was employed, funded by the health service, reflecting the value placed by the health service on the IPE curriculum to be evaluated. Mixed methods were used to evaluate all elements of the curriculum and were inclusive of all stakeholders, students, educators, health service, and patients. Although a theory-based curriculum, researchers missed the opportunity for that theory to initially inform the evaluation but were able to retrospectively apply the Biggs' 3P framework to better understand factors of presage, process, and product (outcome) and how these impacted on the effectiveness of the curriculum and the student experience. The evaluation enabled the identification of early classroom learning as a positive scaffold for later interprofessional inaction in practice placements [7]. Such models which use both quantitative and qualitative approaches afford an evaluation that not only investigates the planned learning outcomes of the curriculum but can also uncover unintended outcomes, explain why these occurred, understand the environment in which they occurred, and how the processes delivered, enabled, or constrained this.

Although often considered a value adding curricular measure, costs associated with an IPE curriculum have been questioned. Researchers in Australia conducted a cost–benefit analysis (CBA) of an IPE program in a residential aged care facility. Although there were significant collaborative learning outcomes for students and social and emotional benefits identified for aged care residents, the cost of the program was mostly borne by the aged care facility and the sustainability of this was questioned without that external funding [78]. Including an economic analysis across a whole curriculum would be more challenging but would significantly support implementation by exploring budgeting methods to ensure return on investment in an interprofessional curriculum [79].

To plan a comprehensive evaluation early on in IPE curriculum development, the following ought to be considered:

- Decide who are the stakeholders and how will they be included in the evaluation?
- Agree as to why the evaluation is being done and what is it measuring.
- Consider what is the learning environment, the T&L process, and the learning and organizational elements of the curriculum?
- Use an evaluation model that adopts a comprehensive approach, and will investigate the presage, the processes, and products of an interprofessional curriculum.
- Consider the use of a theoretical perspective to underpin the evaluation.
- Use an evaluation design that reflects the research question, considering whether quantitative or qualitative data is collected, or a mixed methods evaluation is required and how to do this with a longitudinal approach [69, 80].

Key elements of an interprofessional education curriculum are missed by an outcome focused evaluation with subsequent missed opportunities for improvement. Short term or pre-post initiative evaluation in isolation do not afford an understanding of the effectiveness or impact of an interprofessional education curriculum. A system focused, longitudinal and mixed methods approach is recommended to capture a deeper and constructive evaluation of an interprofessional education curriculum.

5.8 PRODUCT: Sustainability

IPE program sustainability and viability are acknowledged as global challenges that depend on a variety of circumstances related to competing program demands, faculty resources and administrative support and the value placed on an IPE curriculum. Now that collaboration is considered integral to better experience and outcomes for health service users, curricula that prepare collaborative ready graduates must be sustained [81]. At The University of Manitoba in Canada, a systems-based approach to sustainability of the interprofessional curriculum was adopted [82].

Elements for sustainability were considered at the micro, meso, and macro levels. At the micro-level, student engagement and faculty development need to be strengthened along with the development of continuous improvement of the interprofessional T&L resources, informed by theory and a spiral structure of agreed competency development.

Faculty development is so important in the sustainability of an interprofessional curriculum. Just as students require support to learn about, from and with each other, so too faculty require support to build consensus on concepts and behaviors that demonstrate collaborative practice. A qualitative survey study conducted at the University of Otago in New Zealand examined IPE instructors' opinions of the IPE facilitation, what assistance they need, and what variables affected their capacity to continue participating in the program and, consequently, the sustainability of the program. Having provided pre-registration IPE for about 10 years, findings shared that to sustain protected time for participation in IPE delivery, IPE facilitators need both official acknowledgement of their facilitation skills and workload modeling [83].

Essential to sustainability is student and faculty engagement in an IPE curriculum and this requires consensus on purpose and value of interprofessional learning. Sometimes mitigating that consensus, interprofessional competencies found in all uniprofessional frameworks present issues with the standardization of terminology. Mapping of competencies from uniprofessional frameworks to widely adopted or locally developed interprofessional competency frameworks can assist in building consensus of understanding. Development of shared language and definitions of interprofessional competencies would support sustainability by facilitating strengthening of curricula with shared understanding of processes and outcomes across health professions education programs for students and faculty. At the meso level, IPE activities must be fully integrated in curricula and there must be institutional recognition and support either by establishing a funded IPE center or at least the appointment of an IPE faculty lead. Establishing an interprofessional program leadership with dedicated resources and a strategic plan that is reflected in the university's mission and vision is integral to sustainability (Case Study 3). Associated with that institutional commitment to an interprofessional curriculum, funding issues can be a significant hindrance to the sustainability of IPE curricula. Where programs are individually accountable for their budgets there may be challenges with sustaining collaborative learning activities. Three funding models have been suggested for consideration: centralized, blended, and decentralized [79]. Each institution must explore such models to understand which works best and support sustainability of resources while ensuring a return on investment in the IPE curriculum.

At the macro-level, accreditation standards, a dedicated research agenda informed by a continuous improvement evaluation cycle and valued relationships with community partners are all factors upon which the sustainability of an interprofessional curriculum are predicated. In Case Study 5.3 below, an example of strategic steps taken by the University of Maryland Baltimore in the USA to sustain an interprofessional curriculum are illustrated.

Case Study 5.3 University of Maryland Baltimore (UMB) USA
Strong steps for sustainability:

> *Preparing all University students to provide high-quality, affordable health care and human services with a team-based model*

1. Establishment of the Center for Interprofessional Education (CIPE) 2013.
2. University endorsed, vision and Mission statements to provide IPE to prepare collaborative graduates across Health, Law and Human Services programs.
3. Annual funding opportunities for IPE curriculum content development.
4. Faculty awards in support of IPE to build community across university programs.
5. IPE faculty scholars program to expand expertise and experience in IPE development and delivery at UMB.
6. Faculty funding to attend the Interprofessional Education Collaborative (IPEC) Institute (National IPE Center) and support for associated IPE project.
7. CIPE supported annual IPE student activities such as IPE Day and the Interprofessional Patient Management Competition.
8. UMB Faculty Development-Foundation of IPEP course.
9. Annual IPE sustaining funds affording further resourcing to ongoing activities [52].

5.9 Conclusion

Implementation of a novice IPE curriculum is a complex process but an integral component of most modern health profession education programs. To develop collaborative practice ready graduates, students need to develop those competencies that will enable teamwork and effective communication. Constructive alignment of interprofessional learning objectives, teaching and learning activities, and assessment is supported by adoption or development of an interprofessional competency framework. Utilizing an approach such as the modified Biggs' 3P model as presented in this chapter will afford IPE curriculum implementation that considers all stakeholders and elements, includes a comprehensive evaluation to inform continuous quality improvement and sustainability measures.

References

1. World Health Organization. Framework for action on interprofessional education and collaborative practice. Geneva: World Health Organization; 2010.

2. Grymonpre RE, Bainbridge L, Nasmith L, Baker C. Development of accreditation standards for interprofessional education: a Canadian case study. Hum Resour Health. 2021;19(1):12.
3. Moran MC, Steketee C, Forman D, Dunston R. Using a research-informed interprofessional curriculum framework to guide reflection and future planning of interprofessional education in a multi-site context. J Res Interprof Pract Educ. 2015;5:1–13.
4. Centre for the Advancement of Interprofessional Education. Interprofessional education—a definition 2002 [Homepage of Centre for the Advancement of Interprofessional Education (CAIPE)]. http://www.caipe.org.uk/resources/.
5. Reeves S, Freeth D. Re-examining the evaluation of interprofessional education for community mental health teams with a different lens: understanding presage, process and product factors. J Psychiatr Ment Health Nurs. 2006;13(6):765–70.
6. Freeth DS, Hammick M, Reeves S, Koppel I, Barr H. Effective interprofessional education: development, delivery, and evaluation. Hoboken, NJ: Wiley; 2008.
7. Anderson E, Smith R, Hammick M. Evaluating an interprofessional education curriculum: a theory-informed approach. Med Teach. 2016;38(4):385–94.
8. Biggs JB. From theory to practice: a cognitive systems approach. High Educ Res Dev. 1993;12(1):73–85.
9. Frenk J, Chen LC, Chandran L, Groff EO, King R, Meleis A, et al. Challenges and opportunities for educating health professionals after the COVID-19 pandemic. Lancet. 2022;400(10362):1539–56.
10. Freeth D, Reeves S. Learning to work together: using the presage, process, product (3P) model to highlight decisions and possibilities. J Interprof Care. 2004;18(1):43–56.
11. Freeth D, Reeves S, Koppel I, Hammick M, Barr H. Evaluating interprofessional education: a self-help guide. London: Higher Education Academy; 2005.
12. Grace S. Models of interprofessional education for healthcare students: a scoping review. J Interprof Care. 2021;35(5):771–83.
13. Lawlis TR, Anson J, Greenfield D. Barriers and enablers that influence sustainable interprofessional education: a literature review. J Interprof Care. 2014;28(4):305–10.
14. Thistlethwaite JE. Curriculum development in Interprofessional Education in Health. In: Darmann-Finck I, Reiber K, editors. Development, implementation and evaluation of curricula in nursing and midwifery Education. Cham: Springer International; 2021. p. 211–26.
15. Canadian Interprofessional Health collaborative. A national interprofessional competency framework Vancouver, Canada. 2010. http://www.cihc-cpis.com/publications1.html.
16. Interprofessional Education Collaborative Expert Panel. Core competencies for interprofessional collaborative practice: report of an expert panel. Washington, DC: Interprofessional Collaborative; 2011.
17. Reeves S, Fletcher S, Barr H, Birch I, Boet S, Davies N, et al. A BEME systematic review of the effects of interprofessional education: BEME Guide No. 39. Med Teach. 2016;38:656–68.
18. El-Awaisi A, Sheikh Ali S, Abu Nada A, Rainkie D, Awaisu A. Insights from healthcare academics on facilitating interprofessional education activities. J Interprof Care. 2021;35(5):760–70.
19. Anderson ES, Thorpe LN, Hammick M. Interprofessional staff development: changing attitudes and winning hearts and minds. J Interprof Care. 2011;25(1):11–7.
20. Derbyshire JA, Machin AI, Crozier S. Facilitating classroom based interprofessional learning: a grounded theory study of university educators' perceptions of their role adequacy as facilitators. Nurse Educ Today. 2015;35(1):50–6.
21. Nicol P, Forman D. Attributes of effective interprofessional placement facilitation. J Res Interprofession Pract Educ. 2014;4(2).
22. Steinert Y. Learning together to teach together: interprofessional education and faculty development. J Interprof Care. 2005;19(Suppl 1):60–75.
23. El-Awaisi A, AlMukdad S, Jaam M. Opportunities and challenges with student leadership in IPE: a middle eastern perspective. In: Joosten-Hagye D, Khalili H, editors. Interprofessional education and collaborative practice: international approaches at the micro, meso, and macro levels. Solana Beach, CA: Cognella Academic Publishing; 2022. p. 340–56.

24. El-Awaisi A, Anderson E, Barr H, Wilby KJ, Wilbur K, Bainbridge L. Important steps for introducing interprofessional education into health professional education. J Taibah Univ Med Sci. 2016;11(6):546–51.
25. El-Awaisi A, Barr H. East meets west: working together in interprofessional education and practice. J Interprof Educ Pract. 2017;7:72–4.
26. El-Awaisi A, Wilby KJ, Wilbur K, El Hajj MS, Awaisu A, Paravattil B. A middle eastern journey of integrating Interprofessional Education into the healthcare curriculum: a SWOC analysis. BMC Med Educ. 2017;17(1):15.
27. El-Awaisi A, Saffouh El Hajj M, Joseph S, Diack L. Interprofessional education in the Arabic-speaking Middle East: perspectives of pharmacy academics. J Interprof Care. 2016;30(6):769–76.
28. El-Awaisi A, El Hajj MS, Joseph S, Diack L. Perspectives of practising pharmacists towards interprofessional education and collaborative practice in Qatar. Int J Clin Pharmacol. 2018;40(5):1388–401.
29. El-Awaisi A, Saffouh El Hajj M, Joseph S, Diack L. Perspectives of pharmacy students in Qatar toward interprofessional education and collaborative practice: a mixed methods study. J Interprof Care. 2018;32:1–15.
30. McLarnon N, Hutchings M, O'Carroll V, Wetzlmair L-C, Blumenthal S, Boyle L, et al. Rethinking assessment for interprofessional learning during COVID-19: steering a middle course. Br J Midwifery. 2022;30(10):572–81.
31. El-Awaisi A. Qatar—sustaining Interprofessional collaboration in collaborative partnership with other universities. Sustainability and Interprofessional Collaboration. Berlin: Springer; 2020. p. 125–45.
32. QU Health. Mission and vision. Qatar: Qatar University; 2019. http://www.qu.edu.qa/health/about-us/vision-mission.
33. Biggs J, Tang C. Teaching for quality learning at university: what the student does. 3rd ed. Maidenhead: McGraw-Hill/Society for Reserach in Higher Education and Open University Press; 2007.
34. Monash University. Collaborative care curriculum. Melbourne: Monash University; 2022. https://www.monash.edu/medicine/education/ccc.
35. Maddock B, Kumar A, Kent F. Creating a collaborative care curriculum framework. Clin Teach. 2019;16(2):120–4.
36. Division of Health Sciences University of Otago. IPE at Otago: University of Otago; 2022. https://www.otago.ac.nz/healthsciences/staff/ipe/otago109216.html.
37. Aldriwesh M, Alyousif S, Alharbi N. Undergraduate-level teaching and learning approaches for interprofessional education in the health professions: a systematic review. BMC Med Educ. 2022;22:13.
38. Faculty of Health and Behavioural Sciences University of Queensland. Interprofessional Education Brisbane, Australia. University of Queensland; 2022. https://habs.uq.edu.au/interprofessional-education.
39. Milot É, Dumont S, Aubin M, Bourdeau G, Azizah GM, Picard L, et al. Building an interfaculty interprofessional education curriculum: what can we learn from the Université Laval experience? Educ Health (Abingdon). 2015;28(1):58–63.
40. Griffith Health Institute for Development of Education and scholarship. Griffith Health framework for Interprofessional learning. Queensland, Australia; 2018.
41. Herge EA, Hsieh C, Waddell-Terry T, Keats P. A simulated clinical skills scenario to teach Interprofessional teamwork to Health profession students. J Med Educ Curric Dev. 2015;2:JMECD.S18928.
42. Vanier MC, Therriault PY, Lebel P, Nolin F, Lefebvre H, Brault I, et al. Innovating in teaching collaborative practice with a large student cohort at Universite de Montreal. J Allied Health. 2013;42(4):e97–e106.
43. Riskiyana R, Claramita M, Rahayu GR. Objectively measured interprofessional education outcome and factors that enhance program effectiveness: a systematic review. Nurse Educ Today. 2018;66:73–8.

44. Allan CM, Campbell WN, Guptill CA, Stephenson FF, Campbell KE. A conceptual model for interprofessional education: the international classification of functioning, disability and health (ICF). J Interprof Care. 2006;20(3):235–45.
45. Moran M, Bickford J, Barradell S, Scholten I. Embedding the international classification of functioning, disability and health in health professions curricula to enable interprofessional education and collaborative practice. J Med Educ Curric Dev. 2020;7:2382120520933855.
46. Muller J, Snyman S, Slogrove A, Couper I. The value of interprofessional education in identifying unaddressed primary health-care challenges in a community: a case study from South Africa. J Interprof Care. 2019;33(4):347–55.
47. Burgess A, Kalman E, Haq I, Leaver A, Roberts C, Bleasel J. Interprofessional team-based learning (TBL): how do students engage? BMC Med Educ. 2020;20(1):118.
48. Davis BP, Jernigan SD, Wise HH. The integration of TeamSTEPPS into interprofessional education curricula at 3 academic health centers. J Phys Ther Educ. 2019;33(2):134–43.
49. Brewer ML, Barr H. Interprofessional Education and Practice Guide No. 8: team-based interprofessional practice placements. J Interprof Care. 2016;30(6):747–53.
50. Briggs L, Fronek P. Student experiences and perceptions of participation in student-led health clinics: a systematic review. J Soc Work Educ. 2020;56(2):238–59.
51. Oosterom N, Floren LC, Ten Cate O, Westerveld HE. A review of interprofessional training wards: enhancing student learning and patient outcomes. Med Teach. 2019;41(5):547–54.
52. University of Maryland Baltimore. Interprofessional Education. Baltimore: University of Maryland Baltimore; 2022. https://www.umaryland.edu/ipe/.
53. Hudson JN, Croker A. Rural multidisciplinary training: opportunity to focus on interprofessional rapport-building. Rural Remote Health. 2017;17(3):4180.
54. Scott A, Dawson RM, Mitchell S, Catledge C. Simulation-based Interprofessional Education in a rural setting: the development and evaluation of a "remote-in" telehealth scenario. Nurs Educ Perspect. 2020;41(3):187–9.
55. Gum LF, Sweet L, Greenhill J, Prideaux D. Exploring interprofessional education and collaborative practice in Australian rural health services. J Interprof Care. 2020;34(2):173–83.
56. Waller S, Walker L, Farthing A, Brown L, Moran M. Understanding the elements of a quality rural/remote interprofessional education activity: a rough guide. Aust J Rural Health. 2021;29(2):294–300.
57. University of Toronto Center for advancing collaborative healthcare and Education. IPE Core learning activities. University of Toronto; 2022. https://ipe.utoronto.ca/ipe-core-learning-activities.
58. O'Leary N, Salmon N, Clifford AM. 'It benefits patient care': the value of practice-based IPE in healthcare curriculums. BMC Med Educ. 2020;20(1):424.
59. El-Awaisi A, Jaam M, Wilby KJ, Wilbur K. A systematic review of the use of simulation and reflection as summative assessment tools to evaluate student outcomes following interprofessional education activities. J Interprof Care. 2022;36(6):882–90.
60. Blue AV, Chesluk BJ, Conforti LN, Holmboe ES. Assessment and evaluation in interprofessional education: exploring the field. J Allied Health. 2015;44(2):73–82.
61. Rogers GD, Thistlethwaite JE, Anderson ES, Abrandt Dahlgren M, Grymonpre RE, Moran M, et al. International consensus statement on the assessment of interprofessional learning outcomes. Med Teach. 2017;39(4):347–59.
62. Smeets HWH, Sluijsmans DMA, Moser A, van Merriënboer JJG. Design guidelines for assessing students' interprofessional competencies in healthcare education: a consensus study. Perspectives on. Med Educ. 2022;11:316.
63. Thistlethwaite J, Dallest K, Moran M, Dunston R, Roberts C, Eley D, et al. Introducing the individual teamwork observation and feedback tool (iTOFT): development and description of a new interprofessional teamwork measure. J Interprof Care. 2016;30(4):526–8.
64. Crowl AN, Burkhardt C, Shrader S. Potential best practices for assessment of interprofessional team-ready behaviors on APPEs. Curr Pharm Teach Learn. 2020;12(2):156–62.
65. Langlois S. Collective competence: moving from individual to collaborative expertise. Perspect Med Educ. 2020;9(2):71–3.

66. Brown DR, Gillespie CC, Warren JB. EPA 9—collaborate as a member of an Interprofessional team: a short communication from the AAMC Core EPAs for entering residency pilot schools. Med Sci Educ. 2016;26(3):457–61.
67. Havyer RD, Nelson DR, Wingo MT, Comfere NI, Halvorsen AJ, McDonald FS, et al. Addressing the Interprofessional collaboration competencies of the Association of American Medical Colleges: a systematic review of assessment instruments in undergraduate medical education. Acad Med. 2016;91(6):865–88.
68. Margolis A, Shah S, Zorek JA, Kieser M, Martin B. Implementation of the individual teamwork observation and feedback tool to evaluate pharmacy student performance. Am J Pharm Educ. 2022;86(3):8578.
69. Reeves S, Boet S, Zierler B, Kitto S. Interprofessional Education and Practice Guide No. 3: evaluating interprofessional education. J Interprof Care. 2015;29(4):305–12.
70. Thistlethwaite J, Kumar K, Moran M, Saunders R, Carr S. An exploratory review of prequalification interprofessional education evaluations. J Interprof Care. 2015;29(4):292–7.
71. Allen LM, Hay M, Palermo C. Evaluation in health professions education—is measuring outcomes enough? Med Educ. 2022;56(1):127–36.
72. Barr H, Freeth D, Hammick M, Koppel I, Reeves S. Evaluations of interprofessional education. London: United Kingdom Centre for the Advancement of Interprofessional Education; The British Educational Reserach Association; 2000.
73. Freeth D, Hammick M, Koppel I, Reeves S, Barr H. A critical review of evaluations of interprofessional education. London; 2002.
74. Daulton BJ, Weber ZA, Newton AD, Romito L, Manz Friesth BM. Raising the Bar: evolution of a statewide Interprofessional Education program following a 5-year outcomes evaluation. Collab Healthc Interprofession Pract Educ Eval. 2022;12(3).
75. Kent F, Hayes J, Glass S, Rees CE. Pre-registration interprofessional clinical education in the workplace: a realist review. Med Educ. 2017;51(9):903–17.
76. Doucet S, MacKenzie D, Loney E, Godden-Webster A, Lauckner H, Alexiadis P, Andrews C, Packer T. Curricular factors that unintentionally affect learning in a community-based interprofessional education program: the student perspective. J Res Interprofession Pract Educ. 2014;4(2).
77. Darlow B, Brown M, McKinlay E, Gray L, Purdie G, Pullon S. Longitudinal impact of preregistration interprofessional education on the attitudes and skills of health professionals during their early careers: a non-randomised trial with 4-year outcomes. BMJ Open. 2022;12(7):e060066.
78. Nguyen K-H, Seaman K, Saunders R, Williams E, Harrup-Gregory J, Comans T. Benefit–cost analysis of an interprofessional education program within a residential aged care facility in Western Australia. J Interprof Care. 2019;33(6):619–27.
79. Carney PA, Bearden DT, Osborne ML, Driessnack M, Stilp CC, Baggs JG, et al. Economic models for sustainable interprofessional education. J Interprof Care. 2018;32(6):745–51.
80. van Diggele C, Roberts C, Burgess A, Mellis C. Interprofessional education: tips for design and implementation. BMC Med Educ. 2020;20(2):455.
81. World Health Organization. Global competency framework for universal health coverage. 2022.
82. Grymonpre R, Ateah C, Dean H, Heinonen T, Holmqvist M, MacDonald L, et al. Sustainable implementation of Interprofessional Education using an adoption model framework. Can J High Educ. 2017;46(4):76–93.
83. Beckingsale L, Brown M, McKinlay E, Oleary M, Doolan-Noble F. Sustainable interprofessional education programmes: what influences teachers to stay involved? J Interprof Care. 2023;37:637.

Governance of Interprofessional Education and Collaborative Practice

6

Hani Alghamdi and Anthony Breitbach

6.1 Introduction

Devising an integrated system for the governance and control of education, training, and development with a view to designing curricula which are competency based, self-paced, and aligned to workforce needs has become a priority in line with the circumstances we face. It is also vital to produce quality educational, training, and developmental programs that recognize all sectors in society so as to meet the challenges of rapid population growth, economic fluctuations, and environmental degradation. The above changes have necessitated transformation from prevailing models of learning; one such model is IPECP (interprofessional education and collaborative practice). While there is no clear consensus on what IPECP entails there are emerging roles for various disciplines within this approach.

In recent years, there has been an increased focus on interprofessional education (IPE) and collaborative practice (CP) to improve healthcare delivery. IPE gets characterized when two or more students from different specialties learn from each other to achieve a common objective [1]. At the same time, collaborative practice refers to sharing resources and expertise between different health professions to improve patient outcomes [1]. There is mounting evidence that interprofessional education and collaborative practice can enhance patient health outcomes [2]. Systematic reviews of the literature found that IPE interventions were associated with several positive outcomes, including increased knowledge and skills, improved

H. Alghamdi
College of Medicine, King Saud University, Riyadh, Saudi Arabia

A. Breitbach (✉)
Doisy College of Health Sciences, Saint Louis University, St. Louis, MO, USA

M. Y. Alnaami et al. (eds.), *Novel Health Interprofessional Education and Collaborative Practice Program: Strategy and Implementation*,
https://doi.org/10.1007/978-981-99-3420-1_6

communication and teamwork, and reduced medical government and organizational support is essential for the successful implementation of IPE and collaborative practice [3, 4].

Indications that interprofessional education and collaborative practice (IPECP) can enhance patient outcomes and healthcare quality are rising. From studies done, it is evident that there are several mechanisms by which IPECP can improve patient outcomes. A study done on "Analysis of Perceptions of Interprofessional Education" found that IPECP interventions were associated with improvements in a variety of patient outcomes, including mortality, morbidity, length of stay, and patient satisfaction [5]. Guck et al. examined the sustainability of the positive results of IPECP for previously conducted study by the same researchers and they found the original improvements and cost reduction were sustainable for 2 years. The improvement reported in the intervention that utilized IPECP included decreases in patient charges, Emergency Department visits, hemoglobin A1c levels, and hospitalizations [6].

One of the main benefits of IPE is that it can help to prepare healthcare professionals for the increasingly complex and collaborative nature of healthcare delivery. In today's healthcare environment, it is rare for a single healthcare professional to provide all the care a patient needs. Instead, patients are typically cared for by a team of healthcare professionals with different backgrounds and skills [7]. According to Singh and Matthees, IPE can also help address some of the challenges associated with delivering healthcare in a team-based environment. It can help to improve communication and coordination by providing healthcare professionals with the opportunity to learn about and practice working together as a team [8].

An accumulation of evidence supports the importance of CP in improving patient outcomes and reducing healthcare costs. A systematic review of the literature found that IPECP interventions were associated with positive outcomes in terms of improved communication and collaboration, increased knowledge and skills, and changes in attitudes [9]. Organizations such as the World Health Organization (WHO) and the Institute of Medicine (IOM)/National Academies of Science, Engineering and Medicine (NASEM) have recognized the importance of IPECP, and they have issued recommendations for their implementation [10]. The WHO has urged healthcare professional organizations to promote IPECP practice and has developed a framework for action to support these efforts [1].

Although the significant increase in the upstream demand for IPE has been stimulated by the downstream demand for professionals with expertise in interprofessional collaboration (IPC), most IPE programs only involve practitioners who provide direct patient care while those who had administrative and management roles are seldom included [11]. Organizational and government support is critical for developing and implementing interprofessional education and collaborative practice. IPECP can help to improve patient outcomes, reduce healthcare costs, and improve the quality of care. However, there needs to be more purposeful integration between education and healthcare workforce development regarding government/organizations and policy [12]. This gap can be addressed by increasing government and organizational support for IPECP. There are several reasons why government and organizational support is important for IPECP. First, IPECP require a significant investment of resources and their support can help to ensure that these resources are available. Second, IPECP can be complex and challenging to implement, so government and organizational support can help to provide the necessary infrastructure and support to ensure that IPECP is implemented effectively. Finally, IPECP can significantly impact the healthcare workforce, governmental and organizational support can help to ensure that the healthcare workforce is prepared to meet the needs of patients and families.

Government and organizational support for IPECP can take many forms, primarily financial and policy support. Financial support can help to ensure that IPECP programs have the resources they need to be successful while policy support can help to ensure that IPECP programs are implemented effectively, and that the healthcare workforce is prepared to meet the needs of patients and families. Government and organizational support for IPECP are critical for developing and implementing these programs and with their support IPECP programs can achieve their full potential.

The term "governance" refers to systems and procedures that are designed to provide stability, rule of law, integrity, openness, adaptability, diversity, and inclusiveness, as well as empowerment and widespread involvement [13]. In addition, governance refers to the standards, principles, and guidelines that guide the management of public affairs in a truthful, interactive, egalitarian, and responsive manner. Thus, culture and institutional framework in which individuals and stakeholders interact with one another and take part in public affairs generally defines governance.

Good governance enables individuals and organizations to act in the best interests of the institution. Most explicitly, Reddy et al. emphasizes that good governance improves the professional and organizational performance by fostering reliability, efficiency, and openness to new possibilities [14]. Additionally, researchers affirm that governance lowers the propensity of risks by promoting quick and safe growth [15]. Likewise, governance enhances credibility and trust within the institutional frameworks. As such, organizations with good governance exhibit high propensity for succeeding in the competitive entrepreneurial markets.

In light of the growing demand on primary, secondary, and tertiary healthcare services, good governance and effective interprofessional collaboration are essential in maintaining high quality treatment. Effective interprofessional collaboration gets impeded by factors such as governance, perceived hierarchy, and power imbalance between the professionals in the healthcare systems [16]. As a result, poor governance discourages mutual recognition of specialties. Numerous elements have an impact on governance, particularly in the IPECP. Some of the challenges affecting governance include inadequate institutional capacity, poor quality of public services such as healthcare, lack of public demand for improvement, and insufficient government accountability which culminates to corruption and inefficiency in healthcare sector [17].

According to multiple studies, there are several ways through which government can increase interpersonal collaboration in healthcare [18]. For instance, the government can enforce policies that jointly educate specialists, and other medical staff. Reddy et al. assert that the IPECP plays a significant role in jointly training medical practitioners' systems [14]. Through collaborative practice, the firm trains the medical team to close interprofessional gaps by mitigating healthcare inequality concerns.

Besides, addressing accountability issues enables interprofessional teams to collaborate more efficiently and develops stronger working relationships. As a result, this helps the teams to achieve job satisfaction [19]. As such, it improves members' accountability and encourages better teamwork because everyone knows they can rely on one another to get things done effectively.

6.2 Good Governance for IPECP

The concept of IPECP has been around for many years; however, it has taken some time for serious consideration to be given towards interprofessional collaboration within healthcare. The development of interprofessional collaboration in the healthcare delivery system has been a relatively recent phenomenon; and as such there are scant existing resources that may be utilized to support its development. Interprofessional collaboration is an important element in healthcare delivery, but it has yet to achieve real change in the system [20]. This lack of progress has been attributed to lack of focus as well as a lack of support for interprofessional education and training. Since IPECP has not become institutionalized, professionals tend to perceive it as being separate from their everyday practice, which can lead to them having a fragmented outlook on the subject. This can also result from the fact that it is a relatively new concept and not clearly defined. To be able to implement IPECP the governance model should be designed in a way that it will be able to monitor the various activities and program delivery linked to interprofessional education and training [21]. Also, the outputs of these activities should be measured and compared to measure progress in IPECP. If a trial is being implemented in one institution, then it should ideally be replicated in other institutions that are expected to follow similar models.

Good governance for interprofessional education and collaborative practice are essential for achieving positive outcomes from these initiatives. Good governance is a set of principles and practices that ensure that an organization's decisions and resources are used ethically and effectively. Although the governance of IPECP could be a challenge task with the complexity of education and healthcare systems internationally and to bridge the gap between two separately operated systems (i.e., education and healthcare), there are some fundamental principles and practices that should be adopted in order to ensure good governance for IPECP (Fig. 6.1).

First, it is important to define roles and responsibilities among stakeholders, including students, faculty, clinicians, and administrative personnel. This will help ensure that everyone understands their role in the initiative and is held accountable for their part. It is also important to demonstrate transparency and accountability in decision-making and resource allocation. This includes setting clear objectives, developing a process for monitoring progress, and regularly evaluating outcomes.

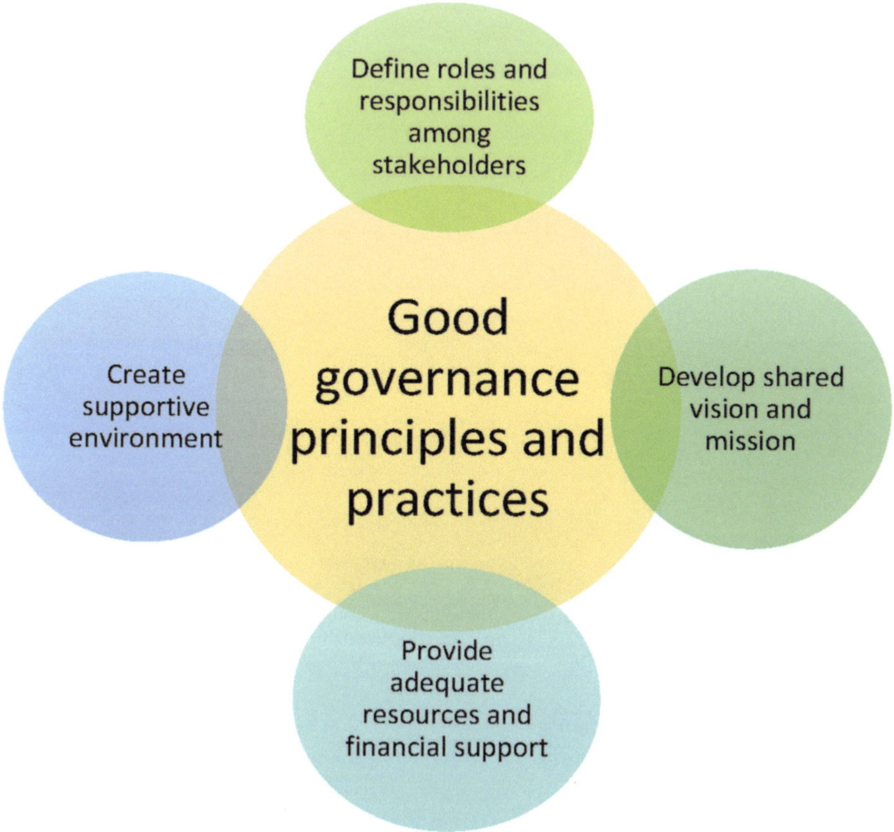
Define roles and responsibilities among stakeholders
Create supportive environment
Good governance principles and practices
Develop shared vision and mission
Provide adequate resources and financial support

Fig. 6.1 Good governance principles and practices

Second, it is essential to develop a shared vision for IPECP that is agreed upon by all stakeholders. This vision should be articulated in a document that outlines the goals and objectives of the initiative and should be reviewed regularly to ensure it remains relevant.

Third, providing adequate resources available for IPECP initiatives is essential. This includes financial and human resources such as faculty, staff, and clinicians. It is also necessary to ensure that resources are allocated equitably and transparently.

Finally, creating an environment of collaboration and cooperation among stakeholders is essential. This involves establishing and maintaining effective communication channels, developing constructive feedback processes, and fostering a culture of respect and collaboration.

A framework for governance should include five key elements: leadership and accountability; clear roles and responsibilities; shared vision and goals; resources and infrastructure; and evaluation and feedback (Fig. 6.2).

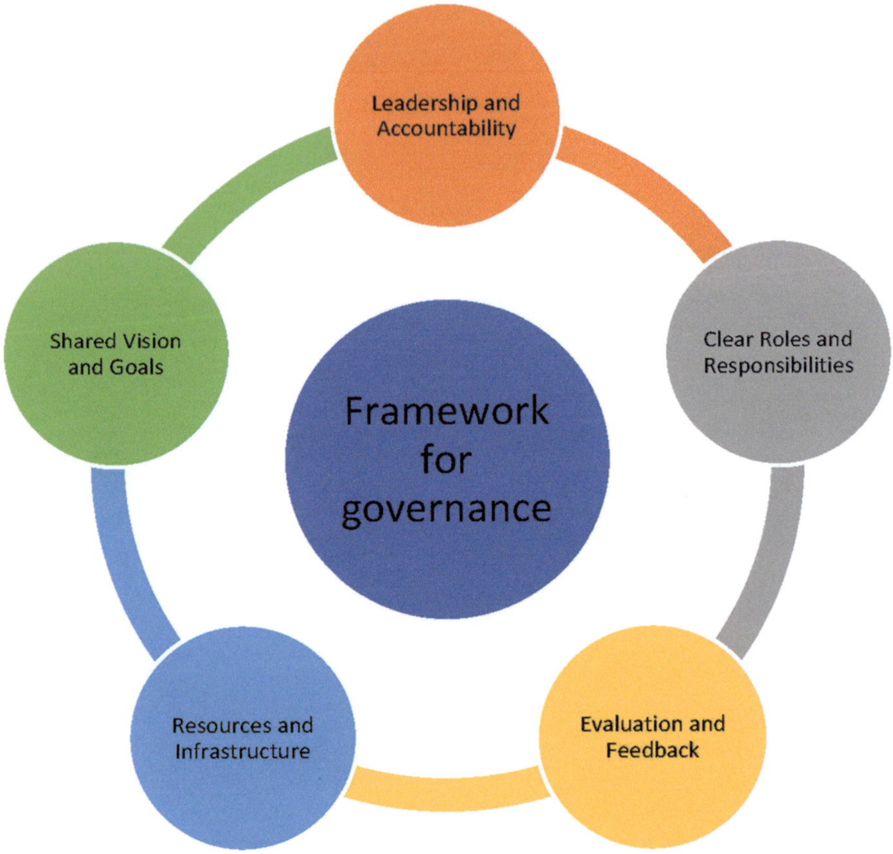

Fig. 6.2 Good governance framework

1. Leadership and Accountability: Leadership is essential for successful IPECP initiatives. Leaders must be accountable for outcomes, define a vision, set goals, and allocate resources. Leaders should be knowledgeable and experienced in IPECP, willing to take risks, make decisions, and set the course for their organization.
2. Clear Roles and Responsibilities: All stakeholders involved in IPECP need to understand their roles and responsibilities to ensure successful outcomes. This includes understanding the scope of practice, the professional boundaries of each profession, and how they overlap in IPECP initiatives.
3. Shared Vision and Goals: All stakeholders should be committed to shared goals. These should be clearly defined, communicated to all stakeholders, and regularly reviewed and updated.
4. Resources and Infrastructure: IPECP initiatives require adequate resources and infrastructure to be successful. This includes human resources, financial

resources, and technology. It is essential to ensure that all stakeholders have access to the resources and infrastructure needed to facilitate IPECP.
5. Evaluation and Feedback: Evaluation and feedback are essential for assessing the impact and effectiveness of IPECP initiatives. This should include quantitative and qualitative measures and involve all stakeholders.

By incorporating these five elements into a governance framework, countries could ensure that IPECP initiatives are successful. Such a framework can help ensure that all stakeholders are held accountable and that resources are allocated appropriately. It can also provide a structure for evaluating the effectiveness of IPECP initiatives and help ensure that they are meeting their goals.

6.3 Governance of IPECP: Saudi Arabia

The Ministry of Education in Saudi Arabia has embarked on an ambitious program of reform to strengthen educational quality, improve efficiency and enhance the relevance of education programs. It is also keen to enhance skills development and the development of human resources which is essential to achieve national objectives. It aims to reduce dependency on expatriate labor which would in turn help the government to achieve its policy objectives. The Ministry of Health (MoH), represented by the primary, secondary, and tertiary care, is actively working to formulate a vision on health services. The perspective of the MoH is aiming to provide healthcare in ways that preserve the dignity of the individual and keep costs low.

Nevertheless, there is no national policy for IPECP in Saudi Arabia at present although the Ministry of Education aimed at encouraging collaboration between education providers which should be key in developing collaborative practice skills. It also aimed at developing competencies in health professionals, and in promoting interagency collaboration across all sectors. The National Centre for Academic Accreditation and Evaluation (NCAAA) was established in Saudi Arabia by the higher education council. The main aim of this establishment was to help acquire quality standards of learning in post-secondary and university programs. Additionally, it was meant to bring confidence to learners, teachers, and parents [22]. For instance, learners could be sure that whatever has been learned in class, any research they conducted, or even the services provided during learning was good interprofessional practice. To ensure these standards are met, NCAAA was responsible for assessing, evaluating, and reviewing the performance of both existing and newly established schools [23]. The accreditation led to positive impacts in the education sector. There were improved learning outcomes in Saudi Arabia, where there was a mandatory issue of course specification before any person could start doing the course. Moreover, accreditation led to program development. Learners felt that medical ethics were more controlled than before and had played a vital role in stimulating a smooth learning curriculum.

The implementation of the policies has so far been relatively weak and there is a general lack of awareness of their existence [24]. Internationally IPECP has become developed in some countries in the Western world because of a growing understanding of organizational change and the influence on education, health, and social welfare systems. The changing nature of professional practice has led to a shift in focus from service provision toward systemic improvement and policy making. Policy makers are now focusing more on relationships between professionals as opposed to their capacity as individuals. The increasing complexity of issues associated with healthcare delivery is also influencing the way policy makers view interprofessional education.

Good governance for interprofessional education and collaborative practice in Saudi Arabia should be guided by a framework that enables the government to ensure quality standards, maximize the impact of interprofessional collaboration, and promote the development of a competent healthcare workforce. This framework should guide the efforts of three main organizations: the Ministry of Education, the Ministry of Health, and the Saudi Commission for Health Specialties to ensure that IPECP initiatives are implemented effectively.

At the Ministry of Education level, the framework should focus on developing a rigorous and comprehensive curriculum for IPE, which should be regularly updated and aligned with the objectives of the Ministry. This curriculum should ensure that students acquire the necessary knowledge, skills, and attitudes to effectively engage in interprofessional collaboration in the healthcare sector. Additionally, the Ministry should create a system of quality assurance and assessment to assess the quality of IPECP initiatives and to ensure that they meet the standards set by the Ministry.

At the Ministry of Health level, the framework should focus on developing mechanisms to ensure that interprofessional collaboration is supported and promoted in the workforce. This should include the development of policies and regulations that facilitate sharing of resources and information between different healthcare professionals and promote collaboration between other healthcare professionals. Additionally, the Ministry should ensure that CP initiatives are implemented with the utmost integrity and that the safety and well-being of healthcare professionals and patients are safeguarded.

Finally, the Saudi Commission for Health Specialties (SCFHS) could bridge the gap between health education and clinical practice. The SCFHS is in charge of supervising and evaluating training programs, as well as establishing controls and standards for health professions practice [25]. The SCFHS could be responsible for regulating IPECP initiatives and ensuring that IPECP initiatives are implemented following the highest standards of quality. The Commission should define the measures that must be met by healthcare professionals involved in IPECP initiatives and ensure that healthcare professionals adhere to these standards. Additionally, the Commission should ensure that IPECP initiatives are appropriately monitored and evaluated to ensure that they are effective and meet the objectives set by the Ministry (Fig. 6.3).

By following this framework, Saudi Arabia can ensure good governance for IPECP initiatives and that these initiatives are implemented following the highest

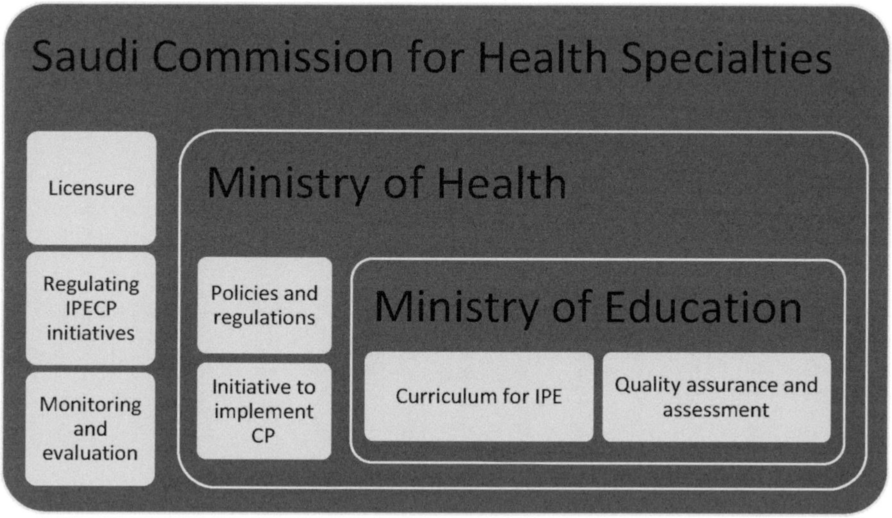

Fig. 6.3 Good governance for IPECP in Saudi Arabia

standards of quality. Additionally, this framework can help to ensure that the healthcare workforce is well-prepared to engage in interprofessional collaboration and that healthcare professionals are working together to provide the best possible care to patients.

6.4 Organizations Supporting Interprofessional Education and Collaborative Practice

In many countries; often due to the lack of centralized governmental structure around medical, nursing, and health professions education; organization and advocacy for Interprofessional Education and Collaborative Practice is coordinated among member organizations that have a mission and vision around IPECP. These groups are organized around differing structures and functions. They are organized at the international, national, and regional levels. Their membership can consist of individuals, academic institutions, healthcare provider organizations, or consortia/networks dedicated to promoting system improvement through interprofessional collaboration. They are also organized by function around: scholarship and research; education and teaching; healthcare delivery; and policy and advocacy. Table 6.1 provides a partial listing of IPECP Organizations.

Table 6.1 IPECP organizations

Organization	Scope/region	Founded	Membership	Website
African Interprofessional Education Network (AfriPEN)	Africa	2015	Individual	https://afripen.org
American Interprofessional Health Collaborative (AIHC)	USA	2009	Individual	www.aihc-us.org
Association of Schools Advancing Health Professions (ASAHP)	USA	1967	Institutional	www.asahp.org
Australasian Interprofessional Practice and Education Network (AIPPEN)	Australia and New Zealand	2010	Individual	https://anzahpe.org/AIPPEN
Canadian Interprofessional Health Collaborative (CIHC)	Canada	2006	Individual	http://www.cihc.ca
Centre for the Advancement of Interprofessional Education (CAIPE)	United Kingdom	1987	Individual and Organizational	http://www.caipe.org.uk
European Interprofessional Practice and Education Network (EIPEN)	Europe	2004	Institutional	http://www.eipen.org
Indian Interprofessional Education Network (IndIPEN)	India		Individual	http://mu.faimerfri.org/indipen
Institute for Healthcare Improvement (IHI)	USA	1991	Individual	www.ihi.org
Interprofessional.Global	Global	2018	Regional Networks	https://interprofessional.global/
Interprofessional Education Collaborative (IPEC)	USA	2010	Organizational	www.ipecollaborative.org
Interprofessional Research.Global	Global	2018	Individual	https://interprofessionalresearch.global/
International Network for Health Workforce Education (INHWE)	Global	2017	Individual	https://inhwe.org/
National Academies of Practice (NAP)	USA	1976	Individual	www.napractice.org
National Academies of Sciences, Engineering and Medicine Global Forum on Innovation in Health Professions Education	USA	1970	Organizational	https://www.nationalacademies.org/our-work/global-forum-on-innovation-in-health-professional-education

Network: Towards Unity for Health (TUFH)	Global	2000	Individual and Organizational	https://tufh.org/
Nordic Interprofessional Network (NIPNET)	Finland, Sweden, Denmark, Norway, and Iceland	2001	Individual and Organizational	www.nipnet.org
Regional Network for Interprofessional Education in the Americas (REIP)	South America, Central America, and Caribbean		Health Ministries	www.educacioninterprofesional.org
Society for Interprofessionalism in Healthcare (IP-Health)	Germany, Austria, and Switzerland	2017	Individual	https://www.ip-health.org
World Health Organization (WHO)	Global	1948	Member Countries	https://www.who.int/

6.5 International Organizations

6.5.1 World Health Organization (WHO)

IPE's formal origins in the World Health Organization (WHO) can be traced to reports from a 1987 Expert Group [26–28] The World Health Organization is "dedicated to the well-being of all people and guided by science, the WHO leads and champions global efforts to give everyone, everywhere an equal chance to live a healthy life." It was established on the 7th of April 1948 by the United Nations. This date is celebrated yearly as World Health Day. The primary headquarters is hosted by the Swiss Federation in Geneva, Switzerland and is home to the WHO's Secretariat and Director-General.

Delegates from all WHO Member States comprise the World Health Assembly and they vote on most priorities and policy decisions. There are also six regional offices and 150 country offices and other offices around the world. This structure is designed to allow the WHO work locally to improve health systems and coordinate response to health threats. Assessed contributions from member countries, calculated as a percentage of GDP, make up less than 20% of the total budget, whereas voluntary contributions, from Member States and other public and private organization covers the rest of the budget, which is monitored by the Independent Expert Oversight Advisory Committee (IEOAC) [29].

Website: https://www.who.int/.

6.5.2 The Network: Towards Unity for Health (TUFH)

The Network, Towards Unity for Health, established in 2000 as an IPE special interest group in the Network for Community-based Medical Education originally began in 1987 as the European Network for the Development of Multiprofessional Education in Health Sciences (EMPE) [26]. TUFH is an international interprofessional community which looks to leverage shared commitment and passion to unite global health leaders towards equity in global health. TUFH combines experience and diversity of thought, with technical/financial resources, so members can push boundaries, learn, share, and innovate on a local, regional, and global scale. TUFH welcomes all institutions and individuals who are passionate around social accountability and global equitable health to join this interprofessional, multicultural, and global community [30].

Website: http://thenetworktufh.org/.

6.5.3 Interprofessional.Global

Interprofessional.Global (IP.Global), the Global Confederation for Interprofessional Education and Collaborative Practice, "facilitates support and exchange between regional interprofessional education and collaborative practice (IPECP) networks, establishes relationships with other like-minded organizations and welcomes and supports new networks sharing the same aims and values" [31] and works with local planning committees to host the All Together Better Health (ATBH) conferences. Preceded by the World Coordinating Committee for Interprofessional Education and Collaborative Practice (WCC), IP.Global was developed at the 2019 ATBH Conference in Auckland, New Zealand and was chartered in the Netherlands in 2021 [26].

Website: https://interprofessional.global/.

6.5.4 International Network for Health Workforce Education (INHWE)

The INHWE is an international interprofessional, and multi-stakeholder network which looks to leverage the expertise of the global health workforce education community to break down silos and address longstanding hierarchies which exist in society and healthcare. There is no cost for membership, and INHWE's Working Groups which are developed around important health workforce education topics focusing on complex, cross cutting issues related to education and training [32].

Website: https://inhwe.org/.

6.5.5 InterprofessionalResearch.Global (IPR.Global)

In 2019, IPR.Global arose from the GRIN2Theory Network, a 2014–2015 collaboration of the from the Global Research Interprofessional Network (GRIN) [33], and In-2-Theory [34], two international IPECP research networks. IPR.Global is a community of practice and scholarship intending to provide leadership and theory-driven, methodologically rigorous IPECP research, as well as advocating for evidence-informed policies and practices to support better health, better care, better cost, and better work experience [35].

Website: https://interprofessionalresearch.global/.

6.6 National-Level Organizations

6.6.1 Centre for the Advancement of Interprofessional Education (CAIPE)

CAIPE was established as a UK-based charity in 1987. It seeks to "promote health and wellbeing and to improve the health and social care of the public by advancing IPE." Members of CAIPE are committed to working collaboratively across health and social care. CAIPE works nationally and globally to promote and develop interprofessional education, learning, research, and practice as well as providing a network for information exchange and discussion through meetings and workshops as well as their official publication, the Journal of Interprofessional Care [26, 36].

Website: https://www.caipe.org/.

6.6.2 Canadian Interprofessional Health Collaborative (CIHC)

IPE was first promoted in Canada in the 1960s but formally developed through the Romanow Commission's call from improved care through new models of training. In 2002, Health Canada, founded *Inter-professional Education for Collaborative Patient Centred Practice* (IECPCPC) [26]. CIHC was established in 2006 and funded by Health Canada with the University of British Columbia and eventually, in 2012, the CIHC became not-for-profit corporation. CIHC has successfully established national interprofessional core competencies and led the development of standards through the Accreditation of Interprofessional Health Education (AIPHE) organization [26, 37]. The CIHC seeks to be a "strong, cohesive voice to amplify and influence a national and global conversation that interprofessional collaborative practices are an essential element of health leadership, workforce strength and resilience, good health outcomes and fiscal accountability" by forming a robust network of partners, leaders, and collaborators [38].

Website: http://www.cihc-cpis.com/.

6.6.3 Indian Interprofessional Education Network (IndIPEN)

IndIPEN looks to provide "national leadership in India moving all health providers, teams and organizations towards improved interprofessional collaboration in health professions education and healthcare practice." IndIPEN's looks to create awareness and significance in the Indian context; stimulate networking of IPECP across stakeholders, share promising IPECP practices in the region; advance interprofessional collaboration in healthcare; and advance IPECP research [39].

6.6.4 American Interprofessional Health Collaborative (AIHC)

AIHC was founded with the mission to "transcend boundaries to transform learning, policies, practices, and scholarship toward an improved system of health and wellness for individual patients, communities, and populations." It co-hosts to the biannual Collaborating Across Borders conference with CIHC. In 2012, with the support of private and public grant funding, the University of Minnesota developed the National Center for Interprofessional Practice and Education. The National Center promotes the concept of the "Nexus" to link IPE to the transformation of the US healthcare delivery system by realigning higher education and healthcare [26]. The American Interprofessional Health Collaborative (AIHC) serves as the professional community of the National Center for Interprofessional Practice and

Education. Through its committees and working groups AIHC members work at all levels to impact policy, develop resources, and share best practices and break down barriers. AIHC and the National Center collaborate to conduct research, mentor, and support colleagues [40]. The National Center has also helped develop initiatives in the USA around interprofessional clinical learning and accreditation [41, 42].

Website: https://aihc-us.org/.

6.6.5 Association of Schools Advancing Health Professions (ASAHP)

Chartered in Washington, D.C. through the Allied Health Professions Personnel Training Act of 1967, ASAHP is a not-for-profit national professional association for administrators, educators, and other stakeholders which was established to respond to a need for an "interdisciplinary and interagency association to relate to improving the quality and quantity of needed workforce in the health occupations and professions." In 2019, the membership voted to change the name of the Association of Schools of Allied Health Professions to the Association of Schools Advancing Health Professions. ASAHP's mission is "to advance health professions education and discovery through interprofessional collaboration, leadership, excellence, and innovation." It is the host organization for the Journal of Allied Health [43].

Website: https://www.asahp.org/.

6.6.6 Institute for Healthcare Improvement (IHI)

The IHI, founded in 1991, is an independent not-for-profit organization dedicated to safety and quality improvements in healthcare [26]. IHI's vision is that "Everyone has the best care and health possible" and their mission is to improve health and healthcare worldwide. The IHI Open School is a library of self-paced online courses for health professionals from around the world, free to students, residents, faculty, and inhabitants of the Least Developed Countries, providing essential training and skills across disciplines in quality improvement, patient safety, leadership, and other topics [44].

Website: https://www.ihi.org/.

6.6.7 Interprofessional Education Collaborative (IPEC)

IPEC was founded in 2009 as a collaborative to "promote and encourage constituent efforts that would advance substantive interprofessional learning experiences to help prepare future health professionals for enhanced team-based care of patients and improved population health outcomes." IPEC's original focus was to create core competencies informing curriculum development for interprofessional collaborative practice in the professions of medicine, nursing, pharmacy, dentistry, and public health, which resulted in its 2011 report. That report was updated in 2016 and a 2023 IPEC Core Competencies revision is now in development. In 2022, IPEC represented 21 national health professions associations whose members deliver health professions educational programs awarding academic degrees which prepare professionals to provide direct care in patient-centered, community- and population-oriented, interprofessional, collaborative practice [45].

Website: https://www.ipecollaborative.org/.

6.6.8 National Academies of Practice (NAP)

NAP was founded in 1981 to advise legislators and government organizations on health and healthcare. In 14 profession-specific academies, Distinguished Practitioners, Scholars and Policy Fellows; along with professional members are nominated by their peers to join this interprofessional group of health practitioners and scholars who are dedicated to supporting "affordable, accessible, coordinated quality healthcare for all." NAP believes that interprofessional collaboration provides a key foundation and in healthcare and preventive care which addresses the whole person. NAP looks to impact the healthcare system by educating/informing health professionals and other stakeholders; facilitating collaborative scholarship; and advocating for interprofessional collaboration in practice and policy. It is the host organization for the Journal of Interprofessional Education and Practice [46].

Website: https://www.napractice.org/.

6.6.9 National Academies of Sciences, Engineering, and Medicine (NASEM)

The National Academies of Sciences, Engineering, and Medicine was originally founded as the National Academies of Sciences in 1863 providing independent advice to inform evidence-based policy, spark innovation, and address key issues to benefit society. The Global Forum on Innovation in Health Professional Education (IHPE Forum) is composed of academic experts and health professionals from 37 member-sponsors from developed and developing countries representing 17 disciplines to host workshops "to network, discuss and illuminate issues for the benefit and promotion of health professional education." Each of these workshops are accompanied by reports of proceedings which include recommendations for policy and practice [47].

Website: https://www.nationalacademies.org/our-work/global-forum-on-innovation-in-health-professional-education.

6.7 Consortia/Regional Networks

6.7.1 European Interprofessional Practice and Education Network (EIPEN)

EIPEN was originally funded by the European Commission's Erasmus program and is now not-for-profit organization with corporate and individual members throughout Europe [26]. EIPEN's aim is to "stimulate and share effective interprofessional training in European higher education, and to improve collaborative practice in health and social care in Europe, to help optimize the quality of care and the quality of life of patients." EIPEN seeks to influence EU and its member states around educational and healthcare policy. They have developed a framework of key competences for interprofessional collaboration and look to: (1) produce tools and publications that underpin interprofessional practice and education; (2) organize biennial conferences, seminars and expert meetings; and (3) support collaborative projects of members [48].

Website: https://www.eipen.eu/.

6.7.2 Regional Network for Interprofessional Education in the Americas (REIP)

REIP is comprised of a large network of organizations characterized by a "strategy of articulation and technical cooperation between educational institutions, professional organizations and Ministries of Health and Ministries of Education, with the objective of promoting interprofessional education and collaborative practice in healthcare in the Region of the Americas." REIP objectives include: proposing policy change around IPE and Universal Health; sharing and disseminating IPE experience and evidence to inform policy, teaching and research; identifying common interests and priorities around IPE to generate shared options for transformation; and promoting intersectoral and multicenter coordination and research in order to improve people's access to health [49].

Website: www.educacioninterprofesional.org.

6.7.3 African Interprofessional Education Network (AFRIPEN)

AfrIPEN was established in 2015 as a consensus-based partnership bringing together individuals, organizations, ministries, and regulatory bodies with the vision to establish interprofessional education and collaborative practice (IPECP) in healthcare workforce and system development in the Africa region. The mission of AfrIPEN is to "advocate for, collaborate on, promote and share good practice of IPECP in the Africa region." [50]. The organization has grown rapidly and currently includes membership across various institutions and countries in the continent and abroad [51].

Website: https://afripen.org/.

6.7.4 Australasian Interprofessional Practice and Education Network (AIPPEN)

IPE began to emerge in Australia in the 1970s in Sydney and Adelaide with some initial government funding. Other initiatives began to take hold in the 1990s and later grew with a focus on rural care with some influence from the UK [26]. Established in 2006, AIPPEN was founded as an Australasian interprofessional practice and education hub for health professionals recognizing the need for an effective interprofessional approach to promote collaboration and teamwork for safe and effective patient care. In 2019, AIPPEN transitioned to a "community of practice for individuals, groups, institutions and organizations across Australia and New Zealand who are committed to researching, delivering, promoting, supporting and researching interprofessional learning, through interprofessional education and practice." [52].

Website: www.anzahpe.org/aippen.

6.7.5 Nordic Interprofessional Network of Europe (NIPNET)

NIPNET was launched at a conference in Aalesund, Norway in 2001 as a network of from educators, practitioners, leaders, managers, and researchers in the areas of healthcare and social services in the Nordic Countries of Denmark, Finland, Iceland, Norway, and Sweden looking to promote the interprofessional learning and collaborative practice [53]. NIPNET is committed to "interprofessional collaboration as a working model in healthcare and health and social services, with the intention to improve quality of care, welfare services and health outcomes; and interprofessional education as learning models to develop interprofessional collaborative competences among health and social care services." [54].

Website: www.nipnet.org.

6.7.6 Society for Interprofessionalism in Healthcare (IP-Health)

IP-Health, established in Berlin in 2017, is an IPECP network of European Countries with the purpose of promoting interprofessionalism in the healthcare at the national and international level by providing information and participating in scientific congresses which promote "holistic, patient-centered cooperation between all healthcare professionals"; and development of programs and projects promoting interprofessional cooperation in science and practice [55].

Website: www.ip-health.org.

6.8 IPECP Organizations in the United States

Interprofessional Education and Collaborative Practice organizations, much like the healthcare system, in the USA are fragmented with multiple organizations with similar missions to promote improved health outcomes through teamwork and collaboration. These organizations (Fig. 6.4) are composed of dedicated individuals with established expertise; however, these groups sometimes act in isolation without a full appreciation of their respective potential synergies.

The primary differences between these organizations are based on their membership structure. Several organizations, IPEC, NASEM Global Forum, and ASAHP, are comprised of other professional organizations/academic institutions. An advantage of this type of membership structure is that they have access to a large group of participants and potential revenue streams. NAP, IHI, and AIHC are largely individual memberships. The structure of the membership differs between these organizations: NAP has honorific roots with most of the members nominated as Fellows into profession-based academies, IHI is dedicated to healthcare system improvement and has different levels of members who are primarily researchers or providers, and AIHC members are primarily academic faculty, administrators, and researchers. Professional identities are retained in several of the organizations (NASEM, IPEC, and NAP) and the others are composed of an intentional interprofessional mix (ASAHP, AIHC, and IHI).

Several groups also have a strong focus on advocacy/policy change. NASEM, ASAHP, NAP, and IHI were all chartered as advisory organizations with the goal of informing policy development. Several have an impact on IPE and health professions education, whether it be through supporting academic institutions (ASAHP),

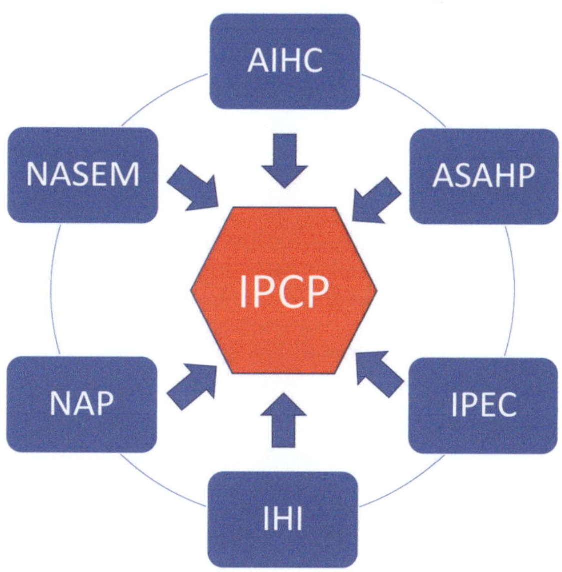

Fig. 6.4 IPECP organizations in the United States

core competency frameworks and faculty development (IPEC), or education and research using their collective expertise (AIHC). Additionally, many of these groups have peer-reviewed vehicles to disseminate information to the public and scholarly community: NASEM Proceedings Reports, Journal of Interprofessional Education and Practice (NAP), Journal of Allied Health (ASAHP), IHI Open School, MedEd Portal and Core Competencies (IPEC) and resources/programming from the National Center for Interprofessional Practice and Education (AIHC).

IPECP organizations in the USA have the mission, structure, and collective expertise to make an appreciable impact. However, due to separate and sometimes competing activities their influence may not be fully realized. It is hoped that these groups can learn about, from and with each other to collaborate in a union of forces that could benefit the system and society moving forward.

6.9 Conclusion

In summary, the development of IPECP has been slow and steady over the past few decades. In Saudi Arabia, the concept is just beginning to take off and there is a need for consistency and support which will encourage cooperation, collaboration, and partnership in the healthcare sector. Governmental organizations and agencies need to create an environment that will be conducive for IPECP to flourish, considering that these bodies are instrumental in expanding partnerships with other stakeholders. For IPECP to be effective it should be institutionalized. This means linking it to other related policies and emphasizing collaboration as well as interagency cooperation. Non-governmental organizations also have an impact by providing resources, programming, and scholarship essential to inform, promote, and advocate for IPECP to the public and policy makers across the world. The role of all parties involved should also be clearly defined through proper work sharing arrangements. Effective leadership helps foster stronger interprofessional relationships while creating a common vision helps to achieve goals.

References

1. World Health Organization. Framework for action on interprofessional education and collaborative practice. Geneva: WHO; 2010.
2. Marshall C, Van Der Volgen J, Lombardo N, Hamasu C, Cardell E, Blumenthal DK. A mixed methods approach to assess the impact of an interprofessional education medical error simulation. Am J Pharm Educ. 2020;84(2):7133.
3. Hammick M, Freeth D, Koppel I, Reeves S, Barr H. A best evidence systematic review of interprofessional education: BEME Guide no. 9. Med Teach. 2007;29(8):735–51.
4. Reeves S, Fletcher S, Barr H, Birch I, Boet S, Davies N, et al. A BEME systematic review of the effects of interprofessional education: BEME Guide No. 39. Med Teach. 2016;38(7):656–68.
5. Mahr KA. Analysis of perceptions of interprofessional education. Chicago, IL: Rosalind Franklin University of Medicine and Science; 2020.
6. Guck TP, Walters RW, Abdul-Greene C, Doll J, Greene MA, McGaha AL. Sustainable and replicable clinical and financial outcomes in an interprofessional education and collaborative practice nexus. J Interprof Care. 2021:1–8.

7. Silverman HJ, Kheirbek RE, Moscou-Jackson G, Day J. Moral distress in nurses caring for patients with Covid-19. Nurs Ethics. 2021;28(7–8):1137–64.
8. Singh J, Matthees B. Facilitating interprofessional education in an online environment during the COVID-19 pandemic: a mixed method study. Healthcare. 2021;9(5):567.
9. Spaulding EM, Marvel FA, Jacob E, Rahman A, Hansen BR, Hanyok LA, et al. Interprofessional education and collaboration among healthcare students and professionals: a systematic review and call for action. J Interprof Care. 2021;35(4):612–21.
10. Institute of Medicine. Measuring the impact of interprofessional education on collaborative practice and patient outcomes. Washington, DC: The National Academies Press; 2015.
11. Morano C, Damiani G. Interprofessional education at the meso level: taking the next step in IPE. Gerontol Geriatr Educ. 2019;40(1):43–54.
12. Aerts N, Anthierens S, Van Bogaert P, Peremans L, Bastiaens H. Prevention of cardiovascular diseases in community settings and primary health care: a pre-implementation contextual analysis using the consolidated framework for implementation research. Int J Environ Res Public Health. 2022;19(14):8467.
13. Governance for Sustainable Human Development. An integrated paper on the highlights of four regional consultation workshops on governance for sustainable human development. United Nations Development Programme. Makati City: United Nations; 1997.
14. Reddy S, Allan S, Coghlan S, Cooper P. A governance model for the application of AI in health care. J Am Med Inform Assoc. 2019;27(3):491–7.
15. John K, Litov L, Yeung B. Corporate governance and risk-taking. J Financ. 2008;63(4):1679–728.
16. Bollen A, Harrison R, Aslani P, van Haastregt JCM. Factors influencing interprofessional collaboration between community pharmacists and general practitioners-a systematic review. Health Soc Care Commun. 2019;27(4):e189–212.
17. Lee JK, Hume AL, Willis R, Boon H, Lebensohn P, Brooks A, et al. Pharmacy competencies for interprofessional integrative health care education. Am J Pharm Educ. 2018;82(6):6302.
18. Wei H, Watson J. Healthcare interprofessional team members' perspectives on human caring: a directed content analysis study. Int J Nurs Sci. 2019;6(1):17–23.
19. Khanbodaghi A, Natto ZS, Forero M, Loo CY. Effectiveness of interprofessional oral health program for pediatric nurse practitioner students at Northeastern University, United States. BMC Oral Health. 2019;19(1):170.
20. Lackie K, Najjar G, El-Awaisi A, Frost J, Green C, Langlois S, et al. Interprofessional education and collaborative practice research during the COVID-19 pandemic: considerations to advance the field. J Interprof Care. 2020;34(5):583–6.
21. Valachovic RW. Integrating oral and overall health care: building a foundation for interprofessional education and collaborative practice. J Dent Educ. 2019;83(2 Suppl):S19–22.
22. Ghadah A. Do the Standards of the National Commission for Academic Accreditation & Assessment (NCAAA) lead to organization excellence. Eur Sci J. 2016;12(34):103.
23. Bougherira MR, Elasmar MH. Impact of academic accreditation on teaching and learning: faculty members' perceptions. J Furth High Educ. 2022;47:167–81.
24. Bashatah AS, Al-Ahmary KA, Arifi MA, Asiri YA, AlRuthia Y, Metwally AS, et al. Interprofessional cooperation: an interventional study among Saudi healthcare teaching staff at King Saud University. J Multidiscip Healthc. 2020;13:1537–44.
25. Specialties SCFH. Wellbeing policy. Saudi Commission For Health Specialties, Riyadh; 2022. https://scfhs.org.sa/sites/default/files/2022-06/Saudi%20Commission%20For%20Health%20Specialties%20Wellbeing%20Policy%20June%202022_0.pdf.
26. Barr H. Interprofessional education: the genesis of a global movement. Farham: CAIPE; 2015.
27. Kantrowitz M, Kaufman A, Mennin S, Fülöp T, Guilbert J-J, et al. Innovative tracks at established institutions for the education of health personnel: an experimental approach to change relevant to health needs. Geneva: World Health Organization; 1987.
28. World Health Organization. Learning together to work together for health: report of a WHO Study Group on Multiprofessional Education of Health Personnel: the team approach. Geneva: World Health Organization; 1988.

29. World Health Organization. About. Geneva: WHO; 2022. https://www.who.int/about.
30. The Network Towards Unity for Health. 2022. http://thenetworktufh.org/.
31. Interprofessional Global. The confederation. 2022. https://interprofessional.global/confederation/.
32. International Network for Health Workforce Education. Our story. 2022. https://inhwe.org/about-us.
33. Thistlethwaite J. Introducing the Global Research Interprofessional Network (GRIN). J Interprof Care. 2013;27(2):107–9.
34. Hean S, Anderson E, Bainbridge L, Clark PG, Craddock D, Doucet S, et al. IN-2-THEORY--Interprofessional theory, scholarship and collaboration: a community of practice. J Interprof Care. 2013;27(1):88–90.
35. InterprofessionalResearch.Global. Our background. 2022. https://interprofessionalresearch.global/background/.
36. Centre for the Advancement of Interprofessional Education. About CAIPE. 2022. https://www.caipe.org/about.
37. Canadian Interprofessional Health Collaborative. A National Interprofessional Competency Framework. Vancouver, BC. 2010.
38. Interprofessional.Global. Canadian Interprofessional Health Collaborative, 2022. https://interprofessional.global/canada/.
39. Interprofessional.Global. Indian Interprofessional Education Network. 2022. https://interprofessional.global/india/.
40. American Interprofessional Health Collaborative. What is AIHC? 2022. https://aihc-us.org/about-us/what-is-aihc.
41. Brandt BF, Kitto S, Cervero RM. Untying the interprofessional gordian knot: the national collaborative for improving the clinical learning environment. Acad Med. 2018;93(10):1437–40.
42. Health Professions Accreditors Collaborative. Guidance on developing quality interprofessional education for the health professions. Chicago, IL: Health Professions Accreditors Collaborative; 2019.
43. Association of Schools Advancing Health Professions. About ASAHP. 2022. https://www.asahp.org/about-asahp.
44. Institute for Healthcare Improvement. History. 2022. https://www.ihi.org/about/pages/history.aspx.
45. Interprofessional Education Collaborative (IPEC). About Us. 2022. https://www.ipecollaborative.org/about-us.
46. National Academies of Practice. Who We Are. 2022. https://www.napractice.org/.
47. National Academies of Sciences Engineering and Medicine. Global forum on innovation in health professional education. 2022. https://www.nationalacademies.org/our-work/global-forum-on-innovation-in-health-professional-education.
48. European Interprofessional Practice and Education Network. EIPEN. 2022. https://www.eipen.eu/.
49. Interprofessional.Global. Regional network for interprofessional education in the Americas. 2022. https://interprofessional.global/south-central-america-caribbean/.
50. African Interprofessional Education Network. What is AFRIPEN? 2022. https://afripen.org/what-is-afripen/.
51. Interprofessional.Global. African Interprofessional Education Network. 2022. https://interprofessional.global/africa/.
52. Interprofessional.Global. Australasian Interprofessional Practice and Education network. 2022. https://interprofessional.global/australasia/.
53. Nordic Interprofessional Network of Europe. About NIPNET. 2022. https://nipnet.org/about/.
54. Interprofessional.Global. Nordic Interprofessional Network of Europe. 2022. https://interprofessional.global/scandinavia/.
55. Interprofessional.Global. Society for Interprofessionalism in Healthcare. 2022. https://interprofessional.global/german-speaking-countries/.

Impact of Interprofessional Education and Collaborative Practice on Healthcare Outcomes: Evidence and Implications

7

Osama Alshogran and Mohammed Almansour

Abbreviations

EM	Emergency medicine
HbA1c	Hemoglobin A1c
HCPs	Health care providers
IPCP	Interprofessional collaborative practice
IPE	Interprofessional education
IPECP	Interprofessional education and collaborative practice
LOS	Length of stay
PCP	Primary care provider
QOL	Quality of life
RCT	Randomized controlled trial
RR	Relative risk
SDH	Social determinants of health
SMD	Standardized mean difference
VBP	Value-based practice

O. Alshogran (✉)
Department of Clinical Pharmacy, Faculty of Pharmacy, Jordan University of Science and Technology, Irbid, Jordan

M. Almansour
Department of Medical Education, College of Medicine, King Saud University, Riyadh, Saudi Arabia

M. Y. Alnaami et al. (eds.), *Novel Health Interprofessional Education and Collaborative Practice Program: Strategy and Implementation*,
https://doi.org/10.1007/978-981-99-3420-1_7

7.1 Introduction

The advances in healthcare systems and the notable complexity of disease conditions emphasize the importance of cooperation between healthcare professionals to practice within the spirit of teamwork as a manner to accomplish optimal patient care. Preparation of future healthcare workers to practice in a collaborative workplace requires understanding of the concept of interprofessional education and collaborative practice (IPECP). This approach involves multiple health professions (two or more) working together to learn with, from and about each other, and has been evolving over time. The model represents an attractive procedure of healthcare services delivery that might alleviate healthcare burden. National and international efforts driven by health academics, social and health care professionals, and policy makers are rising to disseminate the understanding and adopting the conception of IPECP as a central component of patient care. The aims of implementing IPECP can be summarized as improving the learners' knowledge, skills, and attitudes toward collaborative practice, preparing health professions students to work collaboratively in the workforce environment, promoting healthcare professionals' behaviors to better care delivery, encouraging organizational changes to adopt collaborative care, and to ultimately improving health outcomes [1].

Diverse activities have been reported in the literature highlighting the importance of IPECP with variations in the content, setting, the mode of delivery, targeted health professionals or students, duration, and measured outcomes [2]. Examples of activities included in the IPECP programs were based on classroom discussions and debates, workshops, group activities, team discussions of patients' scenarios, online modules, simulations and role play, learning in clinics, professionals co-location, and patient group visits [2, 3]. Most of the conducted studies, however, were focused on team approaches comprising healthcare professionals (HCP) with very limited number involving health professions students. Outcomes measured in these investigations can be broadly categorized under the aspects of clinical parameters (i.e., glycemic control, blood pressure, and cholesterol level), humanistic (patient-reported outcomes such as quality of life (QOL), patient satisfaction, disease knowledge, perception toward the provided care, and self-management), and economic measures (i.e., healthcare cost and utilization) [4]. Other features such as learners (professionals or students) perceptions and attitudes toward IPECP and implementing behavioral or organizational changes because of IPECP interventions were also explored as outcomes [5]. Figure 7.1 depicts the various outcomes that have been assessed within the context of IPECP at the individual and organizational levels.

Giving the expansion and the sustainable growth in the evidence pertained to IPECP empirical testing and implementation, it is critical to synthesize the current knowledge of the effectiveness of IPECP and its anticipated benefits in improving the health and well-being of patients. We searched the major databases such as MEDLINE, Ovid, EMBASE, PsycINFO, Web of Science, Google Scholar, and ERIC for the relevant literature related to IPECP implementation and outcomes. This chapter displays the evidence of the impact of IPECP on health outcomes, healthcare costs, learners' behaviors and perceptions toward collaborative practice,

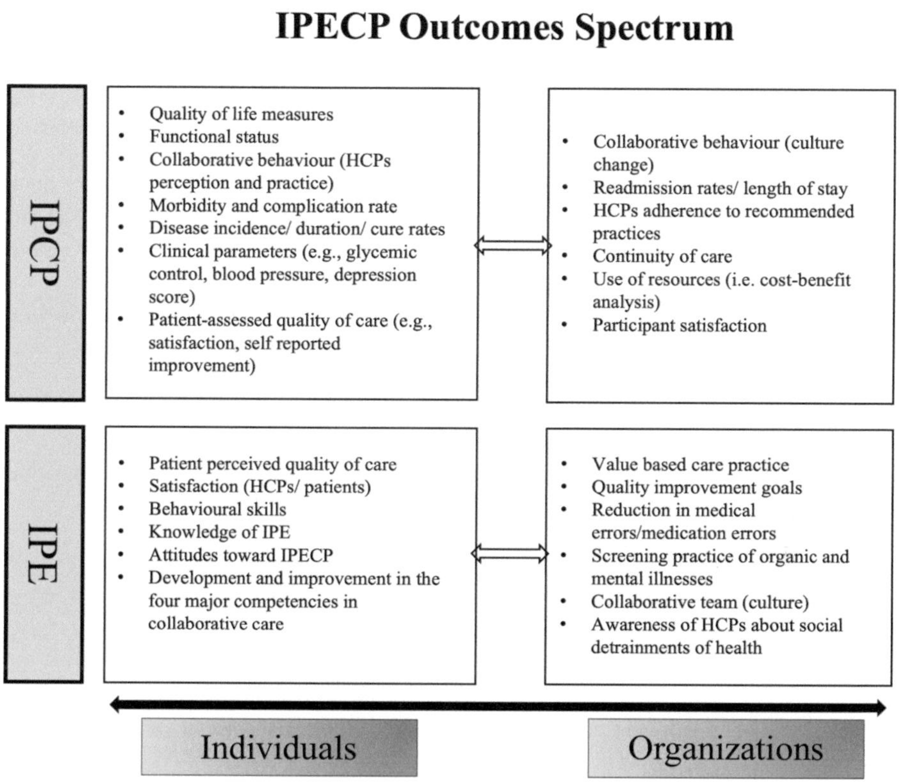

Fig. 7.1 Examples of interprofessional education and collaborative practice (IPECP) health outcomes distributions over individual and organizational levels (horizontal). The figure illustrates the overlap and intersectional reporting of outcomes between Interprofessional Collaborative Practice (IPCP) and Interprofessional Education (IPE). Also, it shows reporting outcomes that are used interchangeably at individual (patients and healthcare providers (HCPs)) and organizational aspects (healthcare institutes)

and healthcare system approaches. As the outcomes reported in the literature were heterogenous, authors attempted the best to present the outcomes based on either interprofessional collaborative practice (IPCP) or interprofessional education (IPE) related interventions.

7.2 Impact of Interprofessional Collaborative Practice (IPCP) on Health Outcomes

The foundational element of IPCP is to work within a team that has shared goals and values, clear roles and responsibilities, and effective communication. The collaboration of healthcare professions of various backgrounds with patients, families, and caregivers is extremely important in achieving optimized healthcare. This is considered a transition from the conventional physician-centered care model. The targeted goal of the implementation of IPCP is to improve the clinical outcomes through the development of multidisciplinary care plan that is directed to provide an optimized, comprehensive, and patient-centered care. A rising body of the literature has been directed toward assessing the impact of integrating IPCP in improving patients' outcomes.

Diabetes mellitus and hypertension are examples of chronic diseases that have been frequently explored in the context of IPCP. This could be related partially to the high disease prevalence worldwide, severe complications, disease burden, increased acute care demands, and the need for an interprofessional healthcare team to control the disease and the associated complications [6]. This team may include physicians (primary care providers (PCPs)), nurses, pharmacists, sociologists, diabetes educators, psychologists, physical trainers, and dietitians among others.

The literature is relatively rich with data on integrating collaborative practice within healthcare workforce and the influence on health outcomes as illustrated in previous review articles [4, 6–10]. Table 7.1 provides examples of such reviews that described the impact of IPCP on health outcomes. Studies included in these reviews were based on a collaborative practice of two care providers or more such as PCPs, nurses, pharmacists, nutritionists/dietitians, psychologists, social workers, and health educators. Various study designs were analyzed including primarily randomized controlled trials (RCTs), case control studies, retrospective/prospective cohorts, and pre/post interventional studies. The results of the individual studies revealed conflicting and limited quantitative evidence related to the impact of IPCP on health outcomes, as some investigations found improvement in clinical and humanistic outcomes [(i.e., hemoglobin A1c (HbA1c), blood pressure, satisfaction, QOL] among patients exposed to team practice, while others demonstrated comparable outcomes to patients exposed to usual care.

To fill some of the gaps in previously mentioned review articles, such as the limited number of professions included, and to incorporate recent clinical trials up to March 2020, a recent systematic review and meta-analysis has been performed to extend our understanding of the effect of IPCP model on health outcomes among patients with uncontrolled diabetes and/or hypertension [2]. The meta-analysis included 39 studies (15 RCTs, 8 cohort, and 16 pre/post interventional studies). The major outcome measures were changes in HbA1c and blood pressure levels. Healthcare team members ranged between 3 and 10 and included part of the following disciplines (physician, pharmacist, behavioral health specialist, diabetes educator, diabetes nurse, diabetes health ambassador, dietitian, nurse high-risk case manager; outreach nurse, patient navigator, program manager, and quality assurance manager). The analysis established that the implementation of interprofessional practice was associated with significant improvements in glycemic control (highest effect for patients with HbA1c ≥9%, standardized mean difference (SMD) = −0.60; 95% CI: −0.80 to −0.40; $p < 0.001$), systolic (SMD = −0.31; 95% CI: −0.46 to −0.17; $p < 0.001$), and diastolic (SMD = −0.28; 95% CI: −0.42 to −0.14; $p < 0.001$) blood pressure readings [2].

The most recent multicenter RCT of IPCP examined the effectiveness of collaborative care provided by a team of physicians, nurses, dietitians, and clinical

Table 7.1 Examples of systematic reviews and meta-analyses of the impact of interprofessional collaborative practice (IPCP) on health outcomes

Author, Year	Patient population	No of studies	Studies design	Primary professions	Examples of interventions	Primary measures	Findings of intervention	Studies duration	Data up to	Countries	Sample size
Atlantis et al. 2014 [6] PMID: 24727428	Comorbid diabetes and depression	7	RCTs	Physician, nurse manager, nurse psychologist case manager	Integrated and collaborative care, supervised case manager, and patient education	Depression scores, HbA1c	Improved depression score and glycemic control	12–52 weeks	Aug-2013	US: 6, Australia: 1	58–417
Reeves et al. 2016 [1] PMID: 28639262	Stroke, COPD, general surgery, other acute care patients	9	RCTs	Any type of health and social care professionals	Team action, interdisciplinary rounds, meetings, management checklists, action plans, team conferencing, professional training	Patient functional status, clinical process or efficiency outcomes or secondary outcomes (collaborative behavior)	• Slight improvement in functional status of stroke patients • Slightly improved HCP adherence to practice recommendations • Slight improvement in the use of healthcare resources	48 weeks	Nov-2015	US: 4, Australia: 2, UK: 1, Belgium: 1, Sweden: 1	29–1854

(continued)

Table 7.1 (continued)

Author, Year	Patient population	No of studies	Studies design	Primary professions	Examples of interventions	Primary measures	Findings of intervention	Studies duration	Data up to	Countries	Sample size
Levengood et al. 2019 [7] PMID: 31227069	Diabetes	35	RCTs	PCPs, nurse, pharmacists	Medication management, education, counseling, development of action plan, patients follow-up and monitoring	HbA1c, BP, lipids, QOL, healthcare use, hospitalization	• Improved glycemic control, blood pressure and lipids level • Increased proportion of patients achieving management targets • Slight improvement in patients satisfaction with care • Slight improvement in medication adherence • Improved QOL and general health. • Less hospital and ED admissions	12 to ≥48 weeks	Oct-2015	US: 25, Canada: 3, UK: 2, Hong Kong, Switzerland, Taiwan, The Netherlands, United Arab Emirates: 1 of each	

Lutfiyya et al. 2019 [8] PMID: 31242239	Primary or hospital care (diabetes, hypertension, asthma, pancreatitis, hyperlipidemia,	20	Clinical trials: 2, pre/post intervention: 10, retrospective cohort: 2, prospective cohort: 1, cross-sectional: 2, sequential-methods, case, or case-control study: 1 each	Physicians, pharmacists and nurses	Patient education, group communication, medication management	Biometrics (HbA1c, BP, etc.), care cost, adherence, healthcare utilization, hospital admission, patient satisfaction	• Improved biometric measures (HbA1c, BP, BMI) • Decreased hospitalizations and ED visits • Improved adherence • Cost savings • Increased in annual outpatients' visits • No effect on patients satisfaction	-	2018	US	2–322,408
Siaw and Lee 2019 [4] PMID: 30369012	Diabetes	16	RCTs	Physicians, pharmacists, diabetes nurse educators, nurses, dietitians, nutritionists, community health workers, peer leaders, health coaches, and health educators	Medication review and optimization, education, counseling, monitoring	Clinical (HbA1c, SBP, lipids), humanistic (patient-reported measures), and economic (healthcare costs and utilization)	• Improved HbA1c and BP • Improved or maintained humanistic • Comparable healthcare costs	12–48 weeks	Jun-2017	US: 6, Brazil: 2, Australia, Canada, Taiwan, Jordan, France, Cyprus, Malaysia, Singapore: 1 of each	48–527

(continued)

Table 7.1 (continued)

Author, Year	Patient population	No of studies	Studies design	Primary professions	Examples of interventions	Primary measures	Findings of intervention	Studies duration	Data up to	Countries	Sample size
McCutcheon et al. 2020 [9]	Primary care setting	51	RCTs: 37, cohort: 14	Physicians, nurses, occupational and physical therapist, mental health professionals, dietitian/nutritionists, pharmacists, and social workers	Medication management, patient education and counseling, disease management, patient care plan, health promotion	Clinical (HbA1c, SBP, lipids), humanistic (patient-reported measures), and economic (healthcare costs and utilizations)	• 27 studies reported positive outcomes, 27 reported no difference, and 1 reported negative impact on mortality • 15 studies reported positive impact on humanistic outcomes • Little or no difference in healthcare cost	6–240 weeks	2013	US: 21, Canada: 7, others: 23	
Lee et al. 2021 [2] PMID: 33576817	Diabetes and hypertension	50 (39 in meta-analysis)	RCTs: 15, prospective cohort: 7, retrospective cohort: 1, pre-post: 16	At least three different health professions including PCPs, and professionals from nutrition, nursing, and pharmacy	Educational sessions, group visits, colocation, face-to-face communication	HbA1c, SBP, and DBP levels	Improved HbA1c, SBP, DBP	12–96 weeks	2018	US: 18, Brazil: 4, Canada: 4, ambulatory care clinic/center/office: 9, community health centers: 8	40–20,524

Wang et al. 2022 [11]	Comorbid diabetes and depression	12	RCTs	PCP with at least one other professional (nurse, pharmacist, psychologist)	Structured medication management, patients follow-up, interprofessional communication	Depression scores, HbA1c, QOL	• Improved depression response, medication adherence, and QOL	12–96 weeks	Oct-20	US: 10, Canada: 1, India: 1	58–417
PMID: 36117873							• No effect on HbA1c				

BMI body mass index, *BP* blood pressure, *COPD* chronic obstructive pulmonary disease, *DBP* diastolic blood pressure, *ED* emergency admission, *HbA1C* hemoglobin A1c, *HCP* healthcare provider, *PCP* primary care provider, *QOL* quality of life, *RCTs* randomized controlled trials, *SBP* systolic blood pressure, *UK* United Kingdom, *US* United States pharmacists on the management of uncontrolled diabetes over a 12-month period at primary care setting [12]. Example of services provided by the team to the intervention group (n = 127) included comprehensive medication management, patient counseling and education, organizing follow-up visits and foot and eye screening, while patients in the control arm (n = 128) received the usual care. The study revealed that the interprofessional collaborative care model resulted in improving the glycemic control and patients' QOL at 6- and 12-month periods, as well as an earlier achievement of improved clinical response (within 3–6 months) as compared to the usual care group (12 months) [12]. The findings suggest the effectiveness and the sustainable benefit of implementing the collaborative practice in diabetes setting.

As mental health disorders are frequently presented in patients with chronic conditions, the impact of IPCP on mental health was also one clinical outcome measure of interest in the literature. The presence of depression in patients with diabetes, as an example of physical and mental comorbidity, might negatively affect the overall health of patients such as glycemic, blood pressure and cholesterol control, increase the development of microvascular and macrovascular complications, and impede the compliance with treatment plan [13]. Thus, there is a need for a collaborative integrated team to manage patients with physical and mental disorders [14]. A recent systematic review and meta-analysis of 12 RCTs published until October 2020 explored the effect of collaborative care on depression outcomes among patients with diabetes and depression, and found that depression treatment response was higher among interventional versus control group at short (≤3 months), medium (3–6 months), and long-term management periods (>6 months), with an overall relative risk (RR) = 1.31, 95% CI: 1.23–1.39 [11]. The same study also showed that collaborative care was associated with improvement in medication adherence but a minor positive impact on QOL (SMD = 0.12, 95% CI: 0.03–0.21). The collaborative care intervention was implemented over a period of 12 weeks to 12 months among the analyzed studies. Besides, the multidisciplinary collaborative team included psychiatrist, diabetologist, and a case manager. Most of these studies were conducted in the US (n = 10), stressing the urgent need for implementing and measuring the positive effects of other collaborative healthcare systems on patients' outcomes worldwide.

Interprofessional consultations in delirium and their impacts on patients outcomes were recently summarized in a systematic scoping review of ten studies [15]. In-hospital setting, other health related outcomes were assessed including delirium incidence and severity, delirium duration, length of stay (LOS) in hospital, and falls. Those studies have found that interprofessional delirium consultation teams, which is a form of IPCP, improved delirium care in hospitals by providing frontline staff with educational resources and patient-specific recommendations. This model of intervention delivery has been shown to be effective in reducing the incidence of delirium, in addition to delirium severity and duration (reported in 7/10 studies). Of the six studies reported evaluation of delirium incidence as an outcome, only one found a significant reduction in the intervention group, three found non-significant effects, while the remaining two revealed no differences between groups. Hospital LOS as an outcome was also measured in 7/10 studies. Only one study found a significant difference in the average LOS in hospital as the intervention group showed decreased LOS significantly from 8.5 to 6.5 days after implementation of Interprofessional Consultative Team intervention approach consisting of five key components: systematic cognitive screening and identification of delirium, interprofessional team consultation, implementation of non-pharmacological strategies, medication management, and staff education and distribution of educational materials [16]. Finally, fall rates among delirious patients were reported in two [17, 18] of the three studies that explored the hospital wide fall rates, and showed a significant reduction of falls after implementation of the consultation process (5.15 vs. 2.49 and 3.58 vs. 2.03 falls per 1000 patient days, respectively). Together, this systematic review revealed enough evidence to suggest that interprofessional consultative delirium teams can help in reducing delirium and its related complications. Despite the benefits of interprofessional consultations in this patient population, the studies included are limited by their sparsity and heterogeneity.

It is worth mentioning that professional multidisciplinary team approach has been also tested in other disease states and showed positive impacts on asthma [19], chronic obstructive pulmonary disease [20], and heart failure [21].

One can describe an example of interprofessional collaboration between two health professions. The integrative service provided by the coordination between physicians and nurses has a tremendous impact on patient care, as roles and responsibilities of nurses are expanding and greatly appreciated in primary care. This has been highlighted and discussed in a review of 11 systematic reviews that described the impact of physician-nurse cooperation in patient care [22]. Multiple outcomes were assessed including patient satisfaction, functional status outcomes, glycemic control, blood pressure control, emergency department visits, and hospitalization rates which are important indicators of health quality. In addition to their impacts on individuals' physical health, utilization of medical services can also act as an indicator for social functioning. Collaboration between nurses and doctors has been shown to improve patient outcomes at various levels of patient satisfaction, blood pressure control, decreased hospitalization, and so on. Interprofessionalism between the two disciplines resulted also in positive effects on a variety of patient pathologies. This study further supports the conclusion that meeting future challenges in primary care requires an integrated interprofessional collaboration among health professionals that are sufficiently educated.

The previously mentioned limitations of variabilities and heterogeneity of IPCP literature were noted also in the systematic review conducted by Kaiser and coworkers [23] assessing patient-reported outcomes presented in 22 studies (16 RCTs, 5 non-randomized studies, and one controlled before-and-after study). Despite those limitations and high risk of biases in most of the studies included, the overall results indicated that IPCP has some positive effect on patient-reported outcomes, including QOL, coping, satisfaction, functional ability and health status, pain, psychiatric morbidity, managing one's own health care, therapeutic relationship, and self-reported treatment success. Nevertheless, there are some studies which did not report any effects and most of the reported estimated effect were imprecise. Authors concluded that future methodically rigorous studies are desirable to answer the question of effectiveness of IPCP on patient-reported outcomes.

As the patient is the core of the collaborative care, exploring patients perspectives and experiences of IPCP is critical. A systematic scoping review of seven studies performed in primary care setting showed positive patient experiences with IPCP activities, including a variety of implementation types [24]. For instance, patients felt that they received excellent care, had healthier relationships with their healthcare providers, and experienced more patient-centered care such as better providers' attitudes, attention, and availability. Interprofessional care made patients feel more like collaborative members of the team. Also, IPCP allowed patients to have greater involvement in managing their conditions(s), treatment plan efficacy, and engagement. Although this review was limited to searching only PubMed for articles related to primary care, it identified the few studies that included patient experience or patient satisfaction outcomes in IPCP literature, and highlighted the role of patient involvement in quality improvement.

Overall, it appears to be a favorable effect of IPCP on health outcomes, nevertheless, the heterogeneity observed among studies in the outcomes and the explicit methodological tools used to measure those outcomes call for further robust investigations about the role of IPCP in improving patients' health. Well-designed RCTs conducted for longer duration, with assessment of morbidity and mortality as long-term outcomes are necessary. Researchers may need to consider other types of complex chronic conditions of public health concern beyond chronic diseases which can further inform the feasibility and validity of IPCP approach in providing patient-centered care.

7.3 Impact of Interprofessional Education (IPE) on Health Outcomes

The concept of IPE occurs when individuals from various health professions working together to learn from, about, and with each other. This looks essential for health professions students to learn professional competencies and to prepare them to practice in an environment enclosed with effective communication, understanding of each other roles and responsibilities, teamwork, respect, and collaborative behavior, aiming at improving patient outcomes. While the idea of IPE looks appealing, the implementation of learning-together approaches to improve health outcomes might be challenging. As described previously, diverse studies have assessed the roles of interprofessional collaborative teams of healthcare members in improving the quality of patient care, nevertheless, the impact of implementing IPE across health professions students on patient-centered care is limited, but growing continuously. Clearly, to prepare students to practice in a collaborate workplace environment, there is an urgent need to offer the IPE within educational programs. Healthcare agencies have been calling repeatedly to offer IPE to healthcare learners to be effective future collaborators. Additionally, international accreditation standards of healthcare academic programs have strongly recommended the integration of IPE within the curricula. Thus, there has been an expanding IPE initiatives and efforts led by students that would be of benefits to clarify the significant role that this style of education might play on patient care.

Many efforts by the researchers were directed to accumulate the reported evidence of the impact of IPE implementations on patients and healthcare outcomes. Reeves and his colleagues keep tracking this growing evidence over years since 2007. In one systematic review, they provided analysis of 15 studies on the IPE impact on different outcomes [25]. The seven studies that reported positive outcomes did so in these areas: communications between patient and healthcare providers, clinical outcomes for people with diabetes, team behaviors in emergency departments, rates of diabetes testing and improved patient outcomes, increased mental health practitioner competencies related to the delivery of patient care, and finally information sharing between operating room teams. Three studies reported that the benefits of IPE lasted for an extended period of time. Furthermore, in their updated review of 2016, a total of 46 studies were analyzed and showed positive impacts on learners' perception of IPE, attitudes toward other health professions, collaborative skills, and the willingness to implement changes to apply and promote IPE in practice, with limited influence on patient care [1].

Similarly, many studies have measured the collaborative practice impacts at the attitude and behavioral level of learners in IPE system toward interprofessional team, environment and readiness to collaborate which match mainly levels 1, 2, and 3 of Kirkpatrick's pyramids of learning impact [26]. That level of impact revealed in Spaulding and coworkers [5] review which highlighted the improvement in attitudes of pre-licensure learners and professionals toward IPE, as well as the increase in the value placed toward a team-based approach to optimizing patient care. Improvement in collaborative behavior was also observed.

The above-mentioned observations in most of the literature focused on the IPE impacts on learners' perceptions and behaviors, rather than the direct health and patients' outcomes, were consistent over years. Students attended IPE programs showed significant improvements in attitudes toward both interprofessional teams and interprofessional learning as revealed in the self-reported effectiveness as a team member and self-perceived confidence, knowledge, and ability to manage long-term conditions [27]. A recent systematic review of 25 studies found that outcomes from IPE interventions were positive for participants in activities and team-based learning [28]. The most commonly used outcome measure in those included studies was the Interprofessional Education Perceptions Scale which showed improvement in students' clinical experiences.

As interprofessional communication is central in collaborative care, one systematic scoping review of 19 studies has clarified the themes of interprofessional training and their impact on communication in emergency medicine (EM) setting [29]. The analyzed studies fell into four themes: (a) indications and outcomes, (b) curriculum and assessment methods, (c) barriers to implementation, and (d) enablers of successful implementation. Outcomes of EM training for different healthcare workers were illustrated at different levels. The host organization experiences outgrowth in a variety of areas, including but not limited to hospital performance levels and reimbursement rates. In addition, reduction in adverse events and errors provided the chance for significant liability cost savings. For participants and colleagues, improvements are seen in attitudes toward teamwork internal communications. There was also increase in safety ideologies present among those studied. Patients themselves witnessed greater satisfaction with quality of staff communication, as well as reduction in issues between staff-patient relations, which often lead to reduced LOS in hospital with improving patients experience while admitted. Training on interprofessional communication occurs in phases. This starts with the use of didactic education which then advances to integrating the physician's new knowledge and skills into practice. Clinical experience follows, resulting in positive attitudes and behaviors toward interprofessional communications.

There are several studies that were designed aiming at exploring the impact of IPE on the interprofessional collaborative competences. Riskiyana and coworkers [30] found that IPE has the potential to improve interprofessional collaborative competences in participants of IPE activities, based on objective assessments. This review showed that IPE can improve collaborative knowledge, skills, and behaviors, as well as the quality of care. In all included 16 studies there were positive impacts of IPE leading to improvement in all domains of the core interprofessional collaborative competences according to (*Interprofessional Education, Expert Panel, 2011*) including value and ethics, roles, and responsibilities, interprofessional communication, and team and teamwork.

Up to the present time, limited evidence exists regarding IPE enhancing the delivery of health services and therefore patient health outcomes. In 2018, an integrative review of 14 studies has synthesized the body of evidence related to the outcomes of incorporating IPE programs about diabetes management across education or clinical settings [3]. The IPE programs in eight of these studies were directed to healthcare professionals and six studies included students of various health professions such as medicine, nursing, pharmacy, dental hygiene, physiotherapy, nutrition, social work, or public health. The IPE program included in this review should include members of two or more health professions learning together about, from, and with each other for the purpose of improving diabetes management. The learning methods in the IPE programs varied between classes, workshops, seminars, project-based, role play, online course, clinical cases, group discussions, and interactive games among others. Learners had the opportunity to practice the gained knowledge through preparing action plans for the team-based projects, testing the knowledge in the work environment, or by visiting patients in clinics. Outcomes measured were primarily related to learners' reaction to the IPE program, acquisition of knowledge about diabetes management, behavioral changes to workplace, and modification of attitudes toward interprofessional care, teamwork, and understanding of other healthcare professionals, with only four studies (two involved students) reported assessing the benefits to patient outcomes [3].

In one of the IPE programs that comprised students, members of the IPE team participated in a curriculum pertaining to diabetes management, supplemented with clinical discussions, and clinic visit to plan and implement the team-based clinical services [3]. Examples of interventions guided by students were medical management, lifestyle assessment, self-management, medication management, and patient education. An evidence of a better healthcare utilization by diabetic patients was provided because of implementing IPE interventions led by students-teams. For instance, improvements in the frequency of blood glucose, HbA1c, blood pressure, microalbumin urea, and lipids monitoring, and more foot examination were reported. Furthermore, increased number of patients with favorable blood pressure and cholesterol levels, and a decline in the number of diabetes management errors were observed. By that date, none of the analyzed studies that explored patient's outcomes reported an improvement in glycemic control (HbA1c) after the IPE implementation.

The gap of measuring IPE impact on patient related outcomes being recognized and there are newer studies, however, that have provided additional evidence of the impact of IPE implementation on patient care. For instance, an interprofessional group of 25 students (physician assistant, medical, and pharmacy programs) and 25 healthcare staff has participated in providing care to diabetic patients collaboratively [31]. The involvement of health professions students in diabetes management program resulted in a significant decline in HbA1c and glucose levels among patients who had HbA1c ≥ 7 at baseline, with negligible improvements in body mass index and annual dental and eye examinations. The number of patients seen by the healthcare provider in clinic per hour was increased suggesting improvement in practice efficiency with the application of IPE. Below we described additional examples.

One case control study has reported that an interprofessional team approach including family medicine professionals and nursing students improved the clinical outcomes in the setting of diabetes [32]. The senior nursing students assisted the medical team in chart reviewing, calling patients for follow-up visits, developing the patient care plan, and patient education about medication adherence, diet, weight management, and exercise. After 1 year follow-up, authors noticed that patients in the intervention group ($n = 58$) showed significant improvement in the HbA1c level, blood pressure control, and completion of urinary microalbumin test, compared to control group ($n = 61$).

The latter findings are promising as we perceive a rising positive impact of IPE on patient outcomes. In fact, part of these observations was supported by a modern pre–post interventional study conducted among diabetic patients in a primary care setting which provided further evidence of efficacy of student-led collaborative practice [33]. In this IPE initiative, an interprofessional team care clinics were formed at primary care settings in Maryland USA in 2014 to provide health professions students from schools of Nursing, Pharmacy, and Social Work with the opportunity to implement IPCP. Patients with uncontrolled diabetes and/or mood disorders were referred to the interprofessional team by the healthcare providers at the primary care setting. In collaboration with regular standard care, a faculty-precepted student-led interprofessional services were provided to patients including patient assessment, medication management, patient education, health promotion, and depression screening among others. The efficacy of implementing IPE on patient care was retrospectively analyzed over a 2-years period (2017–2018) and among 50 diabetic patients. Health outcomes were significantly improved as demonstrated by decreased HbA1c by 2.2% from baseline, a decline in systolic blood pressure, and a 75% decrease in emergency department admissions in the 6 months post-participation, especially among those at higher risk of diabetes complications. Additionally, the pre- and post-completion of Patient Health Questionnaire showed decreased depressive symptoms among a sub-group of patients indicating an improvement in mental health [33].

It is necessary to mention that diabetes and concomitant psychosocial illnesses were not the sole disease conditions that were investigated with respect to IPE. Suen and colleagues have analyzed the existing literature of the impact of students-led health interventions from the perspective of cardiovascular disease, and observed positive effect on patient health [34]. Another disease state that has been investigated with respect to IPE is dementia. The complexity of this disease along with the linked symptoms of impaired memory, personality, and behaviors mandate the need of multidisciplinary team for dementia care. A description of IPE interventions related to dementia showed that the majority were directed toward health and social care practitioners of dementia care, while only two studies involved undergraduate or graduate students [35]. Furthermore, none of these studies had shown benefits on patients' outcomes, with only one study conducted among professionals showed a "very low-low quality" graded evidence of behavioral and organizational changes that support the transfer of learning experience into clinical practice.

It is obvious that the research on IPE that measures health outcomes is limited. The small number of studies, the variations in the setting, design, and implemented services as well as the low quality of the contemporary evidence limit the ability to draw valid conclusions about the efficacy of IPE on patients' outcomes. The challenges toward team-based care models should be recognized and acknowledged. An effective strategy of IPE is indeed a partnership between practicing healthcare professionals and health professions faculty and students, despite the observation that students-led interventions resulted in outcomes that are comparable to professional-led interventions [34]. The implementation of IPE in primary care requires cooperation and willingness of professionals to accept the involvement of students in the delivery of care and to assess various models of IPE in practice. The successful teamwork process requires extensive planning and coordination, setting up clear goals, and effective communication. Healthcare professionals should understand and accept the added value that students may display in the delivery of care in terms of thoroughly reviewing patient information, developing management plans, and patient education and follow-up. Limited resources, space, personnel, and time, the balance between students learning goals and patient satisfaction of health care services, as well as the assurance of the consistency of the delivered care among professionals may act as barriers for successful IPE implementation. Also, we cannot neglect that there is a necessity for: first, studies that compare the effectiveness of IPE interventions against separate profession-specific interventions; second, various study designs such as RCTs, cost–benefit analyses or impact evaluations with qualitative data examining processes related to IPE and changes in practice.

7.4 Impact of Interprofessional Education and Collaborative Practice (IPECP) on Health Cost

Healthcare cost is expected to rise giving the chronicity and complexity of disease conditions and the aging population. It is therefore feasible to understand whether the delivery of IPECP models would be effective in subsiding the cost of health. Assessment of cost is also important to recognize whether the improvements linked to patient health are simultaneously reflected on economic outcomes.

There is a paucity of data describing the impact of IPECP on healthcare cost. Multidisciplinary professional care did not increase the cost of managing uncontrolled diabetes. In fact, studies showed that implementation of IPCP can be associated with cost savings due to, in part, prevention of disease complications, lower medications cost, and less frequent laboratory orders [4]. For instance, one randomized trial that explored a collaborative professional model of physician, dietitian, diabetes nurse educator, and clinical pharmacist in diabetes care found an average cost savings of $91.01 per patient over 6 months in the group received the intervention [36]. This study also showed that the average 6-month diabetes-related expenditures (medications, consultations, and labs) was 15% lower in the intervention arm versus control. In the previously described multicenter RCT, the collaborative care model of professionals resulted in improving HbA1c and QOL in uncontrolled diabetic patients [12]. The same study also investigated the effect of IPCP on direct healthcare cost over 12 months including consultation fees, laboratory and procedures, and medications. The cost-effectiveness of the collaborative care intervention was evaluated from the healthcare institution perspective and the incremental cost-effectiveness ratio was calculated. Results revealed negligible difference between the intervention and control groups regarding the total direct medical costs ($984.8 ± 405.8 for intervention vs. $975.8 ± 374.4 for control, $p = 0.942$), however, the intervention group had significantly lower cost of physician consultations and higher cost of the pharmacist consultations and lab investigations compared to controls. Perhaps, the observed increased in pharmacist consultations were associated with lower medical doctor visits. Implementing IPCP was cost-effective as the costs per 1% improvement in HbA1c and per additional quality-adjusted life years (QALY) were only $40.52 and $920.9 at 1 year, respectively [12]. Multiple previous studies have also demonstrated that integrating pharmaceutical care services to usual care resulted in significant healthcare cost savings [37–39].

To date, little consideration has been given in the literature as to whether implementing IPE is economically favored. The study of Rowe et al. discussed above illustrated that IPE clinics resulted in decreased emergency department visits for diabetic patients [33]. Authors explained that prevention of 12 emergency visits results in a potential cost savings of $13,320, demonstrating the improved economic outcomes of IPE. Another recent study of a collaborative model integrating health professions students (medical and pharmacy) with healthcare professionals directed toward antimicrobial stewardship showed improvement in antibiotic prescription and use in medical intensive care unit setting [40]. Following implementation of interprofessional stewardship program, the total overall expenditures on antibiotics per year was declined, and a significant decrease in antibiotics expenditure per case mix point was observed. Overall, the limited number of studies assessing the economic impact of IPE warrants further investigations that inform about the cost-effectiveness of IPE models.

7.5 Impact of Interprofessional Education and Collaborative Practice (IPECP) on Health System Approach

As described earlier, IPE has been shown to improve communication and collaboration among healthcare professionals which may be leading to better patient outcomes. However, there is still much to learn about how best to support IPE learners, guide the host organization, and oversee the development of IPCP competencies in order to ensure that IPE programs are effective in improving safety and patient experience [29]. Thus, studying this perspective could contribute to the further improvement of healthcare system as a whole. Taking in consideration healthcare systems transformation around the globe, IPECP could be empowered in order to provide better and safer care. As healthcare continues to evolve and face new challenges, the need for effective interprofessional collaboration is becoming increasingly important. By promoting IPECP, healthcare professionals can work together to improve patient outcomes and overall system effectiveness. There is growing evidence that IPECP has the potential to enhance the efficacy of the healthcare system as a whole [1].

One of the key components of an effective healthcare system is high-quality patient safety measures. In 2017, the World Health Organization (WHO) launched the Third Global Patient Safety Challenge: Medication Without Harm, with the goal of reducing severe avoidable medication harm by 50% by 2022 [41]. Implementing IPECP has the ability to positively impact patient safety by improving communication among healthcare providers, leading to better coordination of care and fewer medical errors. A recent systematic review of 31 studies found that medication safety-focused IPE for pre-qualification health professions students is feasible [42]. The IPE activities can be delivered virtually or in simulations, patient encounters, and through classroom settings. Most of the reviewed activities involved medical, pharmacy, and nursing students; a minority involved other types of health professions students. Few activities were integrated into the overall curriculum or part of a wider IPE program strategy. The majority of activities examined were single events that lasted for several hours and reported assessment as a learning tool. Student satisfaction with the activities and their enhanced attitudes toward IP working were commonly reported. The review found limited low certainty evidence that medication safety-focused IPE may improve students' confidence and perceptions of competence for performing technical medication tasks. It also suggested that this approach may lead to increased scores in mediation knowledge tests and improved team performance, though more research is needed on these claims. Because most research employs non-comparative, descriptive study designs, it is difficult to inform that the benefits of IPE are greater than those seen with uni-professional education.

The value-based practice (VBP) as a growing healthcare system approach also intersects with IPECP. In a short report by Merriman and colleagues aimed to explore the relationship between VBP and IPE, suggesting that incorporating the principles of VBP into IPE can improve collaboration between healthcare professionals [43]. This has important implications for how VBP is used within IPE, as well as for inclusion in the preparation and support curriculum for new and established trainers involved in IPE. This report provides a projection of the future of IPE, and how value-based principles can be incorporated into IPE training programs. However, further research is needed to confirm the effectiveness and impact of this perception.

As the healthcare system approach concerning both individual and public health issues, approaching the public health issues of health system and social determinants of health are considered important factors in effectiveness of any healthcare system. A pre–post intervention survey was conducted among 222 third year medical students in order to identify patient issues related to social determinants of health (SDH) such as legal issues that would require consultation [44]. The results showed that the students were more likely to screen patients for SDH issues and refer them to a legal resource after taking the survey. This research is significant because it provides valuable insight into how IPE can be used in a local context prospectively. It also demonstrates how IPE can improve collaboration between healthcare professionals and other community resources, potentially leading to better health outcomes for patients.

Collectively, the research shows that IPECP can have a positive impact on healthcare professionals, their collaborative competence, and the overall functioning of the healthcare system. This highlights the importance of implementing such interventions in order to improve patient care and outcomes. Furthermore, incorporating principles of VBP and addressing social determinants of health can also enhance the effectiveness of IPE, and should be reflected back in improving healthcare system outcomes at the public health and organizational levels.

7.6 Summary and Concluding Remarks

To summarize, this chapter provides an updated overview of literature focusing on the evidence of IPECP impact on healthcare outcomes. We noticed that the literature has been focusing on implementations of IPCP with some advancements in IPE. It is obvious to the readers of this chapter that most of the reported evidence in both IPCP and IPE studies are measuring the human reported outcomes such as perceptions, satisfactions, and self-reported attitudes changes, and relatively positive trend is noticed toward IPECP applications despite the heterogeneity of the evidence. The objective clinical and organizational healthcare outcomes have been addressed scarcely in the literature. Moreover, it will be hard to gage the effect of IPECP interventions on individual and healthcare system outcomes without a clear engaged relationship between education and healthcare systems. To evidently understand the effects of IPECP, targeted studies that examine how well it performs in relation to health and system outcomes are needed. IPE has the potential to improve collaboration between healthcare providers, patient related outcomes, and healthcare systems outcomes, which should prioritize its integration. Future research should focus on strengthening the link between education and healthcare systems, developing a clear conceptual model for IPECP interventions, and examining the impact of IPECP on health and system outcomes. Developing a clear methodological approach to measure precisely the impact of each IPECP interventions on the targeted outcomes is essential step to be taken by the scholars interested in this field. One observation noticed through revising the IPECP literature and highlighted by others is the need for unifying the definitions and taxonomy used when referring to IPECP concepts, interventions, and outcomes. This might help in synthesizing more robust evidence for the upcoming research and reviews. Finally, IPECP evidence in the healthcare system approaches is growing and might be an influential transition in the post pandemic era of health transformation.

References

1. Reeves S, Fletcher S, Barr H, Birch I, Boet S, Davies N, et al. A BEME systematic review of the effects of interprofessional education: BEME Guide No. 39. Med Teach. 2016;38(7):656–68. https://doi.org/10.3109/0142159X.2016.1173663.
2. Lee JK, McCutcheon LRM, Fazel MT, Cooley JH, Slack MK. Assessment of interprofessional collaborative practices and outcomes in adults with diabetes and hypertension in primary care: a systematic review and meta-analysis. JAMA Netw Open. 2021;4(2):e2036725. https://doi.org/10.1001/jamanetworkopen.2020.36725.
3. Kangas S, Rintala TM, Jaatinen P. An integrative systematic review of interprofessional education on diabetes. J Interprof Care. 2018;32(6):706–18. https://doi.org/10.1080/13561820.2018.1500453.
4. Siaw MYL, Lee JY. Multidisciplinary collaborative care in the management of patients with uncontrolled diabetes: a systematic review and meta-analysis. Int J Clin Pract. 2019;73(2):e13288. https://doi.org/10.1111/ijcp.13288.
5. Spaulding EM, Marvel FA, Jacob E, Rahman A, Hansen BR, Hanyok LA, et al. Interprofessional education and collaboration among healthcare students and professionals: a systematic review and call for action. J Interprof Care. 2021;35(4):612–21. https://doi.org/10.1080/13561820.2019.1697214.
6. Atlantis E, Fahey P, Foster J. Collaborative care for comorbid depression and diabetes: a systematic review and meta-analysis. BMJ Open. 2014;4(4):e004706. https://doi.org/10.1136/bmjopen-2013-004706.
7. Levengood TW, Peng Y, Xiong KZ, Song Z, Elder R, Ali MK, et al. Team-based care to improve diabetes management: a community guide meta-analysis. Am J Prev Med. 2019;57(1):e17–26. https://doi.org/10.1016/j.amepre.2019.02.005.
8. Lutfiyya MN, Chang LF, McGrath C, Dana C, Lipsky MS. The state of the science of interprofessional collaborative practice: a scoping review of the patient health-related outcomes based literature published between 2010 and 2018. PLoS One. 2019;14(6):e0218578. https://doi.org/10.1371/journal.pone.0218578.
9. McCutcheon LRM, Haines ST, Valaitis R, Sturpe DA, Russell G, Saleh AA, et al. Impact of interprofessional primary care practice on patient outcomes: a scoping review. SAGE Open. 2020;10(2):2158244020935899. https://doi.org/10.1177/2158244020935899.

10. Reeves S, Pelone F, Harrison R, Goldman J, Zwarenstein M. Interprofessional collaboration to improve professional practice and healthcare outcomes. Cochrane Database Syst Rev. 2017;6:CD000072. https://doi.org/10.1002/14651858.CD000072.pub3.
11. Wang Y, Hu M, Zhu D, Ding R, He P. Effectiveness of collaborative care for depression and HbA1c in patients with depression and diabetes: a systematic review and meta-analysis. Int J Integr Care. 2022;22(3):12. https://doi.org/10.5334/ijic.6443.
12. Xu Y, Tan CWY, Tsou KYK, Tan DHY, Gallagher PJ, Lee JY. Long-term clinical and cost-effectiveness of collaborative care in people with uncontrolled type 2 diabetes mellitus and polypharmacy: a multicenter randomized controlled trial. Prim Care Diabetes. 2022;16(1):188–95. https://doi.org/10.1016/j.pcd.2021.12.013.
13. Owens-Gary MD, Zhang X, Jawanda S, Bullard KM, Allweiss P, Smith BD. The importance of addressing depression and diabetes distress in adults with type 2 diabetes. J Gen Intern Med. 2019;34(2):320–4. https://doi.org/10.1007/s11606-018-4705-2.
14. Huang Y, Wei X, Wu T, Chen R, Guo A. Collaborative care for patients with depression and diabetes mellitus: a systematic review and meta-analysis. BMC Psychiatry. 2013;13:260. https://doi.org/10.1186/1471-244X-13-260.
15. Monaghan C, Martin G, Kerr J, Peters ML, Versloot J. Effectiveness of interprofessional consultation-based interventions for delirium: a scoping review. J Appl Gerontol. 2022;41(3):881–91. https://doi.org/10.1177/07334648211018032.
16. Angel C, Brooks K, Fourie J. Standardizing management of adults with delirium hospitalized on medical-surgical units. Perm J. 2016;20(4):16–002. https://doi.org/10.7812/TPP/16-002.
17. Babine RL, Farrington S, Wierman HR. HELP(c) prevent falls by preventing delirium. Nursing. 2013;43(5):18–21. https://doi.org/10.1097/01.NURSE.0000428710.81378.aa.
18. Ferguson A, Uldall K, Dunn J, Blackmore CC, Williams B. Effectiveness of a multifaceted delirium screening, prevention, and treatment initiative on the rate of delirium falls in the acute care setting. J Nurs Care Qual. 2018;33(3):213–20. https://doi.org/10.1097/NCQ.0000000000000297.
19. Burke H, Davis J, Evans S, Flower L, Tan A, Kurukulaaratchy RJ. A multidisciplinary team case management approach reduces the burden of frequent asthma admissions. ERJ Open Res. 2016;2(3):00039. https://doi.org/10.1183/23120541.00039-2016.
20. Alshabanat A, Otterstatter MC, Sin DD, Road J, Rempel C, Burns J, et al. Impact of a COPD comprehensive case management program on hospital length of stay and readmission rates. Int J Chron Obstruct Pulmon Dis. 2017;12:961–71. https://doi.org/10.2147/COPD.S124385.
21. Huntley AL, Johnson R, King A, Morris RW, Purdy S. Does case management for patients with heart failure based in the community reduce unplanned hospital admissions? A systematic review and meta-analysis. BMJ Open. 2016;6(5):e010933. https://doi.org/10.1136/bmjopen-2015-010933.
22. Matthys E, Remmen R, Van Bogaert P. An overview of systematic reviews on the collaboration between physicians and nurses and the impact on patient outcomes: what can we learn in primary care? BMC Fam Pract. 2017;18(1):110. https://doi.org/10.1186/s12875-017-0698-x.
23. Kaiser L, Bartz S, Neugebauer EAM, Pietsch B, Pieper D. Interprofessional collaboration and patient-reported outcomes in inpatient care: protocol for a systematic review. Syst Rev. 2018;7(1):126. https://doi.org/10.1186/s13643-018-0797-3.
24. Morgan KH, Barroso CS, Bateman S, Dixson M, Brown KC. Patients' experiences of interprofessional collaborative practice in primary care: a scoping review of the literature. J Pat Exp. 2020;7(6):1466–75. https://doi.org/10.1177/2374373520925725.
25. Reeves S, Perrier L, Goldman J, Freeth D, Zwarenstein M. Interprofessional education: effects on professional practice and healthcare outcomes (update). Cochrane Database Syst Rev. 2013;(3):CD002213. https://doi.org/10.1002/14651858.CD002213.pub3.
26. Reeves S, Boet S, Zierler B, Kitto S. Interprofessional education and practice guide No. 3: evaluating interprofessional education. J Interprof Care. 2015;29(4):305–12. https://doi.org/10.3109/13561820.2014.1003637.

27. Darlow B, Coleman K, McKinlay E, Donovan S, Beckingsale L, Gray B, et al. The positive impact of interprofessional education: a controlled trial to evaluate a programme for health professional students. BMC Med Educ. 2015;15:98. https://doi.org/10.1186/s12909-015-0385-3.
28. Guitar NA, Connelly DM. A systematic review of the outcome measures used to evaluate interprofessional learning by health care professional students during clinical experiences. Eval Health Prof. 2021;44(3):293–311. https://doi.org/10.1177/0163278720978814.
29. Ong ZH, Tan LHE, Ghazali HZB, Ong YT, Koh JWH, Ang RZE, et al. A systematic scoping review on pedagogical strategies of interprofessional communication for physicians in emergency medicine. J Med Educ Curric Dev. 2021;8:23821205211041794. https://doi.org/10.1177/23821205211041794.
30. Riskiyana R, Claramita M, Rahayu GR. Objectively measured interprofessional education outcome and factors that enhance program effectiveness: a systematic review. Nurse Educ Today. 2018;66:73–8. https://doi.org/10.1016/j.nedt.2018.04.014.
31. Nagelkerk J, Thompson ME, Bouthillier M, Tompkins A, Baer LJ, Trytko J, et al. Improving outcomes in adults with diabetes through an interprofessional collaborative practice program. J Interprof Care. 2018;32(1):4–13. https://doi.org/10.1080/13561820.2017.1372395.
32. De La Rosa M, Pitts S, Chen PH. An interprofessional collaboration of care to improve clinical outcomes for patients with diabetes. J Interprof Care. 2020;34(2):269–71. https://doi.org/10.1080/13561820.2019.1643297.
33. Rowe GC, Congdon HB, Pittman J, Wiseman R, Shields R. Interprofessional education clinics and improved outcomes for primary care patients with diabetes. J Interprofessional Educ Pract. 2021;24:100441. https://doi.org/10.1016/j.xjep.2021.100441.
34. Suen J, Attrill S, Thomas JM, Smale M, Delaney CL, Miller MD. Effect of student-led health interventions on patient outcomes for those with cardiovascular disease or cardiovascular disease risk factors: a systematic review. BMC Cardiovasc Disord. 2020;20(1):332. https://doi.org/10.1186/s12872-020-01602-1.
35. Jackson M, Pelone F, Reeves S, Hassenkamp AM, Emery C, Titmarsh K, et al. Interprofessional education in the care of people diagnosed with dementia and their carers: a systematic review. BMJ Open. 2016;6(8):e010948. https://doi.org/10.1136/bmjopen-2015-010948.
36. Siaw MYL, Ko Y, Malone DC, Tsou KYK, Lew YJ, Foo D, et al. Impact of pharmacist-involved collaborative care on the clinical, humanistic and cost outcomes of high-risk patients with type 2 diabetes (IMPACT): a randomized controlled trial. J Clin Pharm Ther. 2017;42(4):475–82. https://doi.org/10.1111/jcpt.12536.
37. Brophy L, Williams A, Berman EJ, Keleti D, Michael KE, Shepherd M, et al. Collaborative DTM reduces hospitalization and healthcare costs in patients with diabetes treated with polypharmacy. Am J Manag Care. 2014;20(3):e72–81.
38. Monte SV, Slazak EM, Albanese NP, Adelman M, Rao G, Paladino JA. Clinical and economic impact of a diabetes clinical pharmacy service program in a university and primary care-based collaboration model. J Am Pharm Assoc. 2009;49(2):200–8. https://doi.org/10.1331/JAPhA.2009.08160.
39. Obreli-Neto PR, Marusic S, Guidoni CM, Baldoni Ade O, Renovato RD, Pilger D, et al. Economic evaluation of a pharmaceutical care program for elderly diabetic and hypertensive patients in primary health care: a 36-month randomized controlled clinical trial. J Manag Care Spec Pharm. 2015;21(1):66–75. https://doi.org/10.18553/jmcp.2015.21.1.66.
40. Schmid S, Schlosser S, Gulow K, Pavel V, Muller M, Kratzer A. Interprofessional collaboration between ICU physicians, staff nurses, and hospital pharmacists optimizes antimicrobial treatment and improves quality of care and economic outcome. Antibiotics. 2022;11(3):381. https://doi.org/10.3390/antibiotics11030381.
41. Donaldson LJ, Kelley ET, Dhingra-Kumar N, Kieny MP, Sheikh A. Medication without harm: WHO's third global patient safety challenge. Lancet. 2017;389(10080):1680–1. https://doi.org/10.1016/S0140-6736(17)31047-4.
42. Grimes TC, Guinan EM. Interprofessional education focused on medication safety: a systematic review. J Interprof Care. 2022;37:131–49. https://doi.org/10.1080/13561820.2021.2015301.

43. Merriman C, Chalmers L, Ewens A, Fulford BK, Gray R, Handa A, et al. Values-based interprofessional education: how interprofessional education and values-based practice interrelate and are vehicles for the benefit of patients and health and social care professionals. J Interprof Care. 2020;34(4):569–71. https://doi.org/10.1080/13561820.2020.1713065.
44. Pettignano R, Bliss L, McLaren S, Caley S. Interprofessional medical-legal education of medical students: assessing the benefits for addressing social determinants of health. Acad Med. 2017;92(9):1254–8. https://doi.org/10.1097/ACM.0000000000001581.

Interprofessional Education: Accreditation Standards, Regulatory Policies, and Legal Structures

8

Marie-Andree Girard, Nouf Alrumaihi, and Mohammad Azzam

8.1 Introduction

Health professional education programs have historically been isolated from one another, typically separated either by institution (e.g., technical schools, colleges, and universities) and/or by faculty (e.g., of medicine, nursing, rehabilitation therapy, social work, etc.). These artificial silos represented neither the nature of the health sciences nor the nature of healthcare service delivery, as care for another human being is a holistic endeavor involving an interprofessional team of healthcare workers and patient partnerships, where each team member possesses only a piece of the puzzle leading to the diagnosis, treatment, and management of the patient's illness or disease [1].

For these reasons, institutions have increasingly adopted the *common curriculum approach*, whereby all prelicensure healthcare students are taught the common fundamental sciences (e.g., physiology, anatomy, pharmacology, etc.) and the foundational concepts of patient-centered care (e.g., roles and responsibilities, skills, care continuum, etc.) in tandem. In so doing, institutions have progressively implemented interprofessional education (IPE), through which prelicensure students from diverse health professions regularly learn with, from, and about each other [2],

M.-A. Girard
Faculty of Medicine, University of Montreal, Montreal, QC, Canada

N. Alrumaihi
Health Academy in the Saudi Commission for Health Specialties (SCFHS), Riyadh, Saudi Arabia

M. Azzam (✉)
Curriculum Studies and Studies in Applied Linguistics, Faculty of Education, Western University, London, ON, Canada

M. Y. Alnaami et al. (eds.), *Novel Health Interprofessional Education and Collaborative Practice Program: Strategy and Implementation*, https://doi.org/10.1007/978-981-99-3420-1_8

develop common language, and appreciate the value of their complementary knowledge, skill sets, and future interprofessional collaborative practice (IPCP). These approaches—the common curriculum approach and implementation of IPE—can be viewed as components of the *competency-based education* (CBE) model. In this model, prelicensure students are expected to develop specific competencies (including knowledge, skills, and dispositions) before they can advance to the next stage of their education [3]. Ultimately, this model has the potential to generate post-licensure workers who are *fit-for-purpose* and *fit-for-practice* [3] and can fully use their competence in an interprofessional setting to achieve the World Health Organization's goals of Universal Health Coverage [4].

In the health professions, the dynamics of prelicensure education are inherently distinct from those of post-licensure education. Whereas prelicensure education involves transforming nonspecialized students into qualified individuals who can then become licensed healthcare workers and join the labor market, post-licensure education involves lifelong learning and continual professional development required of healthcare workers until they retire. Further, prelicensure education is mainly controlled by the education sector that *accredits* health professional education programs, while post-licensure education is mainly controlled by regulatory bodies that *regulate* the health professions and healthcare workers' activities. In this chapter, we discuss the importance of both accreditation and regulation—particularly as they relate to IPE and IPCP—and how both can be effectively enacted.

8.2 Accreditation

Accreditation is often misleadingly confused with licensing or certification but they are different processes with different goals (see Table 8.1 for definition). The objective of accreditation is the promotion of best practices for organizations and not individuals, based on a group of best practices worded into accreditation standards [6].

8.2.1 Why Accreditation?

The WHO strongly advocates for IPE-relevant accreditation standards through the National Health Workforce Accounts (NHWA) handbook's *Indicator 3–06: Standards for Interprofessional Education* [7]. It is believed that IPE and IPE-induced IPCP can contribute to meeting the United Nations' health-related Sustainable Development Goals (SDGs) [8] aimed at promoting well-being for all, and two of the WHO's triple billion targets: "1 billion more people better protected from health emergencies" and "1 billion more people enjoying better health and well-being" (p. 1) [9].

Several studies in Australia [10], Canada [11, 12], and the United States [13] have shown that even when IPE is optionally recommended in accreditation standards documents, not holding the respective education programs *accountable* to

Table 8.1 Relevant terminology, as defined by the World Health Organization [5]

Accreditation	Formal process by which a recognized body, usually a non-governmental organization, assesses and recognizes that a health care organization meets applicable pre-determined and published standards. Accreditation standards are usually regarded as optimal and achievable and are designed to encourage continuous improvement efforts within accredited organizations
Certification	Process by which an authorized body, either a governmental or non-governmental organization, evaluates and recognizes either an individual or an organization as meeting pre-determined requirements or criteria. Although the terms accreditation and certification are often used interchangeably, accreditation usually applies only to organizations, while certification may apply to individuals, as well as to organizations
Licensure	Process by which a governmental authority grants permission to an individual practitioner or health care organization to operate or to engage in an occupation or profession. Licensure regulations are generally established to ensure that an organization or individual meets minimum standards to protect public health and safety. Licensure to individuals is usually granted after some form of examination or proof of education and may be renewed periodically through payment of a fee and/or proof of continuing education or professional competence
Regulation	The imposition of external constraints upon the behavior of an individual or an organization to force a change from preferred or spontaneous behavior

those standards usually leads to minimal and/or non-sustainable IPE. Hence, mandating IPE-relevant accreditation standards is necessary, as only through these standards can health professional education programs be held responsible for delivering sustainable IPE and be held accountable to meeting and upholding IPE-specific quality requirements [14].

8.2.2 Accreditation Standards and Different International Experiences

8.2.2.1 The Canadian Experience

Given the importance of IPE and subsequent IPCP towards realizing improved patient-centered care and advanced healthcare delivery systems, the Government of Canada instigated in 2004 the Interprofessional Education for Collaborative Patient-Centered Practice (IECPCP) initiative, which resulted in the formation of the Canadian Interprofessional Health Collaborative (CIHC). Consequently, the CIHC released its *National Interprofessional Competency Framework* [15], which aligned with the WHO's *Framework for Action* [16] and identified six interprofessional competency domains: interprofessional communication; patient-centered care; role clarification; team functioning; interprofessional conflict resolution; and collaborative leadership. The CIHC also led the Accreditation of Interprofessional Health Education (AIPHE) projects [17, 18], making Canada the first country on Earth to cooperatively develop and embed IPE language in the accreditation processes of six health professions: medicine, nursing, occupational therapy, pharmacy, physiotherapy, and social work.

The AIPHE projects [17, 18] were mindful to neither dictate explicit structures and contents to the health professions' accreditation standards nor dictate strict guidelines to how each accrediting body creates their standards and collects evidence of how their respective programs meet and uphold those standards. Rather, AIPHE guiding principles promoted the adoption of common terminology across the professions, highlighted individual domains (Table 8.1) that accreditation standards must address, and emphasized that IPE must be *sustainably* developed, implemented, and evaluated.

When developing accreditation standards domains, the AIPHE projects [17, 18] enacted the guidelines of the Interprofessional Education for Collaborative Patient-Centered Practice Framework [19]. This framework posits that a combination of factors influences whether IPE activities are sustainable—and therefore, effective [20]. First, *faculty* must receive ample development to be properly prepared to facilitate IPE and deliver IPE-relevant, student-centered pedagogy. Further, individual *education* programs must explicitly define IPE-relevant learning objectives and assess their *students'* IPE-relevant capabilities (in both classroom-based and practice-based settings) as they progress through their respective programs. Lastly, *organizational structures must commit* to supporting and allocating adequate *resources* towards the development, implementation, and evaluation of sustainable IPE.

A recent case study [21] of the Canadian accreditation standards documents for 11 regulated health professions in Canada, including those six involved in the AIPHE projects [17, 18], found that nine of the 11 professions' documents contained IPE language to which health professional education programs are held *accountable*. Table 8.2 provides examples of these exemplary accreditation standards.

8.2.2.2 The United States' Experience

The Institute of Medicine (IOM) in the United States had published "Educating for the Health Team" in 1972 to emphasize the importance of having the obligation to engage in IPE and the need for providing interprofessional teams with governmental and professional support. Since then, this term has evolved and subsequent current events and reports further pushed the implementation of IPE and IPCP in the United States.

The creation of the Interprofessional Education Collaborative (IPEC) in 2009 indicated an important commitment to IPE in academia. Comprised of professional associations representing the US colleges and schools of dentistry, medicine, nursing, pharmacy, and public health, IPEC was destined to have a significant impact on IPE and IPCP in the future. IPEC's expert panel published their first report in 2011 [27], in which they highlighted the core competencies for IPE. IPE and IPCP were further advanced by the formation of powerful partnerships focusing on team-based healthcare delivery and the legislation of the Patient Protection and Affordable Care Act [13].

There is a crucial need for healthcare workers to work together and create new models of care. During the past 10 years, the healthcare system in the United States

Table 8.2 Accreditation standards domains identified in the AIPHE projects [17, 18], with examples of exemplary accreditation standards. Used with permission [21]

Domain	Description	Exemplary accreditation standard
Organizational commitment	*Organizational commitment* refers to the administrative structures and processes, preferably at the level of the vice President's office and/or deanship, must foster the development, implementation, and evaluation of interprofessional education	"The university has integrated and endorsed the concept of interprofessional education and collaboration in practice" (p. 16) [22]
Faculty	Faculty members must be supported, encouraged, and prepared to facilitate the development, implementation, and evaluation of interprofessional education	"Preceptors are academically and experientially qualified for their role in assisting interns to achieve the ICDEP" (p. 13) [23]
Students	Students must understand the significance of interprofessional education and demonstrate proficiency in interprofessional competencies	"Students should be exposed to the principles of interprofessional collaboration for the provision of patient care" (p. 30) [24]
Educational program	Educational programs within and across faculties must share a common understanding of IPE and facilitate the development, implementation, and evaluation of interprofessional education throughout the learning continuum for all students	"The program provides opportunities for learners to develop knowledge, skills, and attitudes in using relevant information, communication technology, critical thinking, and clinical reasoning, in the delivery of collaborative client-centered care" (p. 25) [25]
Resources	The human, material, and financial resources that enable the development, implementation, and evaluation of interprofessional education must be supplied	"A report that documents the IPE activities and experiences integrated in the occupational therapy program. The report should describe the program offerings, and include considerations of space, human and learning resources required to deliver IPE" (p. 19) [26]

ICDEP integrated competencies for dietetic education and practice, *IPE* interprofessional education

has become more complex and rapidly developing to be more team-based, with the shift towards a focus on prevention, primary care, and the importance of community of practices. This expanded view has encouraged new models for IPE and IPCP to be developed and implemented.

In order to formalize the different interactions and communication between the accreditors, and to help in information sharing and problem solving, The Health Professions Accreditors Collaborative (HPAC) was founded in 2014 by six accrediting bodies. Since HPAC members have been developing accreditations policies, procedures, and/or standards for IPE in response to the evolving changes in healthcare systems and the development of IPCP competencies. The HPAC members further recognize the importance of accreditation and its significant role in promoting quality IPE that leads to improved healthcare outcomes. Thus, a guidance document was created in 2016 [28] through collaboration with the larger national IPE movement with additional consultation from the National Center and the IPEC.

"The goals of the guidance document are to:

1. facilitate the preparation of health professional students in the United States for interprofessional collaborative practice through accreditor collaboration and,
2. provide consensus guidance to enable academic institutions in the United States to develop, implement, and evaluate systematic IPE approaches and IPE plans, that are consistent with endorsing HPAC member accreditation expectations" [28].

8.2.2.3 The Australian Experience

As it is well known in the academic field that having robust and clear standards and regulations would significantly provide the required support for educational systems to implement IPE, a national approach to regulate the health profession programs and accrediting them was adopted in Australia almost a decade ago [10]. In 2010, a National Registration and Accreditation Scheme (NRAS) was created [29], through which the regulation of all health professions is controlled by the National Board and is supported by the Australian Health Practitioner Regulation Agency (AHPRA). Though the national boards and accreditation authorities have separate and discrete functions, they have corresponding functions under the National Law, e.g., an accreditation authority body accredits a proposed program of study and the National Board approves this program for registration purposes [30].

The WHO *Framework for Action* [16] recognizes the importance to commit to both IPE and IPCP, as both enhance healthcare and patients' outcomes. Accordingly, the *Securing an Interprofessional Future* project was conducted. The project recommended the incorporation of interprofessional practice standards and interprofessional outcomes into the accreditation standards of all Australian health professions and recognizes that meeting these learning outcomes requires the application of IPE pedagogies [31].

Current research literature demonstrates an inconsistent and piecemeal approach to IPE preparation and practice in Australia across all health professions. The Health Professions Accreditation Council Forum (later called the Health Professions Accreditation Joint Forum), which represents Australia's accreditation bodies for regulated health professions, adopted interprofessional learning skills [32] to guide the accreditation processes for health professional education programs [33]. With one exception, these have not yet been formally incorporated into the accreditation criteria. There is an urgent need to consolidate interprofessional competencies of all health professionals at the national level to improve the usefulness and functionality of system-level standards.

8.2.2.4 The Omani Experience

The concepts of IPE and IPCP are relatively new in the Middle East. Though few studies can be retrieved in this matter, most faculty and students have shown positive attitudes towards IPE and the readiness to implement it. Currently, IPE is being promoted in undergraduate education in different colleges including pharmacy, dentistry, medicine, nursing, and other allied health professions [34].

At Sultan Qaboos University (SQU), vital phases were taken towards implementing IPE. A steering committee was formed of faculty from the College of Medicine and the College of Nursing to explore possibilities to implement IPE at SQU. Some challenges were faced due to the rigid structure of the respective curricula with course-specific objectives and outcomes, but both colleges managed to choose two courses with similar objectives in which to initiate IPE. Some challenges have also emerged when it came to assessment, but the steering committee agreed to unify the formative assessment and have different summative assessment for the students of both colleges.

This initiation of IPE at SQU is considered to be in its beginning. However, the steering committee is continually assessing progress and is working towards enhancing IPE implementation providing strategies to support its implementation (Table 8.3).

Table 8.3 Strategies to support the implementation of interprofessional education (IPE) [34]

At the institutional level
1. A strong will and commitment of the university leaders is required. This will allow the healthcare professionals to adapt to the changes required with resources and support provided during its implementation
2.The institution should have supportive institutional policies and commitment to supporting IPE. It should be clearly stated and incorporated into the mission or program learning outcomes of an institution
3. The institution should have a goal for IPE as part of a strategic plan. The clinical affiliations should be trained and informed about IPE and must be involved in the strategic planning process
4. The curriculum should be designed in such a way that the IPE is embedded and linked with its learning activities, outcomes, and assessment of learning
5. The learning outcomes of the students should include competencies of interprofessional collaborative practice, such as teamwork, communication, and advocacy
6. The institution must also consider an office or a champion that will be responsible for coordinating educational activities and identifying barriers to progress
7. The institution's administration should prepare and train faculty members to facilitate IPE
8. The institution's administration should motivate the faculty to use IPE to maximize its implementation
At the faculty level
1. An IPE steering committee with a lead person should be appointed to provide directions and monitor IPE implementation
2. Educators from different professions need to collaborate before the commencement of classes to ensure the delivery of effective IPE. Faculty members can share their best practices in a forum to inform the public on the implementation of IPE
3. A regular review or assessment of the implementation of IPE should be conducted. Feedback and results should be shared with stakeholders through scholarly activities such as research and academic conferences. Various tools to evaluate the extent of integrating IPE in the curriculum can be used

8.2.2.5 The Qatari Experience

IPE is an emerging concept in the Middle East, with many health professional education programs and regulatory bodies constantly striving to meet international accreditation standards and requirements to improve the quality of their educational programs and to ensure that the expected standards of excellence are sustained [35]. Qatar's National Vision 2030 aims to create a world-class, integrated healthcare system that can improve the healthcare outcomes of the Qatar's population [36].

The Qatar Interprofessional Health Council (QIHC) was created in 2009 under the leadership of the Dean of the School of Health Sciences at the College of the North Atlantic–Qatar. Its members come from diverse professional backgrounds in both academic and practice settings. Many meetings have been held since the formation of the council, with a shared goal: the design and integration of IPE within existing curricula. The council's six strategic goals are: knowledge management, capacity development, partnerships, role modeling, curricula reform and development, and research and evaluation [37].

"The following mission, vision, and purpose of the council are:

- **Vision:** To lead the education and development of health care professionals and healthcare systems which exemplify best practices in interprofessional care for the people and State of Qatar and the region.
- **Mission:** The QIHC will focus on embedding interprofessional collaboration in healthcare education and practice. Working with partners locally, regionally, and internationally, the QIHC will lead and foster collaborative interprofessional initiatives.
- **Purpose:** To provide a venue for communication and collaboration regarding interprofessional education and practice" [37].

The Bachelor of Pharmacy degree program in the College of Pharmacy at Qatar University (QU CPH) is the first outside of Canada to be fully accredited by the Canadian Council for Accreditation of Pharmacy Programs (CCAPP). Since 2013, the CCAPP accreditation standards have highlighted the importance that programs implement IPE. As a result, an IPE committee was formed at the QU CPH in 2014 to provide the guidance and support to implement IPE within the pharmacy curriculum, as well as in other professional education programs in the country. The committee was formed by representatives from 14 different programs at four institutions: (1) College of Medicine and College of Health Sciences at Qatar University, (2) Weill Cornell Medical College in Qatar (WCMC-Q); (3) the nursing school at the University of Calgary–Qatar (UC-Q), and (4) the College of North Atlantic–Qatar [35].

Led by the Faculty of Pharmacy, Qatar University hosted the first IPE conference in the Middle East in 2015 [38]. The conference covered various aspects of IPE, including students' perceptions of the effectiveness of IPE and the future plans for IPE in Middle Eastern countries, and pilot studies on IPE teaching methods and IPE evaluation. Some of the topics related to the challenges Middle Eastern countries might face in implementing IPE were also covered.

8.2.2.6 The Saudi Arabian Experience

In 2016, the Saudi Arabian government headed by the Custodian of the Two Holy Mosques, King Salman Bin Abdulaziz, approved Saudi Vision 2030. The determination, efforts, and plans to enhance the health and well-being of the Saudi Arabian population was one of the essential elements of this vision [39]. Improving both health professional education and healthcare systems is essential to provide optimal healthcare. It was suggested that one method to achieve that is through IPE and IPCP [39], which would be enacted through collaborative efforts among accrediting entities, the Ministry of Health, the Ministry of Education, the Saudi Commission for Health Specialties, educational institutions, and the public and private healthcare sectors throughout the country.

Official IPE-relevant standards, policies, and regulations have yet to be identified and approved in Saudi Arabia. The Saudi Commission for Health Specialties, however, has mandated that new health professional education programs must meet specific accreditation standards regarding administrative structure, training capacity, goals and objectives, structure and organization, scholarship, evaluation of trainees' performance, and resources [39].

8.3 Regulation

The legal and policy world is full of these words that are often misused. For example, the definitions of *regulation*, accreditation, and licensing are often confusing (see Table 8.1 for definition). In many health systems, regulating health profession typically involves a legal or policy mandates issued by a regulatory authority (oftentimes, a professional body or government entity) for the objective to maintain high standards of practice for the profession. As such, non-compliance to these mandates may lead to administrative or penal consequences for the individual, as the objective of regulation is the control of unwanted behaviors in individuals, contrary to accreditation [6]. Regarding IPE and IPCP, regulation can either be applied through the care environment or by the healthcare professionals themselves. We will explore the latter first.

8.3.1 Professions Vs Occupation

Differentiating between *profession* and *occupation* is not solely semantic. Mostly, the difference is associated with the level of control or scrutiny a healthcare worker faces in their practice. All healthcare workers practice an occupation—a combination of specialized knowledge and techniques [40]. That being said, not all occupations are considered to be *professions*, by legal standards. From the regulatory perspective, a profession is more than a societal standard [40]. Further, a profession is controlled by an array of different policies and regulations that are determined by different governance bodies, which are also responsible for determining reserved activities, scopes of practice, titles, etc. [41] For IPE and IPCP, this implies that the policies needed to promote IPE and IPCP are different, depending on whether the interprofessional team is mostly comprised of professions, or occupations, or a combination of both.

8.3.2 Why Regulate the Health Professions?

Regulating the professions, by determining their scopes of practice and/or by protecting their titles and/or specific activities, is key to quality healthcare and achieving universal health coverage [4]. As a process, *regulation* is rooted in two philosophical approaches; the first is the regulation of the professions themselves, where the individual healthcare worker is the focus of the control (titles and scopes of practice). The second approach is the regulation of the workers' activities, where the focus is the action done to the patient. These two approaches often coexist, the former being applied to large group of individuals and the latter to specific actions or competencies for a smaller group of healthcare workers.

8.3.3 Regulation of the Professions

The regulation of the professions is necessary to protect the public [42]. As is, it promotes the notion that standardized access to a title and/or a specific scope of practice ensures that healthcare workers have the clinical competence to give the desired care and achieve the desired outcomes [43, 44].

8.3.3.1 Legal Structures

There are two systems that influence the regulation of health professions: the prelicensure and the post-licensure systems. First, the prelicensure system is the interface between the educational system and the professional system. For example, what are the criteria used by the regulator to deem an occupation a regulated profession? Then, once the regulations are determined, how can students access the profession (entry to practice or licensure process)? Once students are licensed professionals, the second system comes into play. In the professional, post-licensure system, the regulators are central and interface with different government bodies. For example, are only titles or both titles and scopes of practice reserved? Are codes of ethics enforced by a disciplinary board? What are the criteria to continually maintain certification?

These regulatory elements from these systems can greatly influence IPE and IPCP, from the determination of IPE in the prelicensure curriculum, to the IPE mandate to allow entry to practice and IPCP mandate in the code of ethics (see Fig. 8.1).

8.3.3.2 Available International Models

There are three main models available for the regulation of the health professions, mostly based on the level of control from the government. The *quasi-regulation*

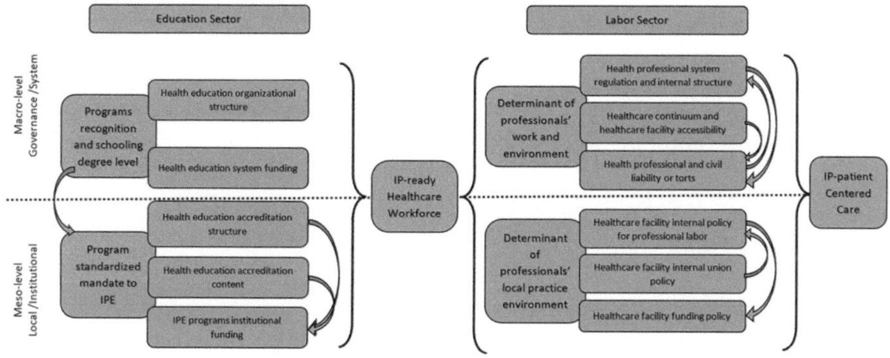

Fig. 8.1 Adapted conceptual model with focus on policy and regulation aspects. (Reproduced with permission from [45]

model is the model with the least involvement from the government, where regulatory bodies or professional associations have the most ownership of the policies that structure their practice. Further, the *co-regulation model* is where there is co-ownership of the regulation and governance of the professions by a regulatory body outside of the government and by the government itself. Finally, the *explicit regulation model* is where the government is the most involved, where the professional associations or regulatory bodies have the least independence and regulatory autonomy [43].

8.3.4 Regulation of Activities

Another way to regulate the professions is through their activities or the care environment. The regulation of specific activities ensures achieving the desired outcomes and minimizing the risk for individual patients. It focuses on a specific clinical competence in a specific context. It can cohabit with the regulation of the professions.

8.3.4.1 Legal Structures

There are two sources for the regulation of activities. First, the healthcare system influences the regulation of professions by determining the practice settings, employment criteria, and even recognition of one profession within the healthcare system [46]. For example, physician assistants, as a profession, are not recognized in all countries or even in all healthcare facilities within the same country, thereby impacting their regulation and presence in the interprofessional teams. Second, the professional system, in addition to regulating scopes of practice, may also regulate specific reserved activities. In combination, these two sources ensure that one care action in a specific setting can only be done by licensed and regulated professionals.

8.3.4.2 Available International Models

There are a few examples available of this approach in different jurisdictions. For example, the Finnish government mandates through its Health Act that primary healthcare systems must be interprofessional by nature—introducing in the fabric of the healthcare system the importance of IPCP [43].

8.4 Summary

Creating accreditation standards for all five domains described by the AIPHE projects [17, 18] (or equivalent) described herein is imperative towards delivering sustainable IPE and IPCP [20]. We hope that accrediting bodies and curriculum developers worldwide can make use of the experience described herein to develop their own accreditation standards and IPE-relevant practices. As per regulation, it is crucial that policymakers and stakeholders act hand in hand to promote a legal environment that fosters IPCP, with healthcare professionals properly trained and prepared to take full advantage of this approach. As an aid to analysis, the following questions can be used as a guide (Table 8.4).

Table 8.4 Reflective questions for policy and legal environment exploration. Reproduced with permission from [45]

Education sector		
Macro level	*Higher education organizational structure*	1. Where are healthcare professionals trained?
		2. How are higher education institutions created?
		3. Do higher education institutions have a governmental mandate to teach IPE?
Meso level	*Higher education accreditation structure*	4. Do higher education healthcare programs have an obligation to be accredited either following a legal obligation or a policy recommendation?
	Higher education accreditation content	5. If education programs/curricula are accredited, are their accreditation standards linked to IPE?
Labor market sector		
Macro level	*Healthcare professional system regulation and internal structure*	1. How are health professions regulated?
		2. How is the scope of practice regulated?
		3. How are health profession regulations enforced within the professional system?
	Healthcare continuum and healthcare facility accessibility	4. How can the patient access specialized care or in-hospital treatment?
		5. How is the in-hospital care episode managed?
		6. How is the continuum of care managed between in-hospital care and community-based care?
	Healthcare professional and civil liability or torts	7. How is the liability or tort system applicable to healthcare professionals or facilities?
		8. How is the "standard of care" determined (how is the action of one professional analyzed by judges or jurists)?
		9. Is there an obligation for liability insurance coverage for healthcare professionals and/or healthcare facilities?

Table 8.4 (continued)

Education sector		
Meso level	*Healthcare facility internal policy for professional labor*	10. What is the employment relationship between healthcare employers (facilities) and healthcare professionals?
		11. How are care activities determined or attributed within one healthcare facility?
	Healthcare facility accreditation structure and content	12. Is there an obligation for healthcare facilities to undergo an accreditation process before accepting patients or give care?
		13. Is there a specific accreditation standard or wording within different standards to mandate interprofessional collaborative practice?

References

1. Zwarenstein M, Reeves S, Perrier L. Effectiveness of pre-licensure interprofessional education and post-licensure collaborative interventions. J Interprof Care. 2005;19(Suppl 1(sup1)):148–65. https://doi.org/10.1080/13561820500082800.
2. Nelson S, White CF, Hodges BD, Tassone M. Interprofessional team training at the prelicensure level: a review of the literature. Acad Med. 2017;92(5):709–16. https://doi.org/10.1097/ACM.0000000000001435.
3. Goldman J, Kitto S, Reeves S. Examining the implementation of collaborative competencies in a critical care setting: key challenges for enacting competency-based education. J Interprof Care. 2018;32(4):407–15. https://doi.org/10.1080/13561820.2017.1401987.
4. World Health Organization. WHO guideline on self-care interventions for health and well-being, 2022 revision. Geneva: World Health Organization; 2022. https://www.who.int/health-topics/universal-health-coverage#tab=tab_1
5. World Health Organization. Health systems strengthening glossary. Geneva: World Health Organization; 2011. https://www.who.int/healthsystems/Glossary_January2011.pdf?ua=1
6. Eaton JS. Is accreditation accountable? The continuing conversation between accreditation and the federal government. Washington, DC: Council for Higher Education Accreditation; 2003. https://www.chea.org/sites/default/files/other-content/CHEAmonograph_Oct03.pdf.
7. World Health Organization. National health workforce accounts: a handbook. Geneva: World Health Organization; 2017. https://apps.who.int/iris/bitstream/handle/10665/259360/9789241513111-eng.pdf?sequence=1.
8. United Nations. Transforming our world: the 2030 agenda for sustainable development. New York: United Nations; 2015. https://sustainabledevelopment.un.org/content/documents/21252030%20Agenda%20for%20Sustainable%20Development%20web.pdf.
9. World Health Organization. Thirteenth general programme of work 2019–2023. Geneva: World Health Organization; 2018. https://apps.who.int/iris/bitstream/handle/10665/324775/WHO-PRP-18.1-eng.pdf.
10. Bogossian F, Craven D. A review of the requirements for interprofessional education and interprofessional collaboration in accreditation and practice standards for health professionals in Australia. J Interprof Care. 2021;35(5):691–700. https://doi.org/10.1080/13561820.2020.1808601.
11. Curran V, Deacon D, Fleet L. Review, assessment and recommendations of accreditation standards, policies, and practices as they relate to interprofessional education for collaborative

patient-centred practice (IECPCP): final report. St. Johns: Centre for Collaborative Health Professional Education, Faculty of Medicine; 2005.
12. Curran VR, Fleet L, Deacon D. A comparative review of Canadian health professional education accreditation systems. Can J High Educ. 2006;36(1):79–102. https://doi.org/10.47678/cjhe.v36i1.183527.
13. Zorek J, Raehl C. Interprofessional education accreditation standards in the USA: a comparative analysis. J Interprof Care. 2013;27(2):123–30. https://doi.org/10.3109/13561820.2012.718295.
14. Gilbert JHV. Abraham Flexner and the roots of interprofessional education. J Contin Educ Heal Prof. 2008;28(Suppl 1(Supplement 1)):S11–4. https://doi.org/10.1002/chp.201.
15. Canadian Interprofessional Health Collaborative. A national interprofessional competency framework. Canadian Interprofessional Health Collaborative. 2010. http://www.cihc-cpis.com/publications1.html.
16. World Health Organization. In: Hopkins D, editor. Framework for action on interprofessional education & collaborative practice. Geneva: World Health Organization; 2010. https://apps.who.int/iris/bitstream/handle/10665/70185/WHO_HRH_HPN_10.3_eng.pdf?sequence=1.
17. Accreditation of Interprofessional Health Education. Interprofessional health education accreditation standards guide. Canadian Interprofessional Health Collaborative; 2011. http://www.cihc-cpis.com/uploads/1/2/4/7/124777443/aiphe_accreditation_standards_guide_phase_2.pdf.
18. Accreditation of Interprofessional Health Education. Principles and practices for integrating interprofessional education into the accreditation standards for six health professions in Canada.
19. D'Amour D, Oandasan I. Interprofessionality as the field of interprofessional practice and interprofessional education: an emerging concept. J Interprof Care. 2005;19 Suppl 1(sup1):8–20. https://doi.org/10.1080/13561820500081604.
20. Grymonpre R, Ateah C, Dean H, Heinonen T, Holmqvist M, MacDonald L, et al. Sustainable implementation of interprofessional education using an adoption model framework. Can J High Educ. 2016;46(4):76–93. https://doi.org/10.47678/cjhe.v46i4.186571.
21. Azzam M, Puvirajah A, Girard M-A, Grymonpre RE. Interprofessional education-relevant accreditation standards in Canada: a comparative document analysis. Hum Resour Health. 2021;19(1):66. https://doi.org/10.1186/s12960-021-00611-1.
22. Canadian Council for Accreditation of Pharmacy Programs. Accreditation standards for Canadian first professional degree in pharmacy programs. Toronto, ON: Canadian Council for Accreditation of Pharmacy Programs; 2018. http://ccapp-accredit.ca/wpcontent/uploads/2016/01/Accreditation-Standards-for-Canadian-First-Professional-Degree-in-Pharmacy-Programs.pdf.
23. Partnership for Dietetic Education and Practice. Accreditation standards for dietetic education programs in Canada. Ottawa, ON: Partnership for Dietetic Education and Practice; 2014. https://www.pdep.ca/library/Accreditation-Policies-and-Standards/PDEP-Accreditation-Standards-for-Dietetic-Educatio.aspx.
24. Commission on Dental Accreditation of Canada. Accreditation requirements for doctor of dental surgery (DDS) or doctor of dental medicine (DMD) programs. Ottawa, ON: Commission on Dental Accreditation of Canada; 2013.
25. Canadian Association of Schools of Nursing. CASN accreditation programs standards. Ottawa, ON: Canadian Association of Schools of Nursing; 2014. https://www.casn.ca/wp-content/uploads/2014/12/2014-FINAL-EN-Accred-standards-March-311.pdf.
26. Canadian Association of Occupational Therapists. Academic accreditation standards and self-study guide. Ottawa, ON: Canadian Association of Occupational Therapists; 2019. https://caot.in1touch.org/uploaded/web/Accreditation/CAOT%20Accreditation%20Self%20Study%20Guide%202017%20English%20rv%202019.pdf.

27. Interprofessional Education Collaborative Expert Panel. Core competencies for interprofessional collaborative practice: report of an expert panel. Washington, DC: Interprofessional Education Collaborative; 2011. https://ipec.memberclicks.net/assets/2011-Original.pdf.
28. Health Professions Accreditors Collaborative. Guidance on developing quality interprofessional education for the health professions. Chicago, IL: Health Professions Accreditors Collaborative; 2019. https://healthprofessionsaccreditors.org/wp-content/uploads/2019/02/HPACGuidance02-01-19.pdf.
29. Australian Government Department Health and Aged Care. National Registration and accreditation scheme. Canberra: Australian Government Department Health and Aged Care; 2019. https://www.health.gov.au/our-work/national-registration-and-accreditation-scheme
30. Australian Health Practitioner Regulatory Agency. Accreditation standards. Melbourne: Australian Health Practitioner Regulatory Agency; 2014. https://www.ahpra.gov.au/Accreditation/Accreditation-standards.aspx
31. The Interprofessional curriculum renewal consortium, Australia. Curriculum renewal for interprofessional education in health. Sydney, NSW: Centre for Research in Learning and Change, University of Technology; 2013. https://nexusipe-resource-exchange.s3.amazonaws.com/AustralianIPECurriculumRenewal_2014.pdf.
32. O'Keefe M, Henderson A, Chick R. Defining a set of common interprofessional learning competencies for health profession students. Med Teach. 2017;39(5):463–8. https://doi.org/10.1080/0142159X.2017.1300246.
33. O'Keefe M. Collaborating across boundaries: a framework for an integrated interprofessional curriculum. Sydney, NSW: Office for Learning and Teaching, Department of Education and Training; 2015.
34. Shakhman LM, Al Omari O, Arulappan J, Wynaden D. Interprofessional education and collaboration: strategies for implementation. Oman Med J. 2020;35(4):e160. https://doi.org/10.5001/omj.2020.83.
35. El-Awaisi A, Wilby KJ, Wilbur K, El Hajj MS, Awaisu A, Paravattil B. A middle eastern journey of integrating Interprofessional education into the healthcare curriculum: a SWOC analysis. BMC Med Educ. 2017;17(1):15. https://doi.org/10.1186/s12909-016-0852-5.
36. General secretariat for development planning. Qatar National Vision 2030. General secretariat for development Planning. 2008. https://www.psa.gov.qa/en/qnv1/Documents/QNV2030_English_v2.pdf.
37. Johnson B, Pyburn R, Bolan C, Byrne C, Jewesson P, Robertson-Malt S, et al. Qatar Interprofessional health council: IPE for Qatar. Avicenna. 2011;2011(1):2. https://doi.org/10.5339/avi.2011.2.
38. First Middle Eastern Conference on Interprofessional Education. Doha, Qatar. Innovations in Global Health Professions Education. 2015.
39. Fallatah HI. Introducing inter-professional education in curricula of Saudi health science schools: an educational projection of Saudi vision 2030. J Taibah Univ Med Sci. 2016;11(6):520–5. https://doi.org/10.1016/j.jtumed.2016.10.008.
40. Abbott A. System of professions: essay on the division of expert labour. Chicago, IL: University of Chicago Press; 1988.
41. Burau V. Governing through professional experts. In: Dent M, Bourgeault IL, Denis J-L, Kuhlmann E, editors. The Routledge companion to the professions and professionalism. Abingdon: Routledge; 2016. p. 109–19.
42. Safriet B. Closing the gap between can and may in health-care providers' scopes of practice: a primer for policymakers. Yale J Reg. 2002;19:310. https://openyls.law.yale.edu/handle/20.500.13051/8007.
43. Girard M-A. Interprofessional collaborative practice and law: a reflective analysis of 14 regulation structures. J Res Interprof Pract Educ. 2019;9(2):1. https://doi.org/10.22230/jripe.2019v9n2a285.

44. Nelson S, Turnbull J, Bainbridge L, Caulfield T, Hudon G, Kendel D, Mowat D, Nasmith L, Postl B, Shamian J, Sketris I. Optimizing scopes of practice: new models of care for a new health care system. Ottawa, ON: Canadian Academy of Health Sciences; 2014. https://cahs--acss.ca/wp-content/uploads/2015/07/Optimizing-Scopes-of-Practice_REPORT-English.pdf.
45. Girard M-A. Interprofessional education and collaborative practice policies and law: an international review and reflective questions. Hum Resour Health. 2021;19(1):9. https://doi.org/10.1186/s12960-020-00549-w.
46. Girard M-A, Régis C, Denis J-L. Interprofessional collaboration and health policy: results from a Quebec mixed method legal research. J Interprof Care. 2022;36(1):44–51. https://doi.org/10.1080/13561820.2021.1891030.

Part III

Interprofessional Education and Collaborative Practice at King Saud University in Riyadh, Kingdom of Saudi Arabia: A Case Study

9 Student-Centered/Self-Directed Learning

Mohammed Yahya Alnaami, Eiad Abdelmohsen Alfaris, Gulam Begum, Mohammed Al Shafaee, and Ciraj Ali Mohammed

9.1 Introduction

Student-centered learning (SCL), also known as learner-centered education, is an approach to education focusing on students' needs, rather than those of others involved in the educational process such as teachers and administrators. The pedagogic shift from the traditional teacher-centered approach, in which the emphasis is on teachers and what they teach, to a student-centered approach, in which the emphasis is on students and what they learn, requires a fundamental change in the roles of the educator from that of a didactic teacher to that of a facilitator, mentor, advisor, or supervisor. This approach has many implications for the design of the curriculum, course content, and interactivity of courses [1, 2]. Self-directed learning (SDL) describes a process by which individuals take the initiative, with or without the assistance of others, in diagnosing their learning needs and formulating learning goals. Furthermore, individuals identify human and material resources for learning,

M. Y. Alnaami (✉)
Department of Surgery, College of Medicine, King Saud University, Riyadh, Saudi Arabia

E. A. Alfaris
Department of Family and Community Medicine, College of Medicine, King Saud University, Riyadh, Saudi Arabia

G. Begum · M. Al Shafaee
Family Medicine, College of Medicine and Health Sciences, National University of Science and Technology, Sohar, Oman

C. A. Mohammed
Medical Education, College of Medicine and Health Sciences, National University of Science and Technology, Sohar, Oman

M. Y. Alnaami et al. (eds.), *Novel Health Interprofessional Education and Collaborative Practice Program: Strategy and Implementation*, https://doi.org/10.1007/978-981-99-3420-1_9

choose and implement appropriate learning strategies, and evaluate learning outcomes [3]. SDL has been recommended as a promising methodology for health science education students to be lifelong learners in this rapidly changing age. However, the concept of SDL continues to be elusive, with students and educators finding difficulty in defining it and agreeing on its worth [4]. In this chapter, our goal is to explore the theory and practice of SCL and SDL, design a blueprint for their inclusion in Health Sciences Colleges (HSCs—Medicine, Dental, Pharmacy, Applied Medical Sciences, Nursing, and Emergency Medical Services) curricula, and design applicable approaches for their implementation. The following sections highlight the strategic steps and initiatives to achieve this goal.

9.2 Strategic Goal 1: Providing High-Quality SCL/SDL Experience for Undergraduate and Postgraduate HSCs Students. That Ensures Best Academic Achievement, Successful Scholarship, Readiness for Employment, and Sustainable Development

This goal is considered to be the first and most important learning goal that constitutes a core issue for learning. It is evident that SCL or SDL is the most effective strategy for best academic achievement [5, 6], as health sciences are witnessing information explosion and continuous renewal. Therefore, old traditional methods such as teacher-centered education might not be effective for millennial learners who are more digital savvy than book readers. Once learning goals of SCL and SDL are achieved, this will pave the way for graduate student to pursue further training and scholarship positions. Those who are familiar with SCL and SDL curricula will find postgraduate training and scholarship easy to adapt with and to become more successful learners [7]. Those who have graduated from student-centered curricula are lifelong learners with talents that employers look for [8].

9.2.1 Objective (Initiative) 1.1: To Provide Means to Get Input from Relevant Stakeholders

The aim of this initiative is to identify all stakeholders who may have a valid input related to SCL/SDL, especially the students, with the strategic plan presented in (Table 9.1). The required timeframe and budget for this and the other initiatives depend on available manpower and resources that will be studied and decided later as a second phase. The way to get input from relevant stakeholders (faculty and students) requires experts who will be able to design and analyze appropriate surveys for students on SCL and SDL achievement and for faculty to get their feedback about these learning strategies. We can use previously published surveys such as the Self-Directed Learning Readiness Scale designed by Gugliemino [9], the Continuing Learning Inventory by Oddi [10], and recent SDL readiness in health science

Table 9.1 Strategic plan for providing means to get input from relevant stakeholders on SCL/SDL

Goal 1: Providing a high-quality student-centered/self-directed learning experience for undergraduate students of HSCs that ensures best academic achievement, successful scholarship, and readiness for employment.			
Objective (1.1): To provide means to get input from relevant stakeholders.			
Initiative (1.1)	**Responsible**	**Accountable**	**Partners**
Identifying all stakeholders who may have a valid input related to learner-centered/self-directed learning.	The T&L Steering Committee and the T&L Units at HSCs.	The VRHS, Deans of HSCs, and the Leadership Committee.	CELT, KSU.
Initiative description			
Getting input from relevant stakeholders involved.			
Requirements and interdependencies			**Stakeholders**
1. Experts to develop and analyze surveys.			Faculty staff, students, employers, and family.
2. Facilitators to administer and collect surveys.			
Action plan			**Estimated time**
1. Developing and adapting students' surveys on self-directed learning achievements (e.g., the Self-Directed Learning Readiness Scale by Gugliemino, the Continuing Learning Inventory by Oddi, and others).			Phase II.
2. Designing and adapting faculty feedback surveys on SCL.			
3. These surveys can be accessed online.			
4. These activities require a 1-day workshop to develop surveys.			
KPIs			**Estimated budget**
1. At least 70% of students' response rate.			Phase II.
2. At least 70% of faculty response rate.			
3. At least 70% of graduates' (interns) response rate.			

SCL student-centered learning, *SDL* self-directed learning, *HSCs* Health Sciences Colleges, *T&L* teaching and learning, *VRHS* vice-rector for health specialties, *CELT* The Center for Excellence in Learning and Teaching, *KSU* King Saud University, *KPIs* key performance indicators

undergraduates [11]. These tools are good to collect information from the learners. However, to collect information from other stakeholders such as teachers, employers, and family, we need to use focus group discussions, interviews, etc. A 1-day workshop involving relevant partners and stakeholders is necessary to develop and agree upon surveys. The items of the surveys should be carefully chosen through the use of standardized procedures to ensure that each respondent can answer the questions at a level playing field to avoid biased opinions that could influence the outcome of the research or study. The process involves asking people for information through a questionnaire, which can be either online or offline. However, with new technologies, it is more preferable to administer surveys using digital media such as social networks, email, or Uniform Resource Locators (URLs). Completed surveys can be also accessed online for ease of administration, collection, and analysis. At least 1 year is required to develop, administer, collect, and analyze surveys on SCL/SDL achievement.

9.2.2 Objective (Initiative) 1.2: To Foster a System That Supports SCL/SDL

This initiative aims to create an environment that supports SCL/SDL, where it can be practiced efficiently at all levels (Table 9.2). This initiative also implies the development of teaching and learning community of students interacting with faculty and potential employers, promotion of open communication, trust, and respect in addressing issues and differences in the students' life experiences. This requires educational support and collaboration among HSCs, e.g., sharing spaces, conferences, workshops, extracurricular activities, etc. This also includes collaborative interactions between students and faculty especially in common areas shared by all HSCs such as research projects, seminars, workshops, and other educational activities. These activities would be further facilitated by providing the necessary resources to achieve this objective including a fully functional online learning management system with a 24-h support desk for both students and teachers, a state-of-the-art health sciences library with an easy access to the literature, small and large group classrooms equipped with all necessary educational tools, available faculty during their office hours for students' reference. A common skills laboratory for all HSCs where students can practice common skills, for example, basic life support, would be ideal for the achievement of this initiative. Also, practical and clinical areas are necessarily to be spacious with areas for small group teaching and student–faculty interactions. The creation of an IT Unit similar to Teaching and Learning (T&L) Units in each HSC was proposed by the IT Deanship for proper networking and facilitation of SCL/SDL. The IT Unit in each HSC also acts as a reference for corresponding faculty and students when pursuing further assistance and IT problem-solving as IT is considered a main resource for T&L. The achievement of SCL/SDL should not be limited to KSU campus but rather collaboration should outreach other universities and health sectors locally or even internationally, e.g., sharing common courses, research, projects, conferences, exchange programs, etc. The development of a scheme to monitor and evaluate cultural and behavioral changes among students and faculty is necessary to measure the achievement and effectiveness of SCL/SDL. The scheme depends on some quality indicators that will be discussed on a subsequent section. Relevant stakeholders include both students and faculty and HSCs administration.

To achieve this initiative, the KPIs and resources outlined in (Table 9.2) can be further explained as follows:

1. Faculty staff in educational institutes and universities are considered the best learning resource for their students throughout history. In addition to their teaching and learning facilitation duties, faculty staff are also encouraged to be available in their office for at least 4 h, which can be split into 2 days/week, for students' inquiries and mentorship, as suggested by the quality deanship.
2. The second important resource for students' learning is a fully functional learning management system with a 24-h support desk for both students and teachers' IT in each HSC at KSU, where they can have easy access to electronic books, journals, lecture notes, reports and reviews, and published theses.

Table 9.2 Strategic plan for fostering a system that supports SCL/SDL

Goal 1: Providing a high-quality student-centered/self-directed learning experience for undergraduate students of HSCs that ensures best academic achievement, successful scholarship, and readiness for employment.			
Objective (1.2): To foster a system that supports SCL/SDL.			
Initiative (1.2)	**Responsible**	**Accountable**	**Partners**
Creating a culture that supports SCL/SDL.	The T&L Steering Committee and the T&L Units at HSCs.	The VRHS, Deans of HSCs, and the Leadership Committee.	CELT, e-Learning and Distance Learning Deanship, and IT Units in each HSC.
Initiative description			
Developing teaching and learning community of students interacting with faculty and potential employers that promotes open communication, trust, and respect in addressing issues and differences in students' life experiences.			
Requirements and interdependencies			**Stakeholders**
1. Educational support and collaboration among HSCs.			Faculty staff, students, and HSCs administration.
2. Interaction among faculty, students, and administration of all HSCs in all educational activities.			
Action plan			**Estimated time**
1. Providing resources for student-centered learning (e.g., faculty office hours, state-of-the-art library, photocopiers, IT resources, etc.)			Phase II.
2. Classrooms designed for small and large groups' education and equipped with all necessary educational tools and internet access.			
3. Providing skills laboratories for formal and informal education.			
4. Clinical practice areas accommodating for learner-centered learning.			
5. Improving faculty and students' encounters by the provision of faculty office hours.			
6. Creating an IT unit in each HSC to support students and faculty to communicate with each other (e.g., intranet) and for other needs.			
7. Developing training and co-operative programs with health sectors outside KSU.			
8. Developing a scheme to monitor and evaluate cultural changes and behavioral implications as a result of the more diverse T&L community with strong interactors with students as part of their T&L experience.			

(continued)

Table 9.2 (continued)

KPIs	Estimated budget
1. Availability of all relevant resources that enhance and promote SCL/SDL.	Phase II.
2. At least 4 h of faculty office hours divided into two parts per week and opened for students' encounters.	
3. Availability of IT units in each HSC college with clear objectives and responsibilities aligned with the T&L units' objectives and responsibilities.	
4. Establishment of educational and training affiliations with other health sectors and universities in the area (e.g., the Ministry of Health, King Saud Bin Abdul-Aziz University, the National Guard, Alfaisal University and KFSH, Princess Nora University, and others).	
5. Degree of adequacy (i.e., a rating) given by expert referees from within and outside KSU on students' interaction with peers, faculty, health staff, patients, community, etc.	
6. Degree of self-confidence and satisfaction for SDL among students based on SDL surveys.	
7. Percentage of activities that involve both students and faculty compared with all other activities in HSCs per year.	
8. Number of health science clubs (centers) that combine both faculty and students as members in HSCs.	
9. Percentage of activities that involve employment sector representatives and beneficiaries in proportion with all activities in HSCs per year.	

SCL student-centered learning, *SDL* self-directed learning, *HSCs* Health Sciences Colleges, *T&L* teaching and learning, *VRHS* vice-rector for health specialties, *CELT* The Center for Excellence in Learning and Teaching, *KSU* King Saud University, *IT* information technology, *KPIs* key performance indicators

3. IT resources should also be complemented by the provision of educational and training facilities, whether in the corresponding HSC and university, or training centers outside KSU, through contractual and scheduled sessions, to enhance students' skills and attitudes.
4. Establishment of measurement tools and external evaluation system to measure and evaluate students' achievement of SCL/SDL.
5. Results of such measurement tools (e.g., surveys) and external evaluation will be compared against national and international educational standards for SCL/SDL achievements by students, to meet quality performance and indicators.
6. SCL/SDL activities should be logged by students and submitted at the end of each course or block to compare it in numbers and percentages with other educational activities.
7. Percentages of activities that involve employment sector representatives and beneficiaries need to be recorded to compare it with all activities in HSCs per year. This will help quality departments in determining the effectiveness of SCL and SDL among students.

The estimated budget for this initiative includes additional resources, which aims to be part of the center of excellence in interprofessional education (CEIPE) resources once established.

9.2.3 Objective (Initiative) 1.3: To Create Exchange Programs Across HSCs

The strategic plan for this initiative is presented in (Table 9.3). Its aim is to develop IPE activities (see Chap. 16). These activities encourage the engagement of both faculty and students in interprofessional health education programs such as courses, research, conferences, campaigns, etc. To achieve this objective, HSCs are required to collaborate with each other to support such core programs. Each HSC can share in the provision of such programs according to available expertise and resources, e.g., the courses "professionalism" and "patient's safety" are currently conducted under the department of medical education, College of Medicine, which are also shared by other HSCs faculty and students. A course in IPE is also proposed by the College of Pharmacy to be added to their curriculum, and the College of Applied/Medical Sciences is preparing to conduct a core course in IT. These courses are also shared by other HSCs. Each HSC should announce such core programs in its corresponding website, the VRHSs, KSU bulletin; and other social media. Highlighting such courses, research projects, conferences, campaigns, and other IPE activities for faculty and students' participation opportunities is an effective way to achieve this initiative. The e-Learning and Distance Learning Deanship at KSU and IT Units in HSCs should facilitate an easy online registration and communication system for such IPE programs. Furthermore, establishment of a separate interprofessional educational center located at the VRHS, or sponsored by any HSC, would be considered an ideal step forward. When it comes to KPIs, the establishment of IPE and

Table 9.3 Strategic plan to create exchange programs across HSCs

<table>
<tr><td colspan="4">Goal 1: Providing a high-quality student-centered/self-directed learning experience for undergraduate students of HSCs that ensures best academic achievement, successful scholarship, and readiness for employment.</td></tr>
<tr><td colspan="4">Objective (1.3): To create exchange programs across HSCs.</td></tr>
<tr><td>Initiative (1.3)</td><td>Responsible</td><td>Accountable</td><td>Partners</td></tr>
<tr><td>Creating exchange programs across colleges to encourage learners to look for interprofessional core courses, research, and other opportunities.</td><td>The T&L Steering Committee and the T&L Units at HSCs.</td><td>The VRHS, Deans of HSCs, and the Leadership Committee.</td><td>The e-Learning and Distance Learning Deanship and the CELT, KSU.</td></tr>
<tr><td colspan="4">Initiative description</td></tr>
<tr><td colspan="4">Developing programs across all HSCs that encourage learners' engagement indifferent learning activities such as interprofessional courses, research, conferences, campaigns, etc.</td></tr>
<tr><td colspan="3">Requirements and interdependencies</td><td>Stakeholders</td></tr>
<tr><td colspan="3">1. Educational support and collaboration among HSCs.</td><td rowspan="2">Faculty staff and students.</td></tr>
<tr><td colspan="3">2. Interaction among faculty, students, and administration of all HSCs in all educational activities.</td></tr>
<tr><td colspan="3">Action plan</td><td>Estimated time</td></tr>
<tr><td colspan="3">1. Developing interprofessional core courses across all HSCs.</td><td rowspan="4">Open (unlimited).</td></tr>
<tr><td colspan="3">2. Highlighting research projects, conferences, campaigns, etc., to all health faculty and students for participation opportunities.</td></tr>
<tr><td colspan="3">3. Developing online registration and communication system for exchange programs.</td></tr>
<tr><td colspan="3">4. Making the teaching, learning, and assessment center at the VRHS as a reference for exchange programs.</td></tr>
<tr><td colspan="3">KPIs</td><td>Estimated budget</td></tr>
<tr><td colspan="3">1. Establishing the Initiative 16.2 (Chap. 16).</td><td rowspan="3">Phase II.</td></tr>
<tr><td colspan="3">2. Establishing online bulletin at the VRHS that announces and links to different interprofessional learning activities.</td></tr>
<tr><td colspan="3">3. Progressive engagement of faculty and students in interprofessional exchange programs throughout the years of implementation (10% first year, 15% second year, 20% third year).</td></tr>
</table>

HSCs Health Sciences Colleges, *T&L* teaching and learning, *VRHS* vice-rector for health specialties, *CELT* Center for Excellence in Learning and Teaching, *KSU* King Saud University, *KPIs* key performance indicators

collaboration among HSCs at any level would be considered an achievement, as part of this initiative. KSU monthly bulletin has been published and accessed by all KSU employers, faculty, and students for many years now. It has a nice design and structure as an electronic and newspaper-like format with a section on health matters. This bulletin can be used at the meantime for all IPE and collaborative announcements as well as links to different learning and training activities until the proposed CEIPE is established and (Phase 2) of the program is operational. Once the latter center is operational, HSC faculty and students' engagement in IPE and other collaborative programs is expected to increase year by year depending on the execution of Chap. 16 goal: "to promote IPE and to develop insights, shared knowledge, and teamwork skills that promote effective collaboration to deliver high and efficient quality care," and its underlying initiatives. The estimated time to achieve this initiative is unlimited as IPE and collaboration among HSCs is a dynamic, and continuous process. The allocated budget for this initiative depends on the operational costs of the bulletin and other related resources, which will be estimated later in (Phase 2).

9.2.4 Objective (Initiative) 1.4: To Foster Team-Based Learning and Extracurricular Team Projects

This initiative is outlined in (Table 9.4). It aims at fostering team-based learning and extracurricular interprofessional team projects that encourage participation and interaction among health sciences students to promote their cognitive, psychomotor, and affective domains in various fields. Team-based learning (TBL) is a student-centered, collaborative learning strategy based on the constructivist learning theory. It is a form of small group learning that gives emphasis to student preparation outside the class and application of knowledge in the class. This creates a framework in which students increasingly hold each other accountable for coming to class prepared and contributing to discussion with their team members and thereby engages in collaborative learning [12, 13]. The nature of TBL lends itself to IPE, with inherent mechanisms that nurture the culture of collaboration among learners from diverse health professions. Interprofessional Team-Based Learning (IP-TBL) essentially involves learning new concepts, developing analytical and reasoning skills, and understanding applications of the concepts. It enables learners from diverse professions to come together and understand and apply the concepts in an interactive way in a safe environment where they are encouraged to make valid arguments to defend their assumptions. Health professions education essentially requires critical thinking and collaborative team work involving learners from various professions to come together. They must exhibit mutual respect and work with a given problem that is contextually relevant to the learner which is linked to the health needs of the population they ought to serve. Interprofessional TBL, besides helping students learn new concepts, also it helps them handle problems better while working as professionals for better patient outcomes. Hence, TBL is increasingly being adopted as an interprofessional educational approach [12, 13]. It involves a cyclical sequence of activities like individual preparation, in-class readiness assurance testing and an application-focused exercise, and team work and immediate feedback embedded in the process [14]. Team-Based Learning involves splitting group of large classes (more than 100 students) with representations from different disciplines into smaller ones (<25 students), incorporating multiple small groups of 7–8 students each, in a single classroom. Students learn how to work in teams through the process of TBL [14].

Table 9.4 Strategic plan for fostering team-based learning (TBL) and extracurricular team projects

Goal 1: Providing a high-quality student-centered/self-directed learning experience for undergraduate students of HSCs that ensures best academic achievement, successful scholarship, and readiness for employment.			
Objective (1.4): To foster team-based learning (TBL) and extracurricular team projects.			
Initiative (1.4)	**Responsible**	**Accountable**	**Partners**
Fostering extracurricular team projects.	The T&L Steering Committee and the T&L Units at HSCs.	The VRHS, Deans of HSCs, and the Leadership Committee.	Deanship for Skills Development, Center for students' Advice and Guidance, and Deanship for Students' Affairs.
Initiative description			
Creating a curriculum for TBL to further enhance SCL/SDL and extracurricular interprofessional programs that encourage participation and interaction among health sciences students to promote their knowledge, skills, and attitudes/values in various fields.			
Requirements and interdependencies			**Stakeholders**
1. Listing all experts on Team-Based Learning in various HSCs to construct a manual on TBL.			Faculty staff and students.
2. Cooperation from HSCs to highlight their extracurricular activities, so they can be easily recognized.			
3. Interaction and support among faculty, students, and administration of all HSCs.			
Action plan			**Estimated time**
1. Highlighting existing TBL curricula and extracurricular programs in each HSC.			Ongoing.
2. Promoting and supporting existing TBL curricula and extracurricular programs and examining how much interprofessional participation these programs can accommodate.			
3. Experts will design a roadmap curriculum/manual for TBL with effective implementation strategies, measurement, and evaluation to be applied by all HSCs (through a 1–2-day workshop).			
4. Creating intercollegiate governance organization for all extracurricular activities (Health Sciences Students' Club).			
5. Developing students' social programs that have input from all colleges.			
6. Supporting and promoting intercollegiate sport programs.			

KPIs	Estimated budget
1. Established instructional curriculum/manual for TBL.	Phase II.
2. At least 50% of the HSC curriculum should involve TBL activities.	
3. At least five extracurricular programs should exist upon surveillance.	
4. At least 50% of these programs have interprofessional participation.	
5. Establishing centralized governance for extracurricular activities.	
6. Establishing at least six new extracurricular social programs.	
7. Establishing a section within the governance structure for sports activities.	

TBL team-based learning, *SCL* student-centered learning, *SDL* self-directed learning, *HSCs* Health Sciences Colleges, *T&L* teaching and learning, *VRHS* vice-rector for health specialties, *KPIs* key performance indicators

9.2.4.1 The Steps Involved in TBL Are as Follows [14, 15]

Step 1: Pre-class Preparation
In this step, students prepare individually before the class with the pre-reading study materials provided to them by the instructor. The pre-reading study material may be in the form of textbook chapters, videos, lecture presentations, articles, etc. with the specific learning objectives.

Step 2: iRAT (Individual Readiness Assurance Test)
Here, each student answers the given multiple-choice questions (MCQs), which can vary from 10 to 20 in numbers from the pre-reading materials provided to them in class. These MCQs should focus on the concepts they need to master in order to be able to solve the Team Application (tAPP) problems.

Step 3: tRAT (Team Readiness Assurance Test)
The same set of MCQs that individual students have answered will be then given to individual teams to solve, which involves team discussion and consensus so as to arrive to an in-class answer. This step uses a typical scratch card as a scoring card wherein the team examines the right answer, which would be hidden by an asterisk sign. This step gives immediate feedback, which helps them improve their decision-making process.

Step 4: Mini Lecture
During this in-class step, the instructor gives clarification on the MCQs for which the team could not find the right answer during tRAT. At the end of the review, students gain confidence that they have adequate knowledge to solve complex problems in the next step, i.e., the Team Application (tAPP).

Step 5: tAPP (Team Application)
The interprofessional teams are presented with scenarios that are relevant to their career/practice but require interventions from diverse health care providers for attainment of positive outcomes. They are asked to find the solution to the given scenario by choosing one of the options provided by the instructor. This happens within the class. This step works on the 4S principle below to ensure that the team activity promotes learning and team development:

1. Significant Problem—A significant case scenario or problem relevant to their practice or carrier is given to the teams. The problem cannot be addressed in silos and can be tackled only by collaborative practice.
2. Same Problem—The same case scenario or problem is given to all the teams.
3. Specific Choice—Teams require to make a most relevant and specific option given.
4. Simultaneous Reporting—All the teams will present their choices simultaneously one after the other.

Step 6: Appeal (Out of Class/Team)

In this step, the team will request the instructor to consider for an alternative answer to the one designated by the instructor as the best option. For this to happen, the appealing team must provide a clear rationale with references as to why they think their chosen option could be considered as good as the "best" option chosen by the instructor.

Step 7: Peer Evaluation

Students should be trained to develop the skill of giving positive feedback about their peers in a constructive format.

9.2.4.2 Steps in Developing TBL Session from the Instructor Perceptive

A backward design beginning with the end in mind is preferred, i.e., this means to start with a clear understanding of your destination is preferred. The first step is to create the application (tAPP) exercise using higher levels of Bloom's Taxonomy. The second step is to create (iRAT) core knowledge needed to solve the application exercise. The third step is to create learning outcomes that match the RATS and select the relevant study material. From the student's perceptive, however, TBL's sequence of steps is forward thinking, which means enabling and guiding students into thinking progressively to address the issue using a collaborative team-based approach.

Group Formation

Transforming a group of diverse individuals into a high-performance team is a difficult task. The primary goal is to create functional teams. In order to achieve this, the group will generally pass through the stages of Forming, Storming, Norming, Performing, and Adjourning as explained by Bruce Tuckman, an educational psychologist using his model of five stages of team development.

Faculty is responsible for the heterogeneous transparent selection criteria of having 7–8 students in one team that would represent various professions such as medicine, dentistry, pharmacy, and nursing. Members in a team have both strengths and weaknesses. When students learn that their assignment to a team is based upon a fair and scientific principle, they value their team members, and realize that each may have some particular strength to bring to the discussion table. The ability to constructively use the strengths while improving upon the weaknesses is also identified as a challenge. A group that overcomes these difficulties will eventually develop the attributes that will effectively allow it to become a functional team [14, 16].

Grading of TBL

TBL can be used for formative or summative assessments. More weightage is given to the team activities, for example, iRAT 25%, tRAT 35%, tAPP 35%, and Peer evaluation 5%. Individual scores are calculated from the Individual Readiness

Assurance Test (iRAT), and the team score is calculated from the Team Readiness Assurance Test (tRAT) and Team application excises (tAPP). Assessing the individual MCQ score and comparing it with team MCQ score will help to determine the level of learning in terms of student understanding, retention, and application of the knowledge. Peer evaluation is done to assess their interprofessional involvement of each member's contribution to the team. Assessment can also include reflective summaries and focus group discussions for ensuring comprehensive learner engagement [14, 17].

TBL Enablers and Barriers

TBL is an instructional strategy that is an ideal fit with IPE. The various elements of TBL facilitate core competencies of IPE and IPCP. The out-of-class activities promote competencies of values/ethics, teamwork, and role clarification in the form of responsibility and accountability. During the pre-class preparation, every member in the team is responsible and accountable for their own learning, honing the skills of self-directed learning. The in-class activities address the competencies of team work and collaboration, effective communication, and shared leadership among the team members. The interdependence built on mutual trust and respect results in the understanding that each team member is unique to achieve desired outcomes. Certain stereotypes and cultural sensitivities have to be taken care of when learners from diverse professions come together, which can often be a challenge. Preparing learning outcomes for an IPE team can be challenging especially while ensuring individual competency during the iRAT. Instead of a single faculty content expert, an IPE session might require multiple faculty staff members [18]. Scheduling IPE sessions always involves logistic issues and incorporating IP-TBL into the curriculum of the professions involved that can be overwhelming right from getting the faculty experts together to preparing learning outcomes, forming teams with the diverse groups of learners, getting the teams to prepare for the out of class activities, and lastly getting the tenets of IPE and collaborative practice together for the in-class application sessions. The faculty who are already used to certain norms in the learning process are likely to pose resistance. A case for extra funding, extra training of faculty, and extra inputs in the curriculum may not go well with many administrators. Therefore, convincing them for a change can also be an arduous task [19–21].

On the other hand, extracurricular team projects require the cooperation among HSCs to announce and highlight all extracurricular activities and make them accessible through KSU bulletin and the VRHSs website. Faculty and students are encouraged to share and participate in these extracurricular activities regardless of the boundaries between HSCs. However, each HSC should control the number of participants and the conduct of its corresponding extracurricular activity. Existing extracurricular programs need to be discussed further by the leadership committee and T&L steering committee members at the VRHSs to see how it can be further promoted to accommodate interprofessional participations. It would be preferred as well that HSC agree upon the creation of intercollegiate governance organization (e.g., Health Sciences Students' Club) for all extracurricular activities. This organization can develop students' social programs that have input from all colleges and promote intercollegiate athletic programs. The KPIs of the strategic planning to achieve this objective are detailed in (Table 9.4). The estimated budget will be decided later in (Phase 2).

9.2.5 Objective (Initiative) 1.5: To Develop Guidelines and Provide Support for Faculty Staff in the Use of SCL/SDL Methods

This initiative aims at developing guidelines and support for faculty staff on how to assist and support learners on SCL/SDL achievements and shift from teacher-centered to learner-centered learning. This requires educational support and collaboration among KSU faculty development programs run by the Deanship for Skills Development, and more specifically by HSCs. Provision of all resources that encourage SCL/SDL is also of paramount importance as discussed earlier in this chapter. To achieve this objective, the T&L Steering Committee needs to develop best practice guidelines for SCL/SDL. This committee can refer to the many reported guidelines in the literature and design new SCL/SDL guidelines that match the strategic plan of the T&L Steering Committee as a whole. In addition to the development of guidelines for SCL/SDL, the T&L Steering Committee needs to ensure its implementation, monitoring, and periodical evaluation. Offering rewards and prizes for best SCL/SDL practices through students' feedback may encourage more practice and innovations for SCL/SDL as it is the case now with the rewards and prizes arranged and given by the Center of Excellence in L&T at KSU for the best innovative projects. Documentation of such SCL/SDL experiences through accredited research projects would also be essential for evaluation and further improvement. Educational research needs to be further emphasized and rewarded by KSU. Further details of this initiative are presented in (Table 9.5).

Table 9.5 Strategic plan for developing guidelines and providing support for faculty staff in the use of SCL/SDL methods

Goal 1: Providing a high-quality student-centered/self-directed learning experience for undergraduate students of HSCs that ensures best academic achievement, successful scholarship, and readiness for employment.			
Objective (1.5): To develop guidelines and provide support for faculty staff in the use of SCL/SDL methods.			
Initiative (1.5)	**Responsible**	**Accountable**	**Partners**
Developing guidelines and providing support for faculty staff in the use of student-centered learning and self-directed learning methods.	The T&L Steering Committee and the T&L Units at HSCs.	The VRHS, Deans of HSCs, and the Leadership Committee.	Deanship for Skills Development, CELT, and the Deanship for Development and Quality, KSU.
Initiative description			
Developing guidelines and support for faculty staff on how to assist and support learners on self-directed achievements and shift from teacher-centered to student-centered learning.			
Requirements and interdependencies			**Stakeholders**
1. Educational support and collaboration among faculty development departments at KSU.			Faculty staff and students.
2. Resources pertinent to student-centered learning.			
Action plan			**Estimated time**
1. Highlighting existing extracurricular programs in each HSC. The T&L Steering Committee will develop best practice guidelines for learner-centered instruction.			Phase II.
2. Ensuring the implementation of these guidelines with continuous monitoring and evaluation.			
3. Teaching credit and rewards for best student-centered instruction based on students' feedback.			
4. Conducting accredited research on student-centered instructional methods.			
KPIs			**Estimated budget**
1. Established guidelines for learner-centered instruction.			Phase II.
2. At least one research paper should be generated from each health science college per year on student-centered effectiveness.			
3. At least three papers of this conducted research should be presented in national and international meetings and get published.			

SCL student-centered learning, *SDL* self-directed learning, *HSCs* Health Sciences Colleges, *T&L* teaching and learning, *VRHS* vice-rector for health specialties, *CELT* The Center for Excellence in Learning and Teaching, *KSU* King Saud University, *KPIs* key performance indicators

9.2.6 Objective (Initiative) 1.6: To Develop Faculty Training and Development Programs in Student-Centered Methodologies

This initiative is presented in (Table 9.6). It aims at faculty preparation and development on SCL/SDL. This implies training and development of faculty on a regular basis in order to master guiding and facilitation skills required for student-centered

Table 9.6 Strategic plan for developing faculty training and development programs in SCL/SDL

Goal 1: Providing a high-quality student-centered/self-directed learning experience for undergraduate students of HSCs that ensures best academic achievement, successful scholarship, and readiness for employment.			
Objective (1.6): To develop faculty training and development programs in learner-centered methodologies.			
Initiative (1.6)	**Responsible**	**Accountable**	**Partners**
Developing faculty training and development programs in learner-centered methodologies.	The T&L Steering Committee and the T&L Units at HSCs.	The VRHS, Deans of HSCs, and the Leadership Committee.	CELT, Deanship for Skills Development, and HSCs.
Initiative description			
Training and developing faculty on a regular basis to master the guiding and facilitation skills required for student-centered education based on needs assessment and training students, parallel to faculty, as self-directed learners.			
Requirements and interdependencies			**Stakeholders**
1. Educational support and collaboration among faculty development programs.			Faculty staff and students.
2. Resources re-allocation and sharing for faculty development programs.			
Action plan			**Estimated time**
1. Conducting needs assessment for faculty and students training related to learner-centered methodology.			Ongoing.
2. Conducting periodic on-site and electronic workshops at KSU level as well as at HSCs level to train faculty to master roles and responsibilities on student-centered instruction.			
3. Collaborating with the Deanship for Skills Development, e-Learning Deanship,			
4. Medical Education Department, etc. at KSU to design local faculty training programs and support them to attend and share in national/international faculty development programs.			
5. Measuring the transfer of learner-centered skills to the workplace through research, students' feedback, peer feedback, etc.			
6. Making use of these outcomes for further improvement.			
7. Recording and storing all on site activities in a database server at the VRHS.			

(continued)

Table 9.6 (continued)

KPIs	Estimated budget
1. Conducting at least one workshop at the beginning of each semester in each HSC on SCL facilitation.	Phase II.
2. Supporting specified faculty in collaboration with the Skills Development Deanship to attend at least one national or one international faculty development program in health profession education per year.	
3. At least one research paper should be generated from all HSCs per year on learner-centered instruction with a copy submitted to the VRHS' database server.	
4. One mandatory orientation course should be conducted each semester for new faculty on "teaching how to teach" and in a learner-centered environment with provision of a certificate on teaching excellence.	
5. At least 75% of faculty staff in each HSC have had structured training on learner-centered instruction by the end of the year.	

SCL student-centered learning, *SDL* self-directed learning, *HSCs* Health Sciences Colleges, *T&L* teaching and learning, *VRHS* vice-rector for health specialties, *CELT* The Center for Excellence in Learning and Teaching, *KSU* King Saud University, *KPIs* key performance indicators education as well as training students parallel to faculty as self-directed learners. Based on needs assessment, these faculty development activities can be recurring and/or changing. This requires educational support and collaboration between the Deanship for Skills Development at KSU and HSCs faculty development programs, and among HSCs with a common central reference to the Interprofessional Health Education Center as discussed earlier. These faculty development programs also require continuous support from KSU administration for resources re-allocation and sharing to serve this objective. Needs assessment of SCL/SDL can be ascertained through surveys administered to both faculty and students. These should be conducted periodically every year. After needs are highlighted, onsite and electronic workshops at the VRHSs level as well as at HSCs level can be designed and conducted to train faculty to master roles and responsibilities on student-centered instruction. In addition to what KSU is offering for its faculty to attend and share in local and international CME activities, faculty development programs (FDPs) in education should also be encouraged and supported by all partners especially at the Deanship for Skills Development at KSU headquarters. Research should be conducted, and faculty, student, and peer feedback in SCL/SDL should be collected to measure and ensure the transfer of this initiative to workplaces. Results of these research and feedback activities should also be used for further improvement, and saved in a common database server located at the VRHS for purposes of documentation and retrieval when needed. The allocated budget will be decided later as (Phase 2).

9.2.7 Objective (Initiative) 1.7: To Create Outreach Programs That Enhance Student-Centered Learning

This initiative is summarized in (Table 9.7). It aims to create programs that allow students to reach to almost all health care and educational facilities at KSU, in the region, or even abroad, as an integral part of their own self-directed learning

Table 9.7 Strategic plan for developing faculty training and development programs in SCL/SDL

Goal 1: Providing a high-quality student-centered/self-directed learning experience for undergraduate students of HSCs that ensures best academic achievement, successful scholarship, and readiness for employment.			
Objective (1.7): To create outreach programs that enhance student-centered learning.			
Initiative (1.7)	**Responsible**	**Accountable**	**Partners**
Creating outreach programs that enhance student-centered learning.	The T&L Steering Committee and the T&L Units at HSCs.	The VRHS, Deans of HSCs, and the Leadership Committee.	Center for Students' Advice and Guidance, Deanship of the Preparatory Year, and Health Care and Educational Facilities outside KSU.

(continued)

Table 9.7 (continued)

Initiative description	
Creating programs that allow students to reach to almost all health care and educational facilities in the region and abroad, as an integral part of their own self-directed learning experience.	
Requirements and interdependencies	**Stakeholders**
1. Cooperation with HSCs to explain their health care and educational facilities on their corresponding websites at KSU.	Undergraduate and postgraduate graduate students and supervising faculty staff
2. Secretarial cooperation of various health care and educational departments.	
3. Cooperation among national and international health care and educational programs.	
Action plan	**Estimated time**
1. Developing programmed visits to health colleges to educate and empower students at the preparatory program to make a career choice that can positively impact personal competencies through their peers.	Phase II.
2. Creating connections with health care sectors across the city/country for employment requirements, needs, opportunities, etc.	
3. Making students' exchange programs possible with national and international universities for electives, courses, graduate and postgraduate programs.	
4. Making graduate and postgraduate students as part of the team from KSU visiting other health/educational sectors within and outside the country that offer exceptional health care and education.	
KPIs	**Estimated budget**
1. Establishing a programmed schedule of preparatory year students to visit HSCs.	Phase II.
2. Establishing an orientation day during summer at the preparatory year for high school graduates.	
3. Establishing an office at the VRHS for health sciences undergraduate and graduates' exchange programs to do internship electives across the city/country; national postgraduate programs through the SCFHS and internationally through the postgraduate program at the VRHS; job opportunities, etc.	
4. Establishing at least one outreach health care and education program through the VRHS to help in fulfilling national needs in these areas.	

SCL student-centered learning, *SDL* self-directed learning, *HSCs* Health Sciences Colleges, *T&L* teaching and learning, *VRHS* vice-rector for health specialties, *CELT* The Center for Excellence in Learning and Teaching, *KSU* King Saud University, *KPIs* key performance indicators

experience. These programs should facilitate the involvement of HSCs students in various educational/experiential and research activities to expand their insights and perceptions to new experiences and see what others are doing. This may give students a holistic view on health problems and issues in the community, so they can direct their study accordingly and even choose their right future career. This direction requires that HSCs start this initiative by disclosing their health care and educational activities on their corresponding websites and KSU bulletin, highlight opportunities for students and even faculty involvement in different educational and experiential and research activities, secretarial cooperation of various health care, and educational departments to facilitate this initiative when students or faculty are inquiring or want to meet responsible bodies, as well as initiating cooperation programs among national and international health care and educational facilities. To achieve this objective, HSCs should develop programmed visits to HSCs to educate and empower students at the preparatory program to make a career choice that can positively impact personal competencies through their peers. HSCs should also cooperate to create connections with health care sectors across the city/country for employment requirements, needs, opportunities, etc. Another way to facilitate SCL/SDL is to make students' exchange programs possible with national and international universities for electives, courses, graduate and postgraduate programs. An example of such exchange programs is the agreement between KSU and Western Ontario University, Ontario, Canada, to make exchange of residents in clinical residency programs where residents can spend at least 2 years outside their mother university, and these years will be counted as part of the training program in either university. Furthermore, after completion of the program, the graduate can set for the Royal College of Physicians and Surgeons of Canada (RCPSC) and the Saudi Commission for Health Specialties (SCFHS) Examinations equally. HSCs should also make opportunities for graduate and postgraduate students to attend and share in conferences and meetings or even be as part of the team visiting other health/educational sectors within and outside the country, which offer exceptional health care and education. Estimated timeframe and budget for this initiative will be decided later as (Phase 2).

9.3 Discussion

Health professional education played a central role in the vast improvements in health care systems and scientific research over the last century. More recent developments, however, including the rapid expansion of health sciences information, the increasing complexity of care, the vast use of IT, and new generations of learners, have posed different challenges to educators and educational institutions. In order to cope with these changes and challenges, education across all health professions needs to be more adaptive, integrated, transformative, and interdependent [22]. These changes and challenges require a type of learning that is mostly student-centered and self-directed. In addition to these general drivers, our program was launched because of major changes and developments at KSU as it is preparing for national accreditation by the National Commission for Academic Accreditation and Assessment (NCAAA) [23] that advocates student-centered and self-directed learning. KSU is also striving to respond to local market demands and needs. Student-centered learning environments have been shown to be effective in higher education [24]. They have been defined specifically within higher education as both a mindset and a culture within a given educational institution and as a learning approach broadly related to, and supported by, constructivist theories of learning. SCL/SDL are characterized by innovative methods of teaching which aim to promote learning in communication with teachers and other learners and which pay careful attention to students as active participants in their own learning and foster transferable skills such as clinical skills [25], problem-solving, critical thinking, and reflective thinking [26, 27]. Also, assessment is different in SCL, which typically involves more formative assessment and less summative assessment than teacher-centered learning [28]. In student-centered learning, students participate in the evaluation of their learning [29]. This means that students are involved in deciding how to demonstrate their learning. Therefore, developing assessment that supports learning and motivation is essential to the success of student-centered approaches. New students' generations are relying more on electronic and internet-driven learning than reading textbooks and journals, which require a curriculum that merges technology and pedagogy with a substantial commitment of resources and recognition of faculty time and change-management issues [30].

9.4 Summary

Student-centered/self-directed learning is the first learning goal in this case study. The strategy for achieving this goal involves seven initiatives. First, to get input from relevant stakeholders involved. Second, to foster a system that supports SCL/SDL. Third, to create exchange programs across HSCs. Fourth, to foster team-based learning (TBL) and extracurricular team projects. Fifth, to develop guidelines and provide support for faculty staff in the use of SCL/SDL methods. Sixth, to develop faculty training and development programs in learner-centered methodologies. Seventh, to create outreach programs that enhance student-centered learning. The strategic details for each initiative were outlined. The estimated time needed to complete each initiative and its budget details depends on studies, meetings, and discussions by relevant stakeholders involved during the implementation process.

References

1. Harden RM, Sowden S, Dunn WR. Some educational strategies in curriculum development: the SPICES model. Dundee: Association for the Study of Medical Education; 1984. (Medical education booklet No 18).
2. Nicklen P, Rivers G, Ooi C, Ilic D, Reeves S, Walsh K, et al. An approach for calculating student-centered value in education – a link between quality, efficiency, and the learning experience in the health professions. PLoS One. 2016;11(9):e016294.
3. Knowles M. "Self-directed learning: a guide for learners and teachers". New York: Associated Press, 1975. 135 pp., paperbound. Group Org Stud. 1977;2(2):256–7.
4. Murad MH, Varkey P. Self-directed learning in health professions education. Ann Acad Med Singap. 2008;37(7):580–90.
5. Miflin BM, Campbell CB, Price DA. A conceptual framework to guide the development of self-directed, lifelong learning in problem-based medical curricula. Med Educ. 2000;34(4):299–306.

6. Hendricson WD, Andrieu SC, Chadwick DG, Chmar JE, Cole JR, George MC, et al. ADEA Commission on Change and Innovation in Dental Education. Educational strategies associated with development of problem-solving, critical thinking, and self-directed learning. J Dent Educ. 2006;70(9):925–36.
7. Zimmerman BJ, Schunk DH, editors. Self-regulated learning and academic achievement: theory, research, and practice. New York, NY: Springer; 1989.
8. Fraser SW, Greenhalgh T. Coping with complexity: educating for capability. BMJ. 2001;323(7316):799–803.
9. Bonham LA. Guglielmino's self-directed learning readiness scale: what does it measure? Adult Educ Q. 1991;41(2):92–9.
10. Oddi LF. Development and validation of an instrument to identify self-directed continuing learners. Adult Educ Q. 1986;36:97–107.
11. Rascón-Hernán C, Fullana-Noell J, Fuentes-Pumarola C, Romero-Collado A, Vila-Vidal D, Ballester-Ferrando D. Measuring self-directed learning readiness in health science undergraduates: a cross-sectional study. Nurse Educ Today. 2019;83:104201.
12. Parmelee DX, Michaelsen LK. Twelve tips for doing effective Team-Based Learning (TBL). Med Teach. 2010;32(2):118–22.
13. Parmelee DX, Hudes P. Team-based learning: a relevant strategy in health professionals' education. Med Teach. 2012;34(5):411–3.
14. Parmelee D, Michaelsen LK, Cook S, Hudes PD. Team-based learning: a practical guide: AMEE guide no. 65. Med Teach. 2012;34(5):e275–87.
15. Guadagnoli JA, Miller TW. Interprofessional education: a team-based learning approach. Med Sci Educ. 2016;26(3):389–95.
16. Black EW, Blue AV, Davidson R, McCormack WT. Using team-based learning in a large interprofessional health science education experience. J Interprofessional Educ Pract. 2016;5:19–22.
17. Nakamura S, Ohtsuki M, Miki Y, Noda T, Suzuki S, Maeno T, et al. Effect of team-based learning in interprofessional education at a health university. Fujita Med J. 2017;3(2):33–9.
18. Chan LK, Ganotice F Jr, Wong FKY, Lau CS, Bridges SM, Chan CHY, et al. Implementation of an interprofessional team-based learning program involving seven undergraduate health and social care programs from two universities, and students' evaluation of their readiness for interprofessional learning. BMC Med Educ. 2017;17(1):221.
19. Lochner L, Girardi S, Pavcovich A, Meier H, Mantovan F, Ausserhofer D. Applying interprofessional Team-Based Learning in patient safety: a pilot evaluation study. BMC Med Educ. 2018;18(48):1–9.
20. Burgess A, Kalman E, Haq I, Leaver A, Roberts C, Bleasel J. Interprofessional team-based learning (TBL): how do students engage? BMC Med Educ. 2020;20(118):1–11.
21. Burgess A, van Diggele C, Matar E. Interprofessional team-based learning: building social capital. J Med Educ Curric Dev. 2020;7:2382120520941820.
22. Frenk J, Chen L, Bhutta ZA, Cohen J, Crisp N, Evans T, et al. Health professionals for a new century: transforming education to strengthen health systems in an interdependent world. Lancet. 2010;376(9756):1923–58.
23. Standards for Program Accreditation. National Center for Academic Accreditation and Evaluation (NCAAA). Kingdom of Saudi Arabia Education & Training Evaluation Commission. 2018. https://www.ncaaa.org.sa/Portal/Accreditation/Institutional/Documents/standards/StandardsforProgramAccreditation.pdf.
24. Wright GB. Student-centered learning in higher education. Int J Learn High Educ. 2011;23:93–4.
25. Tolsgaard MG. Clinical skills training in undergraduate medical education using a student-centered approach. Dan Med J. 2013;60(8):B4690.
26. Attard A, Iorio ED, Geven K, Santa R. Student-centered learning SCL toolkit. Brussels: European Students' Union Report; 2014.

27. Hoidn S. Student-centered learning environments in higher education classrooms. New York, NY: Palgrave Macmillan; 2017.
28. Crumly C. Pedagogies for student-centered learning: online and on-ground. Lanham, MD: Fortress Press; 2014. p. 118.
29. Jahnke I. A way out of the information jungle. In: Coakes E, editor. Technological change and societal growth: analyzing the future. Hershey, PA: IGI Global; 2012. p. 182.
30. Fleiszer DM, Posel NH. Development of an undergraduate medical curriculum: the McGill experience. Acad Med. 2003;78(3):265–9.

Learning Theories 10

Dalal Abdullah Alqahtani, Mohammed Yahya Alnaami, and Eiad Abdelmohsen Alfaris

10.1 Introduction

In recent years, several changes have influenced the healthcare map. These include changes in the number and types of diseases, healthcare systems, and patients. This has led to a need to reassess how tomorrow's healthcare professional should be educated, and it has produced an immediate need to create educational programs with real impact on the learning process and its outcomes [1]. Moreover, many institutes have adopted and implemented major innovations in health professions' education curricula. These changes are mostly pedagogical in nature; that is, they are concerned with how content is taught, as opposed to what is taught. Innovations in health professions education aim to produce competent and motivated learners. The goal of pedagogical reform is to make health colleges more engaging, to enhance learning, and to help our graduates develop the skills they need to become lifelong learners and critical thinkers [2]. Learning can be defined as a process by which individuals gain new knowledge and skills with a relatively permanent change in attitudes, thoughts, feelings, motions, and actions [3]. Learning theory is a framework describing, explaining, and predicting how people learn [3].

D. A. Alqahtani
Oral Medicine and Diagnostic Sciences, College of Dentistry, King Saud University, Riyadh, Saudi Arabia

M. Y. Alnaami (✉)
Department of Surgery, College of Medicine, King Saud University, Riyadh, Saudi Arabia

E. A. Alfaris
Department of Family and Community Medicine, College of Medicine, King Saud University, Riyadh, Saudi Arabia

M. Y. Alnaami et al. (eds.), *Novel Health Interprofessional Education and Collaborative Practice Program: Strategy and Implementation*,
https://doi.org/10.1007/978-981-99-3420-1_10

Learning theories that have been proposed by educational psychologists include the behaviorist, cognitive, social, psychodynamic, and humanistic learning theories. The behaviorist learning theory, first described by Pavlov [4], states that learning depends on a stimulus, e.g., posing a problem (stimulus) would stimulate ways to find solutions. Behaviorist learning can be stimulated by a trigger, problem, or a question. Moreover, Pavlovian conditioning describes that response to stimuli needs to be conditioned (prioritized) by appropriate recipient, learning environment, and prior experience. The constructivist learning theory views learning as a building process in which a learner builds new learning on previous learning of the same subject area. Learners make meaning based on their prior learning, prior experience, and other environmental factors. So, learning is a complex process where different learners may learn/understand the same phenomenon differently based on their prior learning and experience [5, 6].

The cognitive learning theory, after the Russian Psychologist Lev Vygotsky, describes how learning is acquired and stored in the brain. So, the cognitive theory of learning emphasizes what happens to the neural networks (i.e., schemata) of the brain when concepts are learned and how are they stored in the memory [7]. The structure of knowledge described by Bloom [8], revised later by Krathwohl [9], implies that learning develops through several steps as highlighted in (Fig. 10.1). The first and most primitive step is to learn through recognition and recalling knowledge facts by reading, watching, or hearing. The second step is understanding what these facts mean. The third step is applying these facts to real life and practice. The fourth step is analyzing these facts by critically studying each component. The fifth

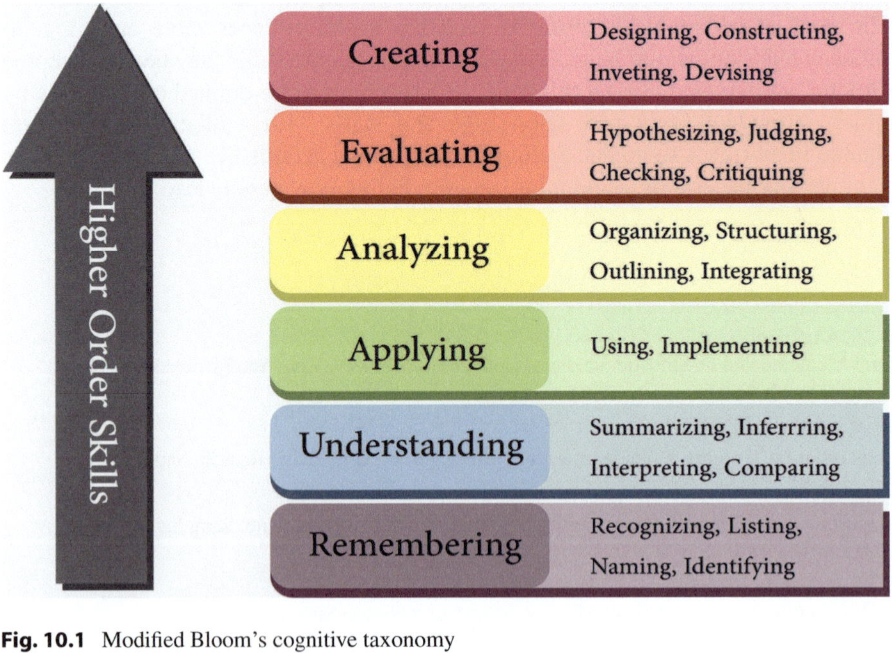

Fig. 10.1 Modified Bloom's cognitive taxonomy

step is to evaluate and judge the value of these facts. The sixth step is to create and invent new knowledge (e.g., through research). The last step is a hierarchy that was added by Bloom's followers.

The social learning theory, which is largely the work of Bandura [10], depends on learning from others who formulate the social context or norms. Albert Bandura also considers the learner's personal characteristics, behavioral patterns, and environment as important complements to the social norms (Bandura's mapping of social learning). Role modeling, which is a perceived behavior to be reinforced by the learner is also part of the social theory. Vicarious reinforcement, however, views other people's emotions and behavior positively, which facilitates learning or negatively inhibits it. The psychodynamic learning theory, based on the work of Freud and his followers, depends on self-desire and preparedness to learn even in stressful and difficult situations and aggressive behavior of others [11]. Motivation, whether internally or externally driven, also plays a major role in the psychodynamic learning theory. Positive motivators enhance learning, while negative motivators inhibit learning. The ego defense mechanisms [3] are ways to protect the self from a perceived threat (or negative motivators). These mechanisms (or tactics) that deal with a perceived threat (verbal or physical) may include:

1. *Denial:* Ignoring or refusing to acknowledge the reality of the threat.
2. *Rationalization:* Explaining or excusing away a threat.
3. *Displacement:* Taking out aggression on other individuals rather than directing anger at the source of the threat.
4. *Depression:* Keeping unacceptable thoughts, feelings, or actions from conscious awareness.
5. *Regression:* Returning to an earlier stage of behavior as a way coping with a threat.
6. *Intellectualization:* Minimizing anxiety by responding to a threat in a detached, abstract manner without feeling or emotion.
7. *Projection:* Seeing one's own unacceptable characteristics or desires on other people.
8. *Reaction formation:* Expressing or behaving the opposite of what is really felt.
9. *Sublimation:* Converting repressed feelings into socially acceptable action.
10. *Compensation:* Making up for weaknesses by excelling in other areas.

The *humanistic learning theory*, described by Rogers [12], Snowman and McCown [13], depends on individuals' needs, feeling about themselves, and desire to grow in positive ways. Humanistically, individuals cannot be denied learning, and they can pursue their own needs based on their socioeconomic class, ethnic background, color, or nationality. Maslow's hierarchy [14] of such needs is summarized in Fig. 10.2. The teacher's role in humanistic learning theory is to assess and encourage changes in the learner's needs, self-concept or belief, and feelings by providing support, freedom to choose, and opportunities for spontaneity and creativity.

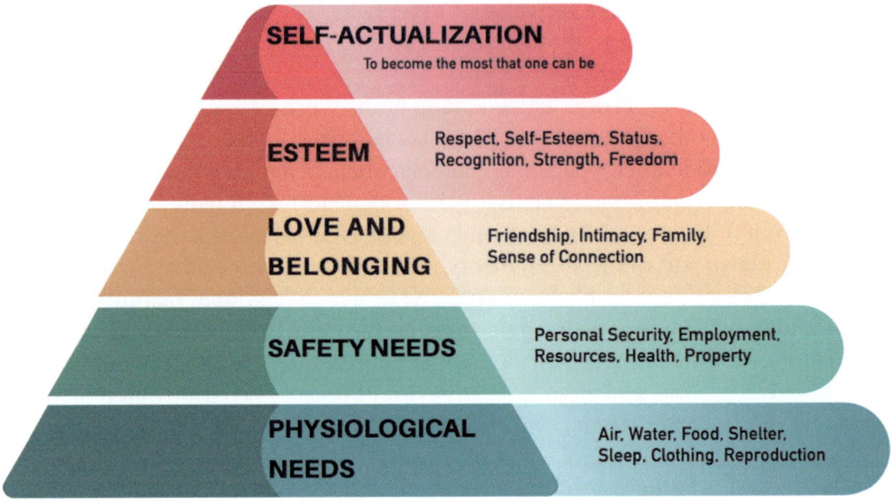

Fig. 10.2 Maslow's hierarchy of needs

10.2 Applying Learning Theories to Health Care

These psychological learning theories can be used singly or in combination according to the situation or context. Some theories might be suitable or applicable for certain individuals, but not for others. Therefore, teachers need to assess personal characteristics of the learner(s) in order to find and apply best learning strategy and environment. Motor skills are also linked to these learning theories, hence mostly described as psychomotor skills learning. Positive attitudes and emotions are integral products of such learning theories if well applied to proper contexts and situations.

Learning theories can be applied at all age groups; however, preschool age may learn best following the cognitive and behaviorist learning theories. Moreover, the social learning theory (where learners interact with social norms) and the constructivist learning theory (where learners build more learning on previous experience) may be more applicable for school age learners. When it comes to graduate (adult) learners, hierarchy learning skills can also be acquired when the psychodynamic learning theory is added to the aforementioned learning theories. The humanistic learning theory must be applied across all age groups. The challenge of adult education is to empower adult learners with the competencies needed to function in a constantly dynamic environment [15]. This highlights the centrality of lifelong learning and critical thinking skills in the new wave of curricular changes, as it reflects the rapidity with which knowledge in the field of health science is evolving. It is often said that much of what is learned will be outdated in less than ten years.

Consequently, the majority of learning occurs after a student graduates, making independent learning skills essential for graduates. At KSU, our goal is to promote learning that utilizes the principles of adult learning to create optimal curricula for the twenty-first-century health sciences student.

10.3 Strategic Goal 2: Promoting Learning that Benefits from the Appropriate Learning Theories in the Right Context Based on Adult Learning Principles

This goal was developed in the early phase of this program after multiple workshops in which key faculty and educators, student representatives, external consultants, and other relevant stakeholders worked together. They agreed upon the need to change how learning occurs, noting that it should be based on adult learning principles. According to these principles, students should be independent and self-directed, have various degrees of life experience, be practical, be goal-oriented, and be motivated more by internal than external factors. As we mentioned earlier, most of HSCs have already moved in this direction, reforming their curricula based on these principles. To support such progress, we propose several initiatives, which are outlined below:

10.3.1 Objective (Initiative) 2.1: To Provide Learning Theory Resources

The strategy for this initiative is presented in Table 10.1. This initiative highlights the importance of providing HSCs with resources on learning theories. This can be accomplished through building and monitoring the collection of suitable references (such as books, journals, and online databases) that can be utilized to enhance teaching and learning in each HSC. Through these resources, faculty and students will have the opportunity to enhance their learning and teaching skills. Collaboration among medical educationists within HSCs is required to gather these resources, as they can be considered the best to select the most appropriate resources based on learning theories that are relevant to the health context and that would support the move toward curricular innovation. The faculty are an important target, and the aim is to enhance their access to information about effective educational tools and to show them the latest research on learning theories. These resources will help improve students to develop their thinking and study skills. Furthermore, it will also help them develop their identities, which Chickering and Reisser [16] define as "the summation of an individual's competence, emotions, autonomy, purpose, integrity, and interpersonal relationships." They argue that identity formation is one of the major goals of the undergraduate's experience. For implementation, not only a must list of educational resources should be prepared, but the progress in the gathering

Table 10.1 Strategic plan for establishing learning theory resources in each health science college (HSC)

Goal 2: Promoting learning that benefits from the appropriate learning theories in the right context based on adult learning principles			
Objective (2.1): To provide learning theory resources			
Initiative (2.1) Building a collection of references (books, journals, online databases, etc.) on appropriate learning theories in each HSC	**Responsible** The T&L Unit/ Medical Education Department in each HSC	**Accountable** The VRHS and Deans of HSCs	**Partners** The T&L Steering Committee, Deanship of Library Affairs, and Deanship of E-learning and Distance Learning
Initiative description Based on the learning theories appropriate for medical education, building and monitoring the establishment of suitable references in each HSC that can enhance teaching and learning			
Requirements and interdependencies 1. Medical educationist collaboration			**Stakeholders** Faculty staff and students
Action plan 1. Providing educational resources that facilitate and support learning 2. Monitoring and evaluating the progress of establishment and utilization of learning resources			**Estimated time** Phase II
KPIs 1. Availability of 70% of intended authoritative references on leaning theories 2. More than 50 % utilization of those references			**Estimated budget** Phase II

T&L teaching and learning, *VRHS* vice-rector for health specialties, *HSCs* health sciences colleges, *KPIs* key performance indicators

and utilization of these resources should be monitored and evaluated as well. The required timeframe and budget for this and the other initiatives depend on available manpower and resources, which will be studied and decided at a second phase.

10.3.2 Objective (Initiative) 2.2: To Develop Guidelines as to the Applicable Learning Theories

This initiative's strategy, presented in (Table 10.2), involves the composition of guidelines regarding relevant learning theories that address dealing with students as adult learners. Knowles [17] identifies several elements that help adults learn. For instance, they need an effective learning climate where they feel safe and comfortable in expressing themselves. They also need to be involved in mutual planning of relevant methods and curricular content, as well as in diagnosing their own needs; this will help trigger internal motivation. Students need to be encouraged to set their own learning objectives, which gives them more control over their learning. They must also learn to identify resources and devise strategies to use the resources to achieve their objectives. Throughout this process, they need support in carrying out

Table 10.2 Strategic plan for developing practical guidelines of the relevant learning theory resources

Goal 2: Promoting learning that benefits from the appropriate learning theories in the right context based on adult learning principles			
Objective (2.2): To develop guidelines as to the applicable learning theories			
Initiative (2.2)	**Responsible**	**Accountable**	**Partners**
Establishing guidelines for health sciences learning theories based on adult learning principles	The T&L Steering Committee and the T/L Unit/Medical Education Department in each HSC	VRHS, Leadership Committee, and Deans of HSCs	CELT and Deanship for Quality and Development, KSU
Initiative description These guidelines should provide general approaches as to how health sciences learning is best implemented in health sciences educational curricula			
Requirements and interdependencies 1. Health profession educationist and educational psychologists' collaboration		**Stakeholders** Faculty staff and students	
Action plan 1. Conducting focus group discussions in each HSC on current use of learning theories 2. Conducting introduction workshop on the appropriate use of learning theories in the right context for health sciences' learning 3. Identifying appropriate learning theories to the particular learning context and competency in each HSC 4. Developing a handbook on the applied aspect of learning theories on health sciences		**Estimated time** Phase II	
KPIs 1. Establishment of database on the current use of learning theories in each HSC 2. >70% of participants are satisfied with the workshop results 3. Production of a handbook on learning theories and practice		**Estimated budget** Phase II	

T&L teaching and learning, *VRHS* vice-rector for health specialties, *CELT* center for excellence in learning and learning, *HSCs* health sciences colleges, *KPIs* key performance indicators

and evaluating their learning. Through feedback and reflection, their critical reflection skills will be developed [18]. The proposed guidelines will outline the general approaches to optimal learning that can be implemented in each HSC. Also, it will provide a link between theory and practice. To write these guidelines, collaboration between health profession educationists and educational psychologists at KSU is required. The proposed action plan for this initiative begins with an assessment of the current teaching and learning practices in each HSC, which will be carried out through focus group meetings with the faculty and students. Based on the results, relevant learning theories will be categorized according to the particular learning contexts and competencies developed in each HSC. Then, a handbook on the application of learning theories in health sciences will be developed.

10.3.3 Objective (Initiative) 2.3: To Develop Workshops for Faculty to Foster Understanding and Practice in the Application of Learning Theories

This initiative's strategy is presented in Table 10.3. In line with the previous initiatives, it aims to enhance learning. This step involves workshops on the appropriate use of learning theories to support teaching and learning practices. These workshops will attempt to show how the gap between educational theory and practice can be bridged. The premise is that by using teaching and learning methods based on educational theories and principles derived from these theories, health profession, teachers can become more effective educators. It will help them develop knowledge, skills, and positive attitudes among their students, thereby improving the next generation of teachers. Ultimately, this should result in better trained health professionals who will provide an even higher level of patient care and improved patient outcomes. This initiative will require planning, implementation, and evaluation. Health professions educationists and external consultants will support this step. Stakeholder satisfaction should be rated over 80% to consider the workshops effective.

Table 10.3 Strategic plan for providing workshops for the faculty on the application of learning theories in teaching and learning

Goal 2: Promoting learning that benefits from the appropriate learning theories in the right context based on adult learning principles			
Objective (2.3): To develop workshops for faculty to foster understanding and practice in the application of learning theories			
Initiative (2.3) Providing workshops on concepts of appropriate use of learning theories in the right context for health sciences education	**Responsible** The T&L Steering Committee and the T/L Unit/Medical Education Department in each HSC	**Accountable** VRHS, Leadership Committee, and Deans of HSCs	**Partners** Deanship for Skills Development and the CELT
Initiative description Conducting workshops on the principles and practice of learning theories in the context of clinical and non-clinical teaching			
Requirements and interdependencies 1. Medical educationist collaboration and external consultants		**Stakeholders** Faculty staff and students	
Action plan 1. Planning and conducting a workshop on learning theories 2. Conducting a workshop on implementation and evaluation		**Estimated time** Phase II	
KPIs 1. More than 80% of increases in knowledge "post-workshop"		**Estimated budget** Phase II	

VRHS vice-rector for health specialties, *T&L* teaching and learning, *CELT* center for excellence in learning and learning, *KSU* King Saud University, *HSCs* health sciences colleges, *KPIs* key performance indicators

10.3.4 Objective (Initiative) 2.4: To Develop and Conduct Introductory Courses for Students to Familiarize Them with the Learning Theories

This initiative's strategy is presented in Table 10.4. As mentioned above, it is important to involve students in learning as theory and practice. For the students to fulfill their role most effectively, their approaches to studying and learning must be grounded on educational learning theories. Understanding the learning process is a key element of the educational learning theory, and it provides a framework for students to plan, create, and learn effectively, as well as for self-assessment. In this light, this initiative provides a path to that end through a course on the psychology of student learning and cognition. Students' learning of the best and most effective study skills will empower them to achieve the required competencies and to succeed in their future careers. It is suggested that this course be introduced in the curriculum during the preparatory year before entry into HSCs. This is meant to prepare students to learn effectively in the years to come.

Table 10.4 Strategic plan for introducing students to the learning theories early on the curriculum

Goal 2: Promoting learning that benefits from the appropriate learning theories in the right context based on adult learning principles			
Objective (2.4): To develop and conduct introductory courses for students to familiarize them with the learning theories			
Initiative (2.4) Introduction course on learning and cognition	**Responsible** The T&L Steering Committee and the T&L Unit/Medical Education Department in each HSC	**Accountable** VRHS, Deans of HSCs, and the Leadership Committee	**Partners** Experts on educational psychology, Preparatory Year Deanship, and Deanship for Students' Affairs
Initiative description Designing a course in the psychology of students' learning and cognition			
Requirements and interdependencies 1. Experts on course design and learning psychology 2. Course approval			**Stakeholders** Faculty staff and students
Action plan 1. Involving experts in developing the course framework in a 3-day workshop at a suitable location outside KSU campus 2. Course curriculum and assessment finalization 3. Implementation of this introductory course on learning and cognition as an interprofessional health education course			**Estimated time** Phase II
KPIs 1. Students scoring more than 60% in the learning theories course 2. More than 80% of students are satisfied with the course			**Estimated budget** Phase II

VRHS vice-rector for health specialties, *T&L* teaching and learning, *KSU* King Saud University, *HSCs* health sciences colleges, *KPIs* key performance indicators

10.3.5 Objective (Initiative) 2.5: To Involve Students in Learning Theories Research

The strategy for this initiative is summarized in Table 10.5. The goal of health professions educational programs is not only to graduate efficient health professionals, but also to train excellent researchers who will be able to plan and run research on sound principles. Involving students in learning theories researches has several purposes such as to allow them to gain considerable knowledge and experience with the research process itself, as well as with best practices in learning; to improve their critical thinking and creativity; and to help them discover new techniques or participate in events that will improve their study skills and, thus, their learning.

In 2002, Rosenstiel and Johnston [19] found in alumni survey that students who were involved in research during their training were three times more likely to successfully complete their postgraduate training, and they were also more likely to become faculty members. Moreover, involving students in research will enhance their self-directed learning skills. Candy [2] identified about 100 qualities associated with self-direction, which included the following traits: methodical and disciplined; logical and analytical; collaborative and interdependent; curious, open,

Table 10.5 Strategic plan for students' involvement in educational research projects

<table>
<tr><td colspan="4">Goal 2: Promoting learning that benefits from appropriate learning theories in the right context based on adult learning principles</td></tr>
<tr><td colspan="4">Objective (2.5): To involve students in research concerning the various learning theories</td></tr>
<tr><td>Initiative (2.5)
Student-oriented educational research projects</td><td>Responsible
The T&L Steering Committee and the T&L Unit/Medical Education Department in each HSC</td><td>Accountable
VRHS, Deans of HSCs, and the Leadership Committee</td><td>Partners
Chair for Medical Education Research, KSU</td></tr>
<tr><td colspan="4">Initiative description
Involving students in research projects focused on learning theories, and how it could relate to students learning</td></tr>
<tr><td colspan="2">Requirements and interdependencies
1. Medical educationist
2. Faculty staff and students from HSCs</td><td colspan="2">Stakeholders
Faculty staff and students</td></tr>
<tr><td colspan="2">Action plan
1. Establishing guidelines with regard to students' involvement in health sciences educational research
2. Designating T&L units in each HSC to list their ongoing and potential researches in health sciences education
3. Establish a database of published and ongoing research in health sciences education at KSU that is updated periodically at the website of the VRHS
4. Drafting letters to the Chairman of the Medical Education Research Chair to review and discuss health sciences research projects prior to publication</td><td colspan="2">Estimated time
Open (unlimited time)</td></tr>
</table>

Table 10.5 (continued)

Goal 2: Promoting learning that benefits from appropriate learning theories in the right context based on adult learning principles	
KPIs	**Estimated budget**
1. Establishment of guidelines concerning student involvement in health sciences educational research 2. At least two researches to be conducted and published per year in each HSC 3. At least 20% of health sciences educational research should involve students 4. At least 20% of educational research publications should be in ISI journals 5. Establishment of a database of published and ongoing researches related to health sciences education	Phase II

T&L teaching and learning, *VRHS* vice-rector for health specialties, *HSCs* health sciences colleges, *KSU* King Saud University, *KPIs* key performance indicators

creative, and motivated; persistent and responsible; confident and competent at learning; and reflective and self-aware. The question here is, "How do we develop these qualities in our students?" Most importantly, students must have the opportunity to develop and practice skills that directly improve self-directed learning. These skills include asking questions, critically appraising new information, identifying their own knowledge and skill gaps, and reflecting on their learning process and outcomes. We believe that involving students in the research experience will improve these skills.

For the implementation of this initiative, the following actions must be undertaken:

- Prepare guidelines to organize student involvement in health sciences educational research.
- Make a list of the ongoing and potential research initiatives in health sciences education at KSU.
- Construct a database of published and ongoing research in health sciences education at KSU, updated periodically at the VRHS website.

10.4 Summary

King Saud University (KSU) students' daily challenges are always growing, and the curriculum should reach a standard that produces competent graduates who are both motivated and lifelong learners.

Our goal is to improve health professional education (HPE) programs and their products through the application of adult and appropriate learning theories. This can be achieved by providing the faculty and students with suitable resources, offering written guidelines on best practices in teaching and learning, conducting workshops, involving students in educational research projects, and introducing students to learning theories early on in their studies.

References

1. Armstrong E, Parsa-Parsi R. How can physicians' learning styles drive educational planning? Acad Med J Assoc Am Med Coll. 2005;80(7):680–4.
2. Candy PC. Self-direction for lifelong learning: a comprehensive guide to theory and practice. San Francisco: Jossey-Bass; 1991.
3. Braungart M, Braungart R, Gramet P. Applying learning theories to healthcare practice. In: Bastable, Gramet, Jacobs, Sopczyk, editors. Health professional as educator. Sudbury: Jones & Bartlett Learning LLC; 2011. p. 55–102.
4. Pavlov IP. Conditional reflexes. New York: Dover Publications [1927], translation by Oxford University Press, 1960.
5. Piaget J. The construction of reality in the child, vol. 82. London: Routledge; 2013.
6. Brooks MG, Brook JG. The courage to be constructivist. Educ Leadersh. 1999;57:18–24.
7. John-Steiner V, Mahn H. Sociocultural approaches to learning and development: a Vygotskian framework. Educ Psychol. 1996;31:191–206.
8. Bloom BS, Engelhart MD, Furst EJ, Hill WH, Krathwohl DR. Taxonomy of educational objectives: the classification of educational goals. In: Handbook I: cognitive domain. New York: David McKay Company; 1956.
9. Anderson LW, Krathwohl DR, editors. A taxonomy for learning, teaching, and assessing: a revision of bloom's taxonomy of educational objectives. Boston: Allyn & Bacon; 2001.
10. Bandura A. Social learning theory. Morristown: General Learning Press; 1971. http://www.asecib.ase.ro/mps/Bandura_SocialLearningTheory.pdf.
11. Cabaniss DL. Teaching psychodynamics in the twenty-first century. J Am Psychoanal Assoc. 2012;60(3):483–92.
12. Rogers C. Freedom to learn. 3rd ed. New York: Merrill; 1994.
13. Snowman J, McCown R. Psychology applied to teaching. 14th ed. Stanford: Cengage Learning; 2015.
14. Maslow AH. A theory of human motivation. Psychol Rev. 1943;50(4):370.
15. Stagnaro-Green A. Personal view applying adult learning principles to medical education in the United States. Med Teach. 2004;26(1):79–85.
16. Chickering AW, Reisser L. Education and identity. San Francisco: Jossey-Bass Publishers; 1969.
17. Knowles MS. The modern practice of adult education: from pedagogy to andragogy. Chicago: Association Press; 1980.
18. Kaufman DM. Applying educational theory in practice. BMJ. 2003;326(7382):213–6.
19. Rosenstiel SF, Johnston WM. Goals, costs, and outcomes of a predoctoral student research program. J Dent Educ. 2002;66(12):1368–73.

11 The Learning Environment

Mohammed Yahya Alnaami, Basil Amarneh,
and Abdullah Alzahrani

11.1 Introduction

A supportive learning environment is well known as an important pillar for successful learning at all levels of education. It improves the experience and quality of students' learning and, where possible, deep approaches to learning [1]. Although they are essential, educational material and facilities are not the sole environmental factors as one might consider. Learners' behavior and emotions, curriculum frameworks, learning approaches, assessment, and learning outcomes are also of paramount importance for a good overall teaching-learning environment. Also, the social, cultural, and political contexts within which a higher education institute operates play major roles and can influence the learning environment anonymously [2]. Another important environmental factor is the staff–student relationship [3]. We all remember examples of "good" and "bad" teachers and how they did influence our learning and learning environment either positively or negatively. Recently, learning environments are getting more concern by educators who have developed ways to measure learning environments quantitatively. A number of instruments have been developed, such as the Dundee Ready Educational Environment Measure (DREEM) [4] for graduate learning environments and the Dutch Residency Educational Climate Test (D-RECT) for postgraduate learning environment, which are considered the best and most reliable examples [5].

M. Y. Alnaami (✉)
Department of Surgery, College of Medicine, King Saud University, Riyadh, Saudi Arabia

B. Amarneh
College of Nursing, King Saud University, Riyadh, Saudi Arabia

A. Alzahrani
College of Applied Medical Sciences, King Saud University, Riyadh, Saudi Arabia

M. Y. Alnaami et al. (eds.), *Novel Health Interprofessional Education and Collaborative Practice Program: Strategy and Implementation*,
https://doi.org/10.1007/978-981-99-3420-1_11

11.2 Strategic Goal 3: Creating a Supportive Learning Environment Where Learners Interact Actively with the Curriculum, Teachers, and Patients in Complex Real-Life Problems

This goal is considered by the learning theme group at the VRHS-KSU as one of the most important learning issues. In order for learners to learn effectively, students need to feel that they belong to the same environment with some sense of security and justice. This cannot be achieved without real interactions with the curriculum, teachers, patients, and other people forming the learning environment. Moreover, motivation is a positive drive for learning if students are becoming responsible and accountable for their acts especially when they are acknowledged of the work done. Teachers are key elements for effective learning by arranging learning material and conduct in a way that engages students' interest and motivation and helps them to connect it to their earlier experience. In addition to these attributes, trust, legitimacy, involvement, and participation in the learning environment are positive motivators for effective learning, especially for postgraduate education and training [6, 7].

11.3 Objective (Initiative) 3.1: To Support and Foster Mentorship Programs

This initiative is presented in Table 11.1. The aim is to support and foster mentorship programs that can help students achieve their learning goals and future perspective. There are many components of mentoring. The required timeframe and budget for this and the other initiatives depend on available manpower and resources, which will be studied and decided later as a second phase.

Mentorship in health education balances three key elements: support, challenges, and a vision of the individual's future career as described by Daloz [8] (Fig. 11.1).

The VRHS at KSU took an initiative by creating a mentorship program lead by specialized experts from HSCs. This program was so successful and later developed to a "Center for Students' Counseling and Guidance," which was not limited to HSCs but for all the three main divisions of the university sciences: health, science, and humanity colleges at KSU. In order to maintain successful mentorship programs, we must work to promote and recognize mentorship as a way of developing mentorship guidelines for mentors, mentees, and educators. The VRHSs and HSCs will have the advantage of being the host of this mentorship program, and the "Center for Students' Counseling and Guidance" is currently led and run mostly by health sciences staff under the umbrella of the Deanship of Student Affairs. The Students' Counseling and Guidance Center at KSU includes the following services:

Table 11.1 Strategic plan for supporting and fostering mentorship programs

<table>
<tr><td colspan="4">Goal 3: Creating a supportive learning environment where learners interact actively with the curriculum, teachers, and patients in complex real-life problems</td></tr>
<tr><td colspan="4">Objective (3.1): To support and foster mentorship programs</td></tr>
<tr><td>Initiative (3.1)
Developing the necessary mentorship guidelines that advocate and support the learning environment</td><td>Responsible
The T&L steering committee, Center for Students' counseling and guidance, and the T&L units/medical education departments, HSCs</td><td>Accountable
VRHS, deans of HSCs, and the leadership committee</td><td>Partners
CELT, deanship of students' affairs, and KSU</td></tr>
<tr><td colspan="4">Initiative description
Creating the necessary tools and means that will maintain the mentorship programs to excel the academic climate in the implementation of the developed mentorship guidelines for mentors, mentees, and educators</td></tr>
<tr><td colspan="3">Requirements and interdependencies
1. Experts in students' mentorship
2. Center for student advising and guidance</td><td>Stakeholders
Faculty and students</td></tr>
<tr><td colspan="3">Action plan
1. Establishing the general guidelines and standards of the mentorship program usage and implementation that can be integrated into the curricula of the different HSCs
2. Establishing the basis for the pairing and shadowing system between the different participating groups (high school students, preparatory year students, and faculty)
3. Creating a mentor and mentee rewarding system that encourages the adoption of the mentorship programs
4. Establishing the necessary follow-up means to:
(a) Ensuring rigorous implementation of the programs
(b) Establishing indicators of success
(c) Using indicators in the rewarding system</td><td>Estimated time
Phase II</td></tr>
<tr><td colspan="3">KPIs
1. Mentorship guidelines established
2. Rewarding system developed</td><td>Estimated budget
Phase II</td></tr>
</table>

T&L teaching and learning, *VRHS* vice-rector for health specialties, *HSCs* Health Sciences Colleges, *KSU* King Saud University, *CELT* Center for Excellence in Learning and Teaching, *KPIs* key performance indicators

11.3.1 Academic Skills and Learning Section

It specializes in helping students improve the skills and strategies required for effective academic work. Services include:

- Free and confidential academic help for all enrolled students.
- Individual consultations, workshops, online courses, podcasts, and handouts.
- Development of academic, critical thinking, communication, and professional skills and strategies foundational to all scholarly activity.

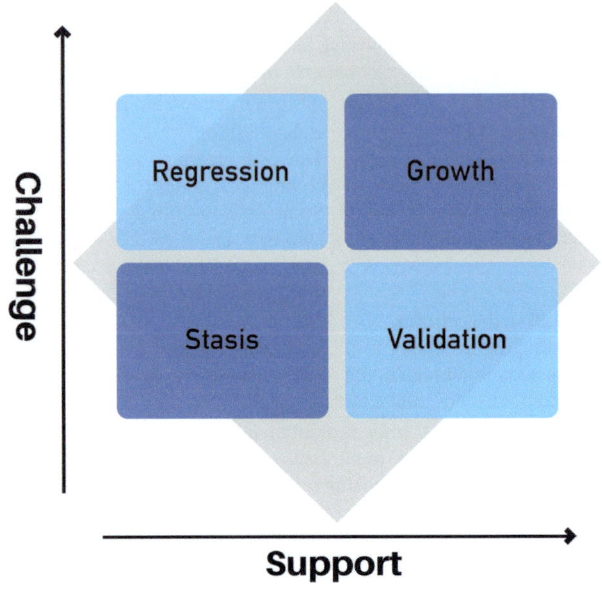

Fig. 11.1 Daloz's model of mentoring relationships

11.3.2 Student Employment and Career Development Section

It provides information on casual, part-time, and graduate employment. Services include:

- Student internships.
- Career counseling.
- Assistance with career planning.
- Resume writing.
- Interview preparation.

11.3.3 Counseling Section

It offers free, confidential services from professionally qualified counselors. Services include:

- Individual appointments.
- Assistance with personal or study related issues.
- Group programs.
- Seminars.
- Webpage resources.
- Urgent appointments available every day.

11.3.4 Disability Services Section

It assists students with disability to participate in their program of study at KSU. Services include:

- Providing advice, support, and adjustment that minimize the impact of disability in education.
- Encouraging independence in learning and self-advocacy.
- Raising awareness and understanding of disability issues with all students and staff.
- Providing advice and support on inclusive education practices.

11.3.5 Statistical Consulting Unit

It provides statistical support for research projects to KSU honors and graduate students. Services include:

- Assistance with the design of experiments and surveys.
- Advice on collection and analysis of data.
- Research collaboration.
- Statistical short courses and training.

11.3.6 Student Information and Guidance Network

New undergraduate and graduate students can register for *Student Information and Guidance Network*, a program to facilitate new students' transition to university life. Services include:

- Social activities and free food.
- Linking to coursework mentors, clubs, societies, networks, and resources.

11.3.7 Students Mobility Program

It manages the inbound and outbound *Study Abroad and Exchange Programs* that enable students to undertake periods of study at an overseas partner institution and those of our partner to study at KSU. Services include:

- Information, nomination, and pre-departure sessions for KSU students and assistance with all the processes associated with going on exchange.
- Advice and assistance to inbound exchange and study abroad students.

11.3.8 University Health Service

KSU offers primary health care to all students at the Deanship of Students' Affairs building and in students' housings. Primary care services at these locations are equipped with clinics that are run by general practitioners (GPs) and a nurse who is also available for health advice and assistance. Also, primary and tertiary health care services are available free for both students and staff at KSU affiliated hospitals at the campus and in Riyadh city. There is a new clinic established for smoking abstinence at KSU main administration building near the central library.

Other services are currently developing such as psychosocial services, preventive guidance, electronic guidance, counseling and guidance at students' housing, public relations, and media.

The vision, missions, goals, actions, governance structure, and further details about the *Students' Center for Counseling and Guidance* are available at KSU website (http://sa.ksu.edu.sa/ar/ccg) [9].

11.3.9 The Guidelines Established for Mentoring, Counseling, and Guidance at KSU Include

- Introduction to students' counseling and guidance.
- Tools for counseling and guidance and their applications.
- Strategies and syllabi for guidance.
- Programs and guidance services aligned to counseling and guidance fields.
- Ethical charter for counseling and guidance in KSA.
- Data gathering tools for guidance.
- Strategies for behavioral change.
- Models for common problems and strategies for guiding and appropriate remedial.

11.3.10 Established Guidelines for Mentors Include

- Common terms within the framework of academic advising.
- Rules governing students' guidance and counseling.
- Skills and qualities of the academic advisor.
- Student's tasks in academic advising.
- Department and department's head tasks in academic advising.
- Students' counseling and guidance center and council tasks.
- Students' counseling and guidance unit tasks in each college.
- Procedural tasks for the academic advisor.
- Calculating the semester and accumulative grade point average for the student.

Learning through shadowing in interprofessional education represents a "training technique", where a student (the shadow) is paired with a leader in the workplace (the host), to enable the shadow a hands-on feel of what it is the career looks like [10]. Ideal setting is exposing a high school student to the actual practice of health science disciplines before application or even during the preparatory year before making final decision about the desired discipline. A student can be paired to another student at a higher level or to a faculty in the desired field depending on the student's needs and aims. Whether this process is useful or not, evidence in the literature is still weak. In a nice review of the literature by Kitsis and Goldsammler [11], data reported from focus groups, interviews, and surveys suggest that shadowing experiences generally increased participants' interest in the specialty or improved participants' confidence in transitioning to a new position, but some articles raised ethical and practical concerns related to shadowing. This shadowing program has not been established officially yet at KSU except through some personal and extracurricular activities.

Establishing a rewarding system for mentoring is essential for the institute and faculty to continue mentoring at a desired level of interest and enthusiasm. Rewarding systems should include at least the followings:

- Use mentoring as criteria for promotion and advancement.
- Consider mentoring activities as teaching activities; faculty should document their mentoring activities on their teaching load and curriculum vitas.
- Stewardship reviews for leaders should evaluate mentoring activities for department or college.
- Establish mentoring awards to best mentor, mentee, department, or college.

Our center for "students' counseling and guidance" took some initiatives in the rewarding system including counting mentoring as a credit unit for promotion and giving awards to the best college and mentors.

Mentoring program evaluation is also necessary to close the loop for the mentoring process. This evaluation process may include:

- handouts for specific details,
- baseline data,
- Performing quantitative and qualitative reviews:
  - recruitment and retention,
  - promotion of junior faculty,
  - career satisfaction.
- Quality and satisfaction surveys done annually for both mentors and mentees.
- Exit interviews.

11.4 Objective (Initiative) 3.2: To Introduce Real-Life Examples and Interactions with Healthcare System in High School and Preparatory Program

This initiative presented in Table 11.2 aims at the creation of an outreach program that explains healthcare education and training to high school and preparatory year students. This initiative is still considered a strategic plan to be materialized soon on

Table 11.2 Strategic plan for introducing real-life examples and interactions with healthcare system in high school and preparatory program

Goal 3: Creating a supportive learning environment where learners interact actively with the curriculum, teachers, and patients in complex real-life problems			
Objective (3.2): To introduce real-life examples and interactions with healthcare system in high school and the preparatory program			
Initiative (3.2) Introducing a new venue of collaboration between the different parties involved in health sciences education (HSE) as well as preparatory education and high schools. Perceiving true insight about roles of the different health science specialties	**Responsible** The T&L steering committee at the VRHS, the T&L units (or medical education departments) at HSCs, and preparatory year administration	**Accountable** VRHS, deans of HSCs, and deanship of the preparatory year	**Partners** Students' affairs deanship, and registration and admission deanship
Initiative description Exposing high school and preparatory year students to real experiences that involve the interaction of the different health care team members in HSCs and in KSU affiliated health care facilities and facilitating a thorough understanding of the expected learning experience in HSCs			
Requirements and interdependencies 1. Formulation of teams from different HSCs 2. Setting site visits programs 3. Scheduling and transportation 4. Surveys data answering by students and faculty		**Stakeholders** Faculty staff, students, and HSCs' administration	
Action plan 1. Peer-observation to facilitate experience sharing between the different groups (faculty members and students) from the different health sciences 2. Developing educative materials about the different health sciences and their different roles in practice 3. Developing a recording of the shared experience to be added to the learning resources 4. Developing evaluation surveys for the participant expectations 5. Tailor visiting programs to the students in the prep year and in the high schools, with the necessary satisfaction evaluation 6. Training mentors and mentees in the cooperative learning nature of the program, which embraces knowledge, leadership, teamwork, and mutual respect of the different health sciences programs		**Estimated time** Summer time and beginning of every academic year	
KPIs 1. Peer-observation is 70% active 2. Educational materials are ready 3. Surveys are filled by ≥70% of students and ≥ 50% of faculty and followed up in 1 year's time		**Estimated budget** Phase II	

T&L teaching and learning, *HSCs* Health Sciences Colleges, *VRHS* vice-rector for health specialties, *KSU* King Saud University, *KPIs* key performance indicators ground at KSU. High school and preparatory year students are usually eager to know about health specialties as a career for their future. This knowledge would be a nice experience if complemented by visiting HSCs and affiliated health care facilities especially by preparatory year student. This will give them an insight to the whole picture of health care specialties. Summer camps are ideal occasions to serve this initiative. Also, if students at this early level of their career undergo some recognized personality character or talents testing, it may help them further on deciding which career one can have as a perfect match. The responsible along with their partner groups will ask each HSC to provide them with a pamphlet or booklet summarizing the college's vision, mission, and strategy toward their faculty, students, and patients including each department and sections. These are mostly available on corresponding webpage of each HSC. A team of faculty nominated by the VRHS representing all HSCs will make a committee named "Learning Environment Task Force." This task force will change every year by another new task force to make the visiting program of newer high school and preparatory year students. This visiting program is a structured program designed by the committee, including faculty teams' tasks, scheduled visit times, transportation arrangements, HSC administration, faculty and students' names responsible for introducing the tariff pamphlets and booklets to visiting students and taking them for a tour in the corresponding HSC departments, laboratories, clinics, and other sections considering breaking them into small groups to avoid overcrowding in one area or section. This visit should take from 3 to 4 h only at a time, allow open discussions, questions and answers, and visiting students will fill a survey for purposes of evaluation and future research to document the benefit and usefulness of this initiative.

A recent study on the effects of summer internship and follow-up distance mentoring programs on middle and high school students' perceptions and interest in health careers shows that these programs have a positive effect on student knowledge of health careers and their attitudes about them [12]. In this study, students took a career interest inventory, completed a scale measuring their self-reported understanding and interest in health careers, and wrote essays about health careers before and after completing 1 week on campus internship on health careers and after 9 months follow-up distance mentoring program where they continued to interact with university faculty by video conference about their career options. Another study done in Southwestern Ontario, Canada, showed the usefulness of a rural secondary school outreach medical mentorship program run by medical students, resulting in more high school students' interest in medical careers [13]. A curriculum pipeline connecting underrepresented minority high school students to medical school is another program that made racial minority students more aware and interested in medical career [14].

11.5 Objective (Initiative) 3.3: To Develop and Provide Learning Resources to Support Real-Life Experiences

This initiative is presented in Table 11.3. Its aim is to encourage leaders in the VRHS and HSCs to support faculty and students with state-of-the-art learning resources to establish an active and competent library that is culturally tailored to

Table 11.3 Strategic plan for developing and providing learning resources to support real-life experiences

<table>
<tr><td colspan="4">Goal 3: Creating a supportive learning environment where learners interact actively with the curriculum, teachers, and patients in complex real-life problems</td></tr>
<tr><td colspan="4">Objective (3.3): To develop and provide learning resources to support real-life experiences</td></tr>
<tr><td>Initiative (3/3)
Encouraging leaders in the VRHSs and HSCs to support faculty and students with state-of-the-art learning resources to facilitate effective teaching and best learning experiences at all levels</td><td>Responsible
The T&L steering committee and the T&L units (or medical education departments), HSCs</td><td>Accountable
VRHS and deans of HSCs</td><td>Partners
CELT, deanship of e-learning and distant learning and clinical skills, and CSSC</td></tr>
<tr><td colspan="4">Initiative description
Establishing an active and competent library that is culturally tailored to meet the real-life experiences for students and encompasses various real class learning resources (digital and video recorded experiences, virtual reality training, electronic resources, and written documents), as well as that acculturates the self-learning motive, in an interdisciplinary environment for all HSCs</td></tr>
<tr><td colspan="3">Requirements and interdependencies
1. Establishing a state-of-the-art virtual library shared by all HSCs
2. Collaboration with CSSC
3. Collaboration with the deanship of e-learning and distance learning
4. Collaboration with the main central library (king Salman library)
5. Collaboration with competitive local and international companies that provide up to date learning resources</td><td>Stakeholders
Faculty staff and students</td></tr>
<tr><td colspan="3">Action plan
1. Developing a classification system that will acknowledge the existing resources and use the newly developed learning resources
2. Providing guidelines that will standardize the development of real-life experiences
3. Regulating a depository system that will have the necessary tools and materials to handle real-life experiences (electronic and traditional)
4. Developing a training package targeting participating faculty members on how to record and use and disseminate existing resources
5. Preparing leaflets and pamphlets that announce the availability of such resources to students
6. Creating a front face library website that can be noticed and simply used by HSCs' students
7. Developing a tool to assess the effectiveness of the learning resources on semester basis</td><td>Estimated time
Phase II</td></tr>
<tr><td colspan="3">KPIs
1. Active classification system for the learning resources is done
2. Guidelines for the new learning resources
3. Establishment of the depository system
4. Training package for faculty is prepared
5. Leaflets and pamphlets are printed
6. Resources online front face is developed
7. Assessment instrument is prepared</td><td>Estimated budget
Phase II</td></tr>
</table>

T&L teaching and learning, *HSCs* Health Sciences Colleges, *VRHS* vice-rector for health specialties, *CELT* Center of Excellence in Learning and Teaching, *CSSC* Clinical Skills and Simulation Center, *KPIs* key performance indicators meet real-life experiences for students and encompasses various real class learning resources (digital and video recorded experiences, virtual reality training, electronic resources, and written documents), as well as that acculturates the self-learning motive, in an interdisciplinary environment for all HSCs. *Responsible* parties include the T&L Steering Committee at the VRHS and T&L Units (Medical Education Departments) at HSCs. Their missions include developing a classification of available learning resources (e.g., references whether books or handouts, journals, electronic material, etc.); develop guidelines that guide the use of such learning resources for the purpose they are matching (e.g., for purpose of doing research, one would find the researched subject in electronic data bases, not in handouts or outdated books!); regulate a depository system in one place ready to accommodate state-of-the-art virtual learning resources that reflect real-life experiences; develop a training package targeting participating faculty members on how to record and use and disseminate existing resources so students can access these resources at any time; prepare leaflets and pamphlets that announce the availability of such resources to students; create a front face virtual library website that can be noticed and simply used by HSCs students; and develop a tool to assess the effectiveness of the learning resources on semester-to-semester basis (e.g., access times, number of users, types of resources commonly used, surveys, etc.). The VRHS and HSCs administration are expected to support these efforts once approved and executed and will be deemed accountable for their success or failure. The *Partners* of this initiative are very crucial to support this initiative and the overall program, and they are expected to cooperate and collaborate with responsible parties to provide advice, expertise, and share experiences to execute this initiative successfully. The Center for Excellence in Learning and Teaching (CELT) operating under the Vice-Rectorship for Academic and Educational Affairs is responsible for setting policies and overall strategic plan in teaching and learning at KSU, monitor their implementation, and reward best 25 researches in health professions education annually. The Deanship of e-Learning and Distance Learning is responsible for all electronic developments at KSU including teaching, learning, and distance learning. The Clinical Skills and Simulation Center (CSSC) is responsible for clinical training and research and educating the future generation of academic clinical leaders through the use of simulation and cutting-edge technology, allowing students, residents, and fellows to practice and become proficient in the basic skills and the cognitive knowledge required to perform prior to entering the clinical areas. Of course, the central library is an important component of this initiative as most of suggested resources are already there; however, KSU faculty and students' library users are overwhelming and sometimes exhausting available resources. Nonetheless, educational companies usually innovate and advertise new technology and learning resources that are sometimes worth trying and eventually buying if proven effective. An exciting experience with a similar objective is the "Critical thinking and Appraisal Resource Library" reported by Castle et al. [15] that promotes the critical thinking about treatment claims needed to help improve healthcare choices.

11.6 Objective (Initiative) 3.4: To Develop Students' Surveys to Gauge Their Interests

This initiative is outlined in Table 11.4. Actually, this is one of the actions of the initiative (3.2) "develop evaluation surveys for the participant expectations." Surveys would assess the potential effects of a career education program on career choice, by measuring career knowledge and interest over time. The most suitable groups to apply this initiative are students at high school and preparatory year levels. As mentioned in initiative (3.2), the students will fill the proposed survey before and after they are exposed to an onsite tariff program (detailed previously) and be followed up after 1 and 5 years. The health science knowledge and interest inventory will be developed from a review of the literature on health science careers. Items to be included in the survey should be carefully invented by a group of expert researchers

Table 11.4 Strategic plan for developing students' surveys to gauge their interests

Goal 3: Creating a supportive learning environment where learners interact actively with the curriculum, teachers, and patients in complex real-life problems			
Objective (3.4): To develop students' surveys to gauge their interests			
Initiative (3.4)	**Responsible**	**Accountable**	**Partners**
Building and adopting a collection of inventories and assessment batteries that can classify the student interests	The T&L steering committee and the T&L units or medical education departments, HSCs	VRHS and deans of HSCs	Deanship of the preparatory year, deanship of e-learning and distant learning, CELT, and deanship of admission/registration, KSU
Initiative description Building a system to help understand and classify students into different interest groups			
Requirements and interdependencies 1. Item analysis specialists			**Stakeholders** Faculty staff and students
Action plan 1. Setting and designing the priorities and the needs of the preparatory year students according to the university available study programs 2. Developing, adopting, and adapting the necessary surveys directed to assess high school and preparatory year students 3. Developing the necessary analyses and reporting system for the used survey tools 4. Placing the generated data in a specially designed data warehouse for future references 5. Creating the necessary referral system based on the results			**Estimated time** Every Year (end of the preparatory year, end of each academic year, and after graduation during the internship)
KPIs 1. Priorities for the necessity of the assessment tools are set 2. The needed surveys are prepared and selected 3. Analysis and reporting system is active 4. Data warehouse is active			**Estimated budget** Phase II

T&L teaching and learning, *HSCs* Health Sciences Colleges, *VRHS* vice-rector for health specialties, *CELT* Center of Excellence in Learning and Teaching, *CSSC* Clinical Skills and Simulation Center, *KSU* King Saud University, *KPIs* key performance indicators who will also validate it before its final use. Surveys are expected to contain items on personal information and permanent address and contact; prior knowledge about health science careers; what students were expecting from the health sciences' academics concerning awareness programs; how they got interested in health sciences career(s); and what they will do in their future (including building knowledge, skills, and attitudes) toward the society and healthcare improvement. In addition to survey items, there should be a room for essay or open-ended reflections on certain important areas including: writing about what they know about health careers; the nature of each career, including working hours, teamwork, and the nature of communication skills needed; the awarded degree and scholarly degrees; and personal characteristics of each career. Conversely, participants who would like to pursue a health career choice are also advised to undergo personality testing (inventory decided by the expert researchers' committee) and match results to appropriate health career. Results of surveys and essays need to be analyzed and reported by expert statistician(s) in addition to the expert researchers' committee chosen for this initiative. The work of surveys and reports can be shared with the *Partners* of this initiative especially the Admission and Registration Deanship as an additional information to students' interviews for appropriate selection and career matching. Moreover, these reports and admission data are saved into a data warehouse for research purposes and future reference.

11.7 Objective (Initiative) 3.5: To Set Standards and Develop Guidelines for Curriculum Development in Support of This Objective

Components of this initiative are outlined in Table 11.5. Health professional colleges are expected to assure that its students learn in an environment that fosters mutual respect, civil behavior, and the values of professionalism, ethics, and humanism. The standards and guidelines for the "Supportive Learning Environment" would be prepared and developed by the expert Ad-hoc group, discussed with HSCs Curriculum Committees, and adopted by the departments. Freedom, though respectfully, in interactions among faculty and student, impacts student learning and satisfaction. Learning in the context of patient care can present special challenges in ensuring a positive learning environment. The Ad-hoc Committee would also prepare a guide for faculty and students with tips on how to handle these challenges. We all have experienced good teachers who made positive learning environments, and they have become role models for us. Meanwhile, we cannot forget bad behaviors and stressful learning environments, which reflected negatively on our learning experience and even hating some good career choices. Therefore, teachers would also need to be an integral part of this initiative with regard to awareness and training in supportive learning environment standards and guidelines. Also, the institution plays a major role in making the learning environment supportive and enjoyable. A standard can be defined as a quality level that needs to be achieved and considered

Table 11.5 Strategic plan for developing students' surveys to gauge their interests

Goal 3: Creating a supportive learning environment where learners interact actively with the curriculum, teachers, and patients in complex real-life problems			
Objective (3.5): To set standards and develop guidelines for curriculum development in support of this objective			
Initiative (3.5) Creating the necessary supporting academic environment through placing specific standards coupled with the working guidelines to be integrated into the curriculum	**Responsible** The T&L steering committee and curriculum committees at HSCs	**Accountable** T&L units (or medical education departments), HSCs	**Partners** Deans of HSCs and CELT, KSU
Initiative description Creating the necessary supportive environment using specific standards and guidelines to help in integrating this goal within health sciences curricula			
Requirements and interdependencies 1. T&L units and medical education departments collaboration 2. Experts in learning environment promotion and development		**Stakeholders** Faculty staff and students	
Action plan 1. Formulating a specific interdisciplinary task group to generate the necessary standards and guidelines (ad-hoc committee) 2. Preparing workshops to educate faculty members in different HSCs on the usage of the developed standards and guidelines 3. Evaluating the achievement of this goal in curriculum development of the various HSCs		**Estimated time** Phase II	
KPIs 1. Standards and guidelines are developed 2. Workshops are prepared and conducted (70% of selected participants have attended) 3. Report extent of achievement of this goal in curricula (minimum 70%)		**Estimated budget** Phase II	

T&L teaching and learning, *HSCs* Health Sciences Colleges, *VRHS* vice-rector for health specialties, *CELT* Center of Excellence in Learning and Teaching, *CSSC* Clinical Skills and Simulation Center, *KSU* King Saud University, *KPIs* key performance indicators

acceptable. If linked to a standard, a guideline can be defined as a guide or way to achieve that standard. Below are some areas to consider when promoting a "supportive learning environment" pertinent to students and faculty and institutions. For example, but not limited to:

Curricular "supportive learning environment" standards pertinent to Students may include:

- Teamwork.
- Self-learning.
- Ethical conduct.

Curricular standards for Teachers to create a respectful workplace and "supportive learning environment" may include:

- Role-modeling.
- Scholarly competency.
- Leadership.

Curricular standards for the Institute may include:

- Equity and fairness.
- Optimal learning resources.
- Recreation.

The corresponding guidelines can be generated from each standard detailing responsibilities and expectations from students, faculty, and the institute. For example, but not limited to:

Teamwork

- Participate in group projects.
- Consider the patient at the center of the team.

Role-modeling

- Model respectful relationships with peers, students, and other team members.
- Supportive.

Equity and fairness

- Admission criteria.
- Outreach programs.

The T&L Steering Committee and Curriculum Committees at HSCs are deemed *responsible* for working together and develop the "supportive learning environment standards and guidelines." The T/L unit (medical education department) will be considered accountable if developed standards and guidelines cannot be implemented in corresponding HSC curriculum. As *partners*, Deans of HSCs play a catalyst role to encourage and advise responsible and accountable parties to develop and implement these standards and guidelines, and the Center of Excellence in Learning and Teaching (CELT) would provide the expertise to help in the development of this initiative.

11.8 Objective (Initiative) 3.6: To Identify and Promote Student Projects That Are Collaborative Across HSCs

This initiative is presented in Table 11.6. It aims to make faculty and students from different disciplines work together in educational research and other projects to get outside corresponding HSC's boundaries, get exposed to real-life problems, and enjoy interprofessional educational projects and collaboration. The CELT offers an annual grant for faculty members, which aims at achieving a stimulating environment for learning and innovation and raising the performance of the teaching and learning processes at the university. Also, the CELT has the Outstanding Students Program (OSP), which offers annual tournament and awards for top 25 students' educational and research projects. The CELT should announce and distribute such

Table 11.6 Strategic plan for identifying and promoting student projects that are collaborative across HSCs

Goal 3: Creating a supportive learning environment where learners interact actively with the curriculum, teachers, and patients in complex real-life problems			
Objective (3.6): To identify and promote student projects that are collaborative across HSCs			
Initiative (3.6) Creating the necessary means to establish a yearly tournament of capstone projects targeting interdisciplinary collaborative work between the students of different HSCs	**Responsible** The T&L steering committee and the T&L units (medical education departments) in HSCs	**Accountable** VRHS, leadership committee, and deans of HSCs	**Partners** CELT
Initiative description Establishing the necessary means to reflect students' interactive, collaborative work			
Requirements and interdependencies 1. Medical and health professional educationists collaboration 2. CELT		**Stakeholders** Faculty staff and students	
Action plan 1. Formulating the necessary guidelines for the interdisciplinary capstone projects tournament, including the guidelines for submission, competing as well as the guidelines for the first place and run-up posters 2. Assigning annual committee to oversee the competition based on the previously established guidelines to accept and classify the submitted projects and posters 3. Announcing a scientific day for the poster session presentations for all the capstone projects from the different HSCs		**Estimated time** Phase II	
KPIs 1. At least 50% of the CELT grants and awards are offered to HSCs 2. Guidelines for interprofessional educational research and projects are developed		**Estimated budget** Phase II	

T&L teaching and learning, *HSCs* Health Sciences Colleges, *VRHS* vice-rector for health specialties, *CELT* Center of Excellence in Learning and Teaching, *CSSC* Clinical Skills and Simulation Center, *KSU* King Saud University, *KPIs* key performance indicators capstone project tournament or awards to all departments and colleges at KSU, encouraging interprofessional educational research and projects collaboration. What is needed at this stage is to enrich such programs through further collaboration between CELT and HSCs educational units and departments. These educational projects and research tournaments and awards offered by the CELT may also need input from all HSCs educational unit and departments with regard to guidelines pertinent to health programs' educational research and projects, which may differ a bit from other science and humanistic programs in some areas, such as teaching and learning in laboratories, clinics, operating theater, emergency, endoscopy, community field projects, etc.

11.9 Summary

Through several meetings and workshops, the T&L Development Theme at the VRHSs tried to highlight important initiatives to fulfill this goal "To create a supportive learning environment where learners interact actively with the curriculum, patients, and teachers in complex real-life problems." Under this goal, one crucial objective is to "support and foster good students' mentorship programs" at KSU in general and at HSCs in specific, especially during early years of their study. The second objective is to "introduce real-life examples and interactions with healthcare system in high school and preparatory program" through onsite and outreach programs. The third objective is to "develop and provide learning resources to support real-life experiences" that include a state-of-the-art virtual library and collaborate with available e-learning and clinical skills and simulation resources. The fourth objective is to "develop students' surveys to gauge their interests" by the task force committee, that changes every year, and expert statisticians. The fifth objective is to "set standards and develop guidelines for curriculum development in support of this goal" by the Ad-hoc Committee and the experts in this field. The last but not exclusive objective is to "identify and promote student projects that are collaborative across HSCs" through collaborations of the medical and health professional educationists and through CELT.

References

1. Entwistle N, McCune V, Hounsell J. Approaches to studying and perceptions of university teaching-learning environments: concepts, measures and preliminary findings. Coventry and Durham: Occasional report 1, © ETL Project, Universities of Edinburgh; 2002; http://www.etl.tla.ed.ac.uk/docs/ETLreport1.pdf.
2. Isba R, Boor K. Creating a learning environment. In: Dornan T, Mann K, Scherpbier A, Spencer J, editors. Medical education: theory and practice. Edinburgh: Churchill Livingstone; 2011. p. 99–114.
3. Tiberius RG, Sinai J, Flak EA. The role of teacher-learner relationships in medical education. In: Norman GR, van der Vleuten CP, Newbel DI, editors. International handbook of research in medical education. Dordrecht: Kluwer Academic Publishers; 2002. p. 462–98.

4. Miles S, Swift L, Leinster SJ. The Dundee ready education environment measure (DREEM): a review of its adoption and use. Med Teach. 2012;34(9):e620–34.
5. Boor KB. The clinical learning climate. S.I.: s.n, 2009; https://research.vumc.nl/en/publications/the-clinical-learning-climate.
6. Lyon PM. Making the most of learning in the operating theatre: student strategies and curricular initiatives. Med Educ. 2003;37:680–8.
7. Lyon PM. A model of teaching and learning in the operating theatre. Med Educ. 2004;38:1278–87.
8. Daloz L. Effective teaching and mentoring. San Francisco, CA: Jossey-Bass; 1986.
9. Students' Center for Counseling and Guidance, King Saud University, Kingdom of Saudi Arabia. http://sa.ksu.edu.sa/ar/ccg.
10. Kusnoor AV, Stelljes LA. Interprofessional learning through shadowing: insights and lessons learned. Med Teach. 2016;38(12):1278–84.
11. Kitsis EA, Goldsammler M. Physician shadowing: a review of the literature and proposal for guidelines. Acad Med. 2013;88(1):102–10.
12. Fernandez-Repollet E, Locatis C, De Jesus-Monge WE, Maisiak R, Liu WL. Effects of summer internship and follow-up distance mentoring programs on middle and high school student perceptions and interest in health careers. BMC Med Educ. 2018;18:84.
13. Robinson MA, Douglas-Vail MB, Bryce JN, van Zyl TJ. Medical school outreach and mentorship for rural secondary school students: a pilot of the Southwestern Ontario medical mentorship program. Can J Rural Med. 2017;22(2):62–7.
14. Derck J, Zahn K, Finks JF, Mand S, Sandhu G. Doctors of tomorrow: an innovative curriculum connecting underrepresented minority high school students to medical school. Educ Health (Abingdon). 2016;29(3):259–65.
15. Castle JC, Chalmers I, Atkinson P, Badenoch D, Oxman AD, Austvoll-Dahlgren A, et al. Establishing a library of resources to help people understand key concepts in assessing treatment claims-the "critical thinking and appraisal resource library" (CARL). PLoS One. 2017;12(7):e0178666.

12 Professionalism

Dalal Abdullah Alqahtani, Eiad Abdelmohsen Alfaris, Kelechi Ogbuehi, Ramprasad Vasthare, Prajna Nayak, and Ciraj Ali Mohammed

12.1 Introduction

An essential aspect of health professional education (HPE) is to graduate competent practitioners who have the appropriate attitude toward professionalism. This is because it affects their future career in dealing with patients, the quality of care they provide and, eventually, health and disease outcomes [1]. It has been recognized that the knowledge and clinical skills (hard skills) are not the only skills needed to succeed in the health care profession, but there is a need to other skills

D. A. Alqahtani (✉)
Oral Medicine and Diagnostic Sciences, College of Dentistry, King Saud University, Riyadh, Saudi Arabia

E. A. Alfaris
Department of Family and Community Medicine, College of Medicine, King Saud University, Riyadh, Saudi Arabia

K. Ogbuehi
College of Applied Medical Sciences, King Saud University, Riyadh, Kingdom of Saudi Arabia

R. Vasthare · P. Nayak
Manipal College of Dental Sciences, Manipal Academy of Higher Education, Manipal, India

C. A. Mohammed
Medical Education, College of Medicine and Health Sciences, National University of Science & Technology, Sohar, Oman

M. Y. Alnaami et al. (eds.), *Novel Health Interprofessional Education and Collaborative Practice Program: Strategy and Implementation*,
https://doi.org/10.1007/978-981-99-3420-1_12

named (soft skills) such as ethical and professionalism skills, in addition to communication skills. This change in perspective got the attention of health profession educators by incorporating those skills in health sciences curricula. In KSU, curricular reforms have been initiated in a number of HSCs in order to assure excellence in education. This reform has recognized professionalism as a prominent issue that needs to be addressed in educational programs. However, teaching and assessing professionalism are still difficult tasks. It was previously thought that professionalism was an innate character of an individual that could not be taught. Professionalism now is considered one of the most important competencies to be learned at all levels of HPE. In recent years, the importance of professionalism teaching and assessment in HPE is widely emphasized. But this has changed with time, and now there is much focus in developing professionalism through formal education. Nevertheless, the best practices in teaching and assessment of professionalism are still unclear. This could be explained that there is still ambiguity in defining professionalism. As a result, it is hard to be measured. Identifying the attributes that formulate the professional act is central to curriculum developers because it would guide them in choosing the appropriate methods of professionalism instruction and assessment. Although professionalism is multifaceted and has multiple definitions, still most of its attributes have some elements of reflection and/or self-assessment. Wilkinson et al. [2] reviewed systematically the published definitions of professionalism in order to select the best tools for its assessment. They stated that there are many tools, and they classified into themes and subthemes. The major themes were: "adherence to ethical practice principles," "effective interactions with patients and with people who are important to those patients," "effective interactions with other people working within the health system," "reliability," and commitment to autonomous maintenance and continuous improvement of competence self, others, and systems.

At KSU, our goal is to develop professionalism among learners by selecting the right teaching and assessment methods. The following section discusses the strategic steps and initiatives proposed to achieve this goal.

12.2 Strategic Goal 4: Building Learners' Self-Awareness of Values, Attitudes, and Beliefs That Influence Their Learning Achievement and Actions to a High Caliber Professional Career

In the early stages of this program, this goal was developed through a planned process that involved conducting multiple workshops among key faculty members, educators, consultants, student representatives, and other relevant stakeholders. They discussed the need for developing the professional character in the learner, and they proposed several initiatives to achieve this goal, which are outlined below:

12.3 Objective (Initiative) 4.1: To Set Standards for Learning Achievements in Order to Create Awareness of These Issues

This initiative's strategy is presented in Table 12.1. It sets the standards for learning achievements: to enhance students' self-awareness of their performance and to know about themselves in order to manage their limitations during their efforts to

Table 12.1 Strategic plan for developing standards for students' learning achievements

Goal 4: Building learners' self-awareness of values, attitudes, and beliefs that influence their learning achievement and actions to a high caliber professional career			
Objective (4.1): To set standards for learning achievements in order to create awareness of these issues			
Initiative (4.1) Setting standards for learning achievements in order to create awareness of these issues	**Responsible** The T&L steering committee and vice-deans for quality assurance at HSCs	**Accountable** VRHS, deans of HSCs; and T&L units (medical education departments) at HSCs	**Partners** CELT and deanship for quality development, KSU
Initiative description Assuring high caliber professional performance through self-awareness of the values, attitudes, and beliefs by setting standards for their achievement derived from and constant with the learning goals and mission of the program			
Requirements and interdependencies 1. Collaboration among educational quality assurance departments at HSCs and faculty staff 2. Partners' support with expertise and materials			**Stakeholders** Faculty staff, students, and patients
Action plan 1. Specifying values, attitudes, and beliefs that undergraduate students need to be aware of according to the college's mission and cultural circumstances 2. These values, attitudes, and beliefs should be developed in a more integrative and interdisciplinary fashion at the postgraduate level 3. Training faculty to be good role models in adopting these qualities to their daily practice. This will definitely be reflected on their students 4. Developing students and faculty surveys to measure the extent of their awareness on values, attitudes, and beliefs 5. These guidelines should be documented and stored in relevant database at VRHSs			**Estimated time** Phase II
KPIs 1. At least 75% of students are aware of the values, attitudes, and beliefs required by HSCs mission and goals 2. At least 75% of postgraduate students in various programs are adopting these values, attitudes, and beliefs in their daily practice based on patients' surveys, students' surveys, etc. 3. Demonstration of high-quality professional attitude by majority of faculty staff (≥85%) at HSCs based on students' and patients' surveys 4. At least 85% of faculty staff in each HSC have had structured training in demonstrating values, attitudes, and beliefs 5. Publication of at least one research paper addressing this goal by each HSC (~50% of these should be cited in peer reviewed journals)			**Estimated budget** Phase II

T&L teaching and learning, *HSCs* Health Sciences Colleges, *VRHS* vice-rector for health specialties, *CELT* Center of Excellence in Learning and Teaching, *KSU* King Saud University, *KPIs* key performance indicators

learn. Standards act as specific motivational processes that encourage students to pay more attention to their performance [3]. It has been found that students who are aware of their performance show more self-control upon their learning [4]. These effects are called reactivity that implies metacognition (knowing about knowing). Students who set specific goals for themselves demonstrated superior achievement and perceptions of self-efficacy [5].

Certainly, self-awareness is not enough when the learner lacks the basic skills, but it generates the readiness necessary for learner change. Zimmerman [6] describes those learners as self-regulated learners. He said, "These learners monitor their behavior in terms of their goals and reflect on their increasing effectiveness." This enhances their self-satisfaction and motivation to continue to improve their methods of learning. Therefore, they are more likely "to succeed academically and to view their futures optimistically." Self-regulation is an essential skill for learners because it is part of life-long learning skills. Educationists and quality experts need to assure high caliber professional performance through self-awareness of the values, attitudes, and beliefs and setting standards for their achievement.

The proposed action plan for this initiative begins with identifying the values, attitudes, and beliefs that students need to be aware of according to the college's mission and cultural circumstances to support their learning achievement and professional development. This would be followed by writing the suitable guidelines and training the faculty to be role models in adopting these qualities to their daily practice. Examples of these standards include leadership, teamwork, ethical conduct, scientific inquiry, clinical reasoning and judgment, critical analysis, decision-making, coping with uncertainty, etc. To write these standards, collaboration between educational quality assurance departments at HSCs and the support of faculty are required. The required timeframe and budget for this and the other initiatives depend on available manpower and resources, which will be studied and decided as a second phase.

12.4 Objective (Initiative) 4.2: To Develop Ethical Values and Codes of Ethics for Students and Faculty and Aligning These for IPECP

This initiative's strategy is presented in Table 12.2. Ethics are the moral virtues or obligations that direct professional conduct and judgment. Incorporating both rationality and belief, ethics makes much of spirit, rather than law. It is rational because it makes us pursue three basic questions: (1) What should be done? (2) Why should that be done? (3) How should that be done? Conversely, it also relies on belief since an action can be good or bad, right or wrong, based on the moral value attached to it.

Codes of ethics: For the past several years, health professions educational activities have been identified as significant development but frequently an absent aspect in the academic preparation for IPE and collaborative practice. When health professionals collaborate, they can collectively express a greater commitment to patients and optimize care delivery. Professionals are so-called if they conduct ethically, and

Table 12.2 Strategic plan for developing ethical values and codes of ethics for students and faculty and align these for IPE

Goal 4: Building learners' self-awareness of values, attitudes, and beliefs that influence their learning achievement and actions to a high caliber professional career			
Objective (4.2): To develop ethical values and codes of ethics for students and faculty and to align these for IPE			
Initiative (4.2) Developing ethical values and codes of ethics for students and faculty staff and aligning these for IPE	**Responsible** The T&L steering committee at the VRHS and the T&L units (medical education departments) at HSCs	**Accountable** VRHSs and deans and vice-deans of quality assurance in HSCs	**Partners** CELT, student affairs deanship, and quality deanship at KSU
Initiative description Developing ethical values and codes of ethics for students and faculty and aligning these for IPE			
Requirements and interdependencies 1. Collaboration among health professionals and experts in ethics 2. Collaboration among various ethical bodies and committees 3. Collaboration among experts in ethics and experts in IPE		**Stakeholders** Faculty staff, students, patients, and society	
Action plan 1. Creating a task force committee to review the current code of ethics documents for students and faculty members at HSCs and producing a report accordingly 2. Producing common ethical curricula and codes of ethics for all HSCs 3. Assuring the communication of these codes to students and faculty members 4. Incorporating ethical values curricula and codes of ethics in HSCs curricula along with the IPE and collaborative practice curricula		**Estimated time** Phase II	
KPIs 1. Availability of codes of ethics for students and faculty staff 2. At least 75% of HSCs adopt common ethical values and codes of ethics 3. At least 25% of IPE curricula have ethical values and applications		**Estimated budget** Phase II	

IPE interprofessional education, *T&L* teaching and learning, *HSCs* Health Sciences Colleges, *VRHS* vice-rector for health specialties, *CELT* Center of Excellence in Learning and Teaching, *KSU* King Saud University, *KPIs* key performance indicators

that distinguishes their standing as professionals. In health professional practice, what ought to be done differs with circumstances. Thus, there is a need to streamline and lay down the DOs and DONTs in such circumstances. In this regard, many organizations around the world have issued "Codes of Ethical Conduct" to integrate ethics during health care delivery [7].

There are five fundamental principles that serve as the foundation of codes [8]:

1. *Beneficence:* It is the principle of promoting patients' welfare and acting to their benefit. This emphasizes the primary commitment of a health care professional, which is a service to the patient and to the community. Likewise, health care professionals also have a commitment to use their knowledge and expertise in various avenues like:
   (a) Community service.
   (b) Governing of the profession.
   (c) Research and development.
   (d) Reporting the signs of abuse and neglect.
   (e) Professional demeanor in the workplace.
2. *Non-maleficence:* Patient's protection from any impairment and damage is upheld by this principle. Professionals need to keep their knowledge and skill updated, know their limitations, and ensure careful and mindful handling of the case. They need to be acquainted about:
   (a) Second opinion.
   (b) Personal impairment.
   (c) Patient abandonment/patient referral.
   (d) Infection control.
   (e) Appropriate use of auxiliary personnel.
3. *Respecting the patient:* This principle incorporates two important virtues.
   (a) Patient autonomy: Health care professionals have an obligation to respect the rights of sovereignty and confidentiality. Hence, this involves patient involvement in decision-making and management according to his/her desires within the bounds of standard treatment. They have to protect the patient's confidentiality and safeguard the confidentiality of patient records.
   (b) Informed consent: It is a process of communication where patients receive information about recommended treatments to appropriate "informed" decisions. It is fundamental to both ethics and law and is often overlapped. Health care professionals must be aware of applicable laws, regulations, and standards regarding the nature, scope, and depth of informed consent and refusal discussions.
4. *Justice:* This principle upholds health care professionals' duty to be fair in their communications with patients, colleagues, and society. Various situations to be looked over during their practice include:
   (a) Patients with disabilities.
   (b) Patients with infectious diseases.
   (c) Emergency services.
   (d) Contingent fees.
5. *Veracity/truthfulness*: Health care professionals have a responsibility to be trustworthy and truthful in their dealings with people. Health care professionals have to represent the care rendered to their patients accurately. They have to be cautious in the following situations:
   (a) Unsubstantiated representations.

(b) Treatment dates and procedures.
(c) Fee representation.
(d) Reporting adverse reactions.
(e) Marketing or sale of products or procedures.
(f) Professional announcements.
(g) Advertising.

Aligning ethics in IPECP: Health care professionals from various disciplines come together to render patient-centered care. In addition, within the multidisciplinary teams, they ought to make decisions. Any lapse in communication and collaboration can lead to professional errors. Second, various professional perspectives may lead to conflicts within the team.

World Health Organization calls for "learning together to work together" that facilitates effective teamwork to ascertain safe and effective treatment and care to patients.

Merits of learning ethics through IPE: The aims and objectives of ethics and IPE are alike. Both intend to improve care and compassion toward patients, including ethical teaching fosters learning ethical and professional values. These values form an important component in decision-making and communicating with patients, which otherwise differs among different professionals. There is a need to synthesize the complexity of information and impressions that can then be delivered to patients. Health care professionals need to recognize and collaboratively address and resolve ethical dilemmas.

Content of ethics curricula [9]*:*

1. Ethical principles.
2. Professional codes of ethics.
3. Legal issues.
4. Approaches in dealing with ethical dilemmas.
5. Personal values.

These are explained further as follows:

1. *Ethical principles.* These principles assist in:
   (a) Interests of patients and populations are given utmost significance in the interprofessional health care delivery.
   (b) Maintain confidentiality during provision of team-based care.
   (c) Embrace the professional multiplicity and individual differences.
   (d) Sustain proficiency in one's own profession.
2. *Professional code of ethics*: Professional organizations lay down the "Codes of Ethics" to be pursued in certain situations. Students need to gain familiarity with their respective professional codes of ethics to guide their professional attitudes and behaviors.

3. *Legal issues*: Though conduct in many circumstances does not attract legal scrutiny, there is a thin line of demarcation between ethical and legal bearing. Students have to be equipped to differentiate between them.
4. *Approaches in dealing with ethical dilemmas*: A framework or methodology to guide ethical decision-making in clinical practice has to be incorporated. This includes identifying resources and evaluating alternative courses of action in dealing with ethical dilemmas.
5. *Personal values*: Students need to be trained to identify their personal values and explore the implications for patient care.

Conflict management: Conflict is to be expected when two or more professions are coming together, comprising professionals with differing mindsets and personality types. When expected, preparation is that very thorough, which results in improved communication, enhanced qualities, and experiences translating to improved networking, relationships, and enrichment of lives.

It is better to be prepared for conflict in the formative stages of IPE and IPCP activities rather than address it toward the end as a summative process. The goal is to minimize the issues of conflict for healthier outcomes by mutual discussion, respect, and understanding of the working of each profession and professional. Benefits will eventually be delivered to the patient and translated to enhanced quality of life, health outcomes, and longevity of life.

There have been classical areas in the field of interprofessional ethics which have seen a major conflict of thought processes regarding the accountability between working professionals and have been listed in the literature as case scenarios.

Area 1: Patients having a particular religious' sect, which prohibits acceptance of another's blood. That is, they refuse blood transfusion in the most demanding of situations. How should this be addressed and who should be accountable?

Area 2: A neonatology Intensive Care Unit scenario, where the neonate admitted for epilepsy, has fallen out of the crib door which was accidentally kept open resulting in a serious head injury. How should this be addressed and who should be held accountable?

Management of conflicts needs to be addressed with due sensitivity in relation to the type of conflict, people involved, and the work environment. Issues when addressed with due concern for ethical issues of the collaborating professions and professionals ensure a foundation on which further structures can be planned and implemented.

It is affirmed the professional role within an organization, as a code of ethics, should be developed for both learner and faculty. Not that only, but indeed ethics education should be integrated within curriculum [10, 11]. This is to provide future health care professionals with a sufficient set of skills to deal with ethical issues. There should also be faculty development programs for instructors to have formal training in ethics. There is a general belief that medical schools lack the capable faculty to teach medical ethics. Smith et al. [12] affirm that "one of the major barriers to teaching clinical ethics is the faculty's perception that they lack expertise."

For the development of this initiative, collaboration between health profession educationists among heath science colleges is required. Clinical ethics consultation and clinical ethics committees have various roles and functions in different institutes. They can provide healthcare personnel with advice and recommendations regarding the best course of action (code of ethics) [13]. The proposed action plan begins with reviewing the current codes of ethics in each HSC and produces a revised, and, may be, a unified version that will be communicated to students and faculty members. This can be done through health sciences curriculum committees and faculty development programs at HSCs.

12.5 Objective (Initiative) 4.3: To Support Mentorships for Students

According to the KSU designed strategic plan, the strategy of this initiative has been planned as shown in Table 12.3. In line with the Initiative 3.1 "support and foster mentorship programs" presented in Chap. 3, we will discuss the depth of the

Table 12.3 Strategic plan for supporting mentorships for students

Goal 4: Building learner's self-awareness of values, attitudes, and beliefs that influence their learning achievement and actions to a high caliber professional career			
Objective (4.3): To support mentorships for students			
Initiative (4.3) Establishing the culture of mentorship for students	**Responsible** The T&L steering committee and the T&L units (medical education departments) in each HSC	**Accountable** VRHS, leadership committee; and deans of HSCs	**Partners** Center for Students' counseling and guidance and CELT, KSU
Initiative description Developing facilitative tools and establishing means of the mentorship culture among faculty staff and students for everlasting trust relationship			
Requirements and interdependencies 1. Experts in students' mentorship 2. Center for Students' counseling and guidance			**Stakeholders** Faculty staff and students
Action plan 1. Establishing programs and workshops that address mentorship to assist in faculty awareness and provide positive attitudes toward assisting others 2. Establishing the guidelines that control mentor–mentee relationship 3. Developing tools to assess students' expectations from mentorship			**Estimated time** Phase II
KPIs 1. Workshops and programs planned are conducted (at least for 70%) 2. Guidelines for the mentor–mentee relationship are established 3. Students' expectations are listed			**Estimated budget** Phase II

T&L teaching and learning, *HSCs* Health Sciences Colleges, *VRHS* vice-rector for health specialties, *CELT* Center of Excellence in Learning and Teaching, *KSU* King Saud University, *KPIs* key performance indicators

relationship between the mentor and the mentee by highlighting the importance of cultivating mentorship culture and creating the suitable environment and system for this relationship. Mentoring has different forms of students' support inclusively described by Megginson [14] as "off line help by one person to another in making significant transitions in knowledge, work or thinking." Therefore, a mentor is "someone who helps another person to become what that person aspires to be." The mentor helps the learner "mentee" to adapt to new situation such as new college, personal circumstances, etc. Mentoring has different models and types: one-to-one mentoring, co-mentoring/peer mentoring, and group mentoring. Mentoring can also be formal where a mentee chooses his/her mentor or informally when a student looks for guidance and help from another person. Starting a new health science program is a stressful situation for students posing challenges that need to be overcome not only by the students themselves but also with the help of their organization. Mentoring actually provides the students with this support as it guides them through critical periods of their education where knowledge, skills, and attitudes are acquired.

This initiative, in addition to what is suggested in Initiative 3.1, provides the tools and means of successful mentor–mentee relationship. The responsible for the execution of this initiative will need to recruit experts in mentoring from KSU and may be from outside the university, in collaboration with the Center for Students' Counseling and Guidance, to form a task force committee. This committee will conduct faculty and student awareness programs and workshops in HSCs, highlighting the importance of mentoring and nature of the mentor–mentee relationship. To succeed in activating mentorship programs, the support and cooperation of the faculty and departments are also required. Not each faculty member is supposed to be a mentor; those who are enthusiastic and interested in mentoring are the candidates to be mentors. The first and most important character of a good mentor is the willingness to be a mentor. Other important characteristics include: to be non-judgmental, good listener, honest, empathetic, feedback provider, accessible, dedicating with time for mentoring, and optimistic [15]. Regarding the proposed action plan to establish this initiative, it starts with educational programs for all the stakeholders (faculty members and students), this is to create a positive culture toward mentoring. Also, those programs need to be complemented with guidelines that describe the nature of successful mentoring relationship. The guidelines that control mentor–mentee relationship are already established at the "Center for Students' Counseling and Guidance," but need to be implemented successfully in each department through the T&L units (medical education departments) at HSCs. The accountable for establishing this initiative are the VRHSs as a legislative body; Deans as authoritative and top administrative persons; and the Leadership Committee as the liaison for the implementation of the guidelines and mentorship programs in various departments. The Partners for this initiative are "Center for Students' Counseling and Guidance" and CELT that will provide the experts and materials for this initiative. Students' expectations from mentorship are best judged after establishing and merging in mentorship programs, using many tools especially through surveys and personal interviews [16, 17].

12.6 Objective (Initiative) 4.4: To Train Faculty Staff to be Role Models

This initiative's strategy is presented in Table 12.4. In line with the aim of the previous initiative in building learners' self-awareness of values, attitudes, and beliefs of professional performance, this objective brings the importance of role modeling, or

Table 12.4 The strategic plan for training faculty in role modeling

<table>
<tr><td colspan="4">Goal 4: Building learner's self-awareness of values, attitudes, and beliefs that influence their learning achievement and actions to a high caliber professional career</td></tr>
<tr><td colspan="4">Objective (4.4): To train faculty to be role models</td></tr>
<tr><td>Initiative (4.4)
Improving faculty behaviors as role models of professional behaviors through training</td><td>Responsible
The T&L steering committee and the T&L units (medical education departments) in HSCs</td><td>Accountable
Leadership committee and deans of HSCs</td><td>Partners
Deanship for skills development and CELT</td></tr>
<tr><td colspan="4">Initiative description
Training faculty to role model appropriate professional behaviors in their interactions with students, peers, seniors, and staff with emphasis on excellence, integrity, compassion, interpersonal relationships, communications, mutual respect, and ethics</td></tr>
<tr><td colspan="2">Requirements and interdependencies
1. Consultants/experts to develop and facilitate courses and workshops for faculty about professionalism
2. Instruments to assess role modeling of professional behaviors by faculty</td><td colspan="2">Stakeholders
Faculty staff, both undergraduate and postgraduate HSCs students, and patients</td></tr>
<tr><td colspan="2">Action plan
1. Strengthening an environment that emphasizes and values professional behaviors through development of guidelines to recognize and reward exemplary faculty role models
2. Increasing faculty education about professionalism through workshops and courses using videos, films, directed reading, experiential learning, small group discussion, case scenario, role plays, etc., through faculty development programs
3. Promoting reflection in action and on action by faculty
4. Utilizing instruments such as 360 evaluations, student portfolios, and reflections to assess role modeling of professional behaviors by faculty and providing feedback on performance to faculty</td><td colspan="2">Estimated time
Phase II</td></tr>
<tr><td colspan="2">KPIs
1. At least 70% of HSCs faculty have attended workshops or courses on teaching, assessing, and providing feedback about professionalism
2. At least 50% of faculty are recognized as role models through awards</td><td colspan="2">Estimated budget
Phase II</td></tr>
</table>

T&L teaching and learning, *HSCs* Health Sciences Colleges, *CELT* Center of Excellence in Learning and Teaching, *KPIs* key performance indicators teaching by example. Indeed, "Role modeling" is at the heart of professional character formation. Excellence in professional practice is learned in and through experience and critical reflection on its expression in the clinical encounter. Knowledge and skills are essential but putting them together in a competent and caring response to patients' needs is learned in personal interaction and role modeling [18]. Role modeling is educational methodology that teaches students in different settings, in the lecture room, outpatient clinics, and rounds [19]. It has been shown that it is one of the influential methods, and faculty should be aware that their attitudes and behaviors affect students' actions. Also, it has been found that role models affect students' choice of specialty and career [20, 21]. Therefore, this initiative is important in providing the faculty with needed training to utilize this method to benefit with students' learning.

In developing the professional behavior, the literature focuses on building self-reflective skills and professional identity. Those skills start to develop since students enter the school. The role of faculty is essential in creating those skills [22]. Yet, there is deficiency in faculty' role modeling and their professional character influence. In a survey administered among second-year students and senior clerks in Canadian medical schools [23], it was found that 25% of second-year students and 40% of senior clerks did not agree that their faculty were good role models in teaching physician–patient relationship. In addition, more than half of second-year students and senior clerks did not agree that their faculty appreciated human contact with them or were helpful with students who had difficulties. Thus, it is essential to focus on this fundamental aspect of faculty's professional character formation for the benefit of both faculty staff and learners.

The action plan for this initiative is to encourage the environments of professional behavior through development of guidelines to recognize and reward exemplary faculty role models. This is also done by training faculty through experiential learning, small group discussions, workshops and courses using videos, films, directed reading, case scenarios, and role plays. In addition, we can employ stimulation of reflection in action and on action by faculty, using evaluative instruments such as 360 surveys, student portfolios, and reflections to assess role modeling of professional behaviors by faculty, and providing feedback on performance to faculty.

12.7 Objective (Initiative) 4.5: To Train Faculty in Giving Feedback in This Area

The strategy for this initiative is summarized in Table 12.5. In continuation with the pervious initiative, faculty should also be trained in providing students with effective feedback regarding their professional behavior. Feedback is an essential part of learning and developing professional behavior [24]. It helps students to self-reflect, raise self-awareness, and plan for future learning and practice [25]. A study on the relationship between trainees and supervisors in medicine shows that feedback,

Table 12.5 Strategic plan for training faculty in giving constructive feedback

Goal 4: Building learner's self-awareness of values, attitudes, and beliefs that influence their learning achievement and actions to a high caliber professional career			
Objective (4.5): To train faculty in giving feedback in this area			
Initiative (4.5) Improving faculty capacity to provide feedback to students about their professional behaviors through training	**Responsible** The T&L steering committee and the T&L units (medical education departments) in HSCs	**Accountable** Leadership committee and deans of HSCs	**Partners** CELT and deanship for skills development at KSU
Initiative description Training faculty in providing appropriate constructive feedback to students' professional behaviors			
Requirements and interdependencies 1. Consultants/experts to develop and facilitate workshops on providing feedback to students 2. Developing instruments to assess professional behaviors of students (or use one or more of the existing valid and reliable instruments such as LAMPS, nurse practitioners' roles and competencies scale, and perceived faculty competency inventory)			**Stakeholders** Faculty staff and students (undergraduate and postgraduate)
Action plan 1. Developing techniques for teaching professionalism sensitive to the learner's level 2. Promoting reflection in action and on action by students about professionalism 3. Utilizing instruments such as continuous evaluation of professional behaviors using rating scales, 360 evaluations, student portfolios, and reflections to assess students' professional behaviors 4. Providing effective feedback based on observation and evidence using suitable techniques			**Estimated time** Phase II
KPIs 1. Students' professional behaviors formally assessed 2. Interprofessional course on professionalism is established (at least in four out of the six HSCs)			**Estimated budget** Phase II

T&L teaching and learning, *HSCs* Health Sciences Colleges, *CELT* Center of Excellence in Learning and Teaching, *LAMPS* learner's attitude of medical professionalism scale, *KPIs* key performance indicators

when given in a constructive way, influences trainees positively and makes them see their specialty and themselves positively and confidently [26]. Nevertheless, there is a general lack of practice in that area, and feedback is not conveyed by faculty to students frequently or effectively. A survey found that feedback given by consultants to pre-registration house officers is rudimentary. It is recommended, "The educational supervisor should help with both professional and personal development and be aware of the pre-registration house officer's individual needs … provide feedback on their clinical progress … and should personally undertake and not delegate their tutorial functions" [27].

12.8 Objective (Initiative) 4.6: To Suggest Methods of Reflective Practice

This initiative's strategy is presented in Table 12.6. It has been recognized that reflective practice has a beneficial effect on the student's professional development with recent evidence showing its role in the appraisal and revalidation process for health care professionals "Tomorrow's Doctors" [28]. The concept of reflective practice was introduced by Schön [29] as a process that would support an individual's skills in a specific discipline. Schön defines reflective practice as analytical and effortful thinking process considering self-experiences in applying knowledge to practice. It enables students to review and improve their own performance and become self-directed learners [30]. Also, it helps students to realize consonance between their own individual performances and those of successful professionals. Following the introduction of reflective practice concept by Schön [29], many

Table 12.6 Strategic plan for suggesting methods of reflective practice

<table>
<tr><td colspan="4">Goal 4: Building learner's self-awareness of values, attitudes, and beliefs that influence their learning achievement and actions to a high caliber professional career</td></tr>
<tr><td colspan="4">Objective (4.6): To suggest methods of reflective practice</td></tr>
<tr><td>Initiative (4.6)
Promoting reflective practice among students using appropriate methods</td><td>Responsible
The T&L steering committee and the T&L units of medical education departments in each HSC</td><td>Accountable
VRHSs, leadership committee, and deans of HSCs</td><td>Partners
CELT and deanship for skills development</td></tr>
<tr><td colspan="4">Initiative description
For students' professional development, reflective practice is an important skill to be learned that would enhance students' self-awareness and regulation</td></tr>
<tr><td colspan="2">Requirements and interdependencies
1. Collaboration among health profession educationists
2. Collaboration among HSCs
3. Developing 10 vignettes for students and faculty reflective practice</td><td colspan="2">Stakeholders
Faculty staff and students</td></tr>
<tr><td colspan="2">Action plan
1. Creating a task force committee that would look into the suitable methods for enhancing reflection among faculty and students
2. Running a trial on some courses to test student and faculty responses
3. Modifying based on feedback and expand to a strategy</td><td colspan="2">Estimated time
Phase II</td></tr>
<tr><td colspan="2">KPIs
1. More than 70% satisfaction from faculty and students in applying reflection in/on educational practice</td><td colspan="2">Estimated budget
Phase II</td></tr>
</table>

T&L teaching and learning, *HSCs* Health Sciences Colleges, *VRHS* vice-rector for health specialties, *CELT* Center of Excellence in Learning and Teaching, *KPIs* key performance indicators schools, colleges, and other educational programs introduced this concept into their curricula and designed professional development programs to their student and faculty based on this concept.

In this program, reflective practice is one of the initiatives to achieve excellence in learning and teaching of professionalism. The appropriate methods for developing reflective practice among teachers and students would be used, and the challenges that face educators should be identified and managed properly. Reflection is not an intuitive process, and simulating students to reflect efficiently is not easy. Philip [31] states that, "By its nature reflective practice is difficult to teach, difficult to encourage and not a process that students and indeed some staff are entirely comfortable with." Currently, there are two main methods to engage students in reflective practice: using portfolios and the process of mentoring by Davies [30]. There are also other approaches in teaching and assessment that would encourage reflection such as: self-assessment, peer-assessment, group-work, effective feedback, and peer-tutoring [31].

12.9 Summary

Developing professionalism into the learning behavior is part of the curriculum and instructional agenda. It takes structural steps with horizontal integration among courses and longitudinal approach along the program years. At KSU, our goal is to improve health profession education programs, so it would graduate professionals with the appropriate values, attitudes, and beliefs that would influence their learning achievement and actions to a high caliber professional career. This can be accomplished by the support of developing achievement standards, code of ethics, mentoring, positive role modeling, feedback, and reflective practice.

References

1. Jha V, Bekker HL, Duffy SR, Roberts TE. A systematic review of studies assessing and facilitating attitudes towards professionalism in medicine. Med Educ. 2007;41(8):822–9.
2. Wilkinson TJ, Wade WB, Knock LD. A blueprint to assess professionalism: results of a systematic review. Acad Med. 2009;84(5):551–8.
3. Ames C, Archer J. Achievement goals in the classroom: students' learning strategies and motivation processes. J Educ Psychol. 1988;80(3):260–7.
4. Shapiro ES, Cole CL. Self-monitoring in assessing children's problems. Psychol Assess. 1999;11(4):448–57.
5. Zimmerman B, Schunk D. Reflections on theories of self-regulated learning and academic achievement. In: Zimmerman B, Schunk D, editors. Self-regulated learning and academic achievement: theoretical perspectives. London: Tylor and Francis e-Library; 2008. p. 273.
6. Zimmerman BJ. Becoming a self-regulated learner: an overview. Theory Pract J. 2002;41(2):64–70.
7. Machin LL, Bellis KM, Dixon C, Morgan H, Pye J, Spencer P, et al. Interprofessional education and practice guide: designing ethics-orientated interprofessional education for health and social care students. J Interprof Care. 2018;33(6):608–18.

8. American Dental Association. Principles of ethics and code of professional conduct. Washington, DC: ADA; 2020; https://www.ada.org/about/principles/code-of-ethics.
9. Naidoo S, Turner KM, McNeill DB. Ethics and interprofessional education: an exploration across health professions education programs. J Interprof Care. 2019;34(6):829–31.
10. Campbell AV, Chin J, Voo TC. How can we know that ethics education produces ethical doctors? Med Teach. 2007;29(5):431–6.
11. Hafferty FW, Franks R. The hidden curriculum, ethics teaching, and the structure of medical education. Acad Med. 1994;69(11):861–71.
12. Smith S, Fryer-Edwards K, Diekema DS, Braddock CH 3rd. Finding effective strategies for teaching ethics: a comparison trial of two interventions. Acad Med. 2004;79(3):265–71.
13. Rasoal D, Skovdahl K, Gifford M, Kihlgren A. Clinical ethics support for healthcare personnel: an integrative literature review. HEC Forum. 2017;29(4):313–46.
14. Megginson D. Mentoring in action: a practical guide (2nd edition). Development and learning in organizations. Hum Resour Manag Int Dig. 2006;14:1.
15. Mckimm J, Jollie C, Hatter M. Mentoring: theory and practice. Preparedness to Practice Project, Mentoring Scheme, 2007; http://www.faculty.londondeanery.ac.uk/e-learning/feedback/files/Mentoring_Theory_and_Practice.pdf.
16. Bell-Ellison BA, Dedrick RF. What do doctoral students value in their ideal mentor? Res High Educ. 2008;49(6):555–67.
17. Elcigil A, Sari HY. Students' opinions about and expectations of effective nursing clinical mentors. J Nurs Educ. 2008;47(3):118–23.
18. Kenny NP, Mann KV, MacLeod H. Role modeling in physicians' professional formation: reconsidering an essential but untapped educational strategy. Acad Med. 2003;78(12):1203–10.
19. Ficklin FL, Browne VL, Powell RC, Carter JE. Faculty and house staff members as role models. J Med Educ. 1988;63(5):392–6.
20. Babbott D, Levey GS, Weaver SO, Killian CD. Medical student attitudes about internal medicine: a study of U.S. medical school seniors in 1988. Ann Intern Med. 1991;114(1):16–22.
21. Lieu TA, Schroeder SA, Altman DF. Specialty choices at one medical school: recent trends and analysis of predictive factors. Acad Med. 1989;64:622–9.
22. Wright S, Wong A, Newill C. The impact of role models on medical students. J Gen Intern Med. 1997;12:53–6.
23. Maheux B, Beaudoin C, Berkson L, Côté L, Des Marchais J, Jean P. Medical faculty as humanistic physicians and teachers: the perceptions of students at innovative and traditional medical schools. Med Educ. 2000;34(8):630–4.
24. Nicol DJ, Macfarlane-Dick D. Formative assessment and self-regulated learning: a model and seven principles of good feedback practice. Stud High Educ. 2006;31(2):199–218.
25. Devi V, Mandal T, Kodidela S, Pallath V. Integrating students' reflection-in-learning and examination performance as a method for providing educational feedback. J Post Grad Med. 2012;58(4):270–4.
26. Paice E, Moss F, Heard S, Winder B, McManus C. The relationship between pre-registration house officers and their consultants. Med Educ. 2002;36:26–34.
27. Wilson DH. Education and training of preregistration house officers: the consultants' viewpoint. BMJ. 1993;306:194–6.
28. Turner MA, Kelly M, Leftwick P, Dogra N. Tomorrow's doctors and diversity issues in medical education. Med Teach. 2014;36(9):743–5.
29. Schön DA. The reflective practitioner: how professionals think in action. Qual Soc Work J. 2009;8(1):124–9.
30. Davies S. Embracing reflective practice. Educ Prim Care. 2012;23(1):9–12.
31. Philip L. Encouraging reflective practice amongst students. Planet. 2006;17:37–9.

Faculty Development and Promotion 13

Dalal Abdullah Alqahtani, Eiad Abdelmohsen Alfaris, and Naghma Naeem

13.1 Introduction

Faculty members are the most important resource of any academic institution. As such, faculty development programs are essential in supporting and improving the educational excellence of this invaluable resource. Wilkerson and Irby [1] state, "Academic vitality is dependent upon faculty members' interest and expertise; faculty development has a critical role to play in promoting academic excellence and innovation."

While it was once assumed that a competent health care practitioner would naturally be an effective teacher, it is now acknowledged that preparation for teaching is necessary [2]. By developing faculty members' skills in teaching, mentorship, research, and leadership, educational institutions can achieve their goals and visions. Although the responsibility for such development falls largely on the faculty members themselves, institutional leaders also bear the moral and professional responsibility to support the growth of those faculty members they have recruited and hired

D. A. Alqahtani (✉)
Oral Medicine and Diagnostic Sciences, College of Dentistry, King Saud University, Riyadh, Saudi Arabia

E. A. Alfaris
Department of Family and Community Medicine, College of Medicine, King Saud University, Riyadh, Saudi Arabia

N. Naeem
College of Medicine, King Saud University, Riyadh, Kingdom of Saudi Arabia

M. Y. Alnaami et al. (eds.), *Novel Health Interprofessional Education and Collaborative Practice Program: Strategy and Implementation*, https://doi.org/10.1007/978-981-99-3420-1_13

[3]. This is important especially with the increasing complexity of healthcare delivery and the need to develop new approaches to teaching and learning that would foster students' learning in diverse settings.

At KSU, our goal is to enable faculty to meet their goals as scholars and teachers so as to achieve innovation and educational excellence. The following sections discuss the strategic steps and initiatives proposed to achieve this goal.

13.2 Strategic Goal 5: Promoting and Supporting Distinguished and Innovative Educational Excellence and Scholarship Among Faculty

Based on multiple meetings, seminars, and workshops among the key faculty members, educators, consultants, student representatives, and other relevant stakeholders, this goal was developed. The goal was founded on the crucial role of faculty members in HSCs on achieving educational excellence by preparing and training them in the latest principles of learning and teaching strategies. Several initiatives were proposed to achieve this goal. These are outlined below:

13.3 Objective (Initiative) 5.1: To Collaborate with the Deanship of Skills Development

This initiative's strategy is presented in Table 13.1. It states the need for collaboration with Skills Development Deanship to reach the ultimate goal, which is to support distinguished and innovative educational excellence and scholarship among faculty. Missions of the Skills Development Deanship include drawing up the future

Table 13.1 Strategic plan for collaboration with the Deanship of Skills Development

Goal 5: Promoting and supporting distinguished and innovative educational excellence and scholarship among faculty			
Objective (5.1): To collaborate with the deanship of skills development			
Initiative (5.1) Collaboration with deanship of skills development to build faculty's capacity to realize the university's mission of excellence in education and scholarship	**Responsible** T&L steering committee and T&L units (medical education departments) in HSCs	**Accountable** VRHS and deans of HSCs	**Partners** Deanship of skills development and CELT
Initiative description Faculty skills development is a continuous activity, whereby universities sustain faculty vitality. This can be achieved by cultivating professional and personal development of faculty at all levels. Collaboration between different entities involved in faculty development is therefore essential. Collaboration should aim to provide contemporary vision of educational leadership, facilitate academic collaborations and educational innovations across the university, and harness the full capacity of faculty to achieve excellence in educational scholarship			

Requirements and interdependencies	**Stakeholders**
1. Experts and consultants in faculty skills development	Faculty staff
Action plan	**Estimated time**
1. Developing policies, practices, and an infrastructure of systems that assures needs-based faculty development 2. Advancing a culture of university-wide academic excellence 3. Promoting university-wide culture of professionalism	Ongoing
KPIs	**Estimated budget**
1. Collaboration established and working	Phase II

T&L teaching and learning, *HSCs* Health Sciences Colleges, *VRHS* vice-rector for health specialties, *CELT* Center of Excellence in Learning and Teaching, *KPIs* key performance indicators

strategies necessary to raise the skills of faculty members to achieve excellence and creativity in teaching and learning and developing faculty members' ability to design and develop courses and transform them into electronic content. Faculty development is an ongoing effort whereby universities sustain faculty vitality [4]. This can be achieved by cultivating professional and personal development of faculty at all levels. Collaboration between different entities involved in faculty development is therefore essential. Collaboration should aim to provide contemporary vision of educational leadership, facilitate academic collaborations and educational innovations across the university, and invest on the full capacity of faculty to achieve excellence in educational scholarship. The required timeframe and budget for this and the other initiatives in this section depend on available manpower and resources, which will be studied and decided as a second phase.

13.4 Objective (Initiative) 5.2: To Develop and Support the Utilization of Educational Materials by Faculty Members

According to the KSU designed strategic plan, the strategy of this initiative has been planned as shown in Table 13.2. It suggests the need for developing educational materials that would support faculty members in improving their teaching skills.

In line with the previous initiative (2.1) in Chap. 10 "provide learning theory resources," educational resources are vital for faculty development, since it offers not only literature findings, but also practical ideas and tips that faculty members can use throughout their teaching practice. These resources might be digital or non-digital and can be used for learning, education, or training. Non-digital educational materials may include textbooks, journals, and course-materials on CDs or other forms of storage. Digital educational materials may include portals that provide relevant links or URLs, curricular material developed by other faculty or institutions, encyclopedia, data archives, videos and films, images or visual materials, simulations and animations, personal online diaries (blogs), mailing list/forums, online book, presentation, publication, how-to articles, reference resources and manual, etc.

Table 13.2 Strategic plan for developing and providing faculty members with educational resources

Goal 5: Promoting and supporting distinguished and innovative educational excellence and scholarship among faculty			
Objective (5.2): To develop and support the utilization of educational materials by faculty members			
Initiative (5.2) Build a central repository of educational resources for faculty	**Responsible** The T&L steering committee, vice-deans academic affairs of HSCs, and the T&L units (medical education departments) in HSCs	**Accountable** VRHS and deans of HSCs	**Partners** Deanship of library affairs, deanship of e-learning, and CELT
Initiative description An educational resource may be defined as any entity, non-digital or digital that may be used for learning, education, or training. Non-digital educational material may include textbooks, journals, course-materials on CDs and DVDs, educational games, etc. Digital educational materials may include portals that provide relevant links or URLs, curricular material developed by other faculty or institutions, encyclopedia, data archives, videos and films, images or visual materials, simulations and animations, personal online diaries (blogs), mailing list/forums, online book, presentations, publications, how-to articles, reference resources, etc.			
Requirements and interdependencies 1. Medical educationist collaboration 2. Sharing and unifying core educational resources for all HSCs		**Stakeholders** Faculty and students	
Action plan 1. Providing a list of educational materials that facilitate and support learning 2. Building a repository of educational materials 3. Monitoring the progress of establishment of repository and utilization of educational materials		**Estimated time** Phase II	
KPIs 1. Availability of 70% of intended educational material 2. More than 50% of faculty utilization of those materials		**Estimated budget** Phase II	

T&L teaching and learning, *HSCs* Health Sciences Colleges, *VRHS* vice-rector for health specialties, *CELT* Center of Excellence in Learning and Teaching, *CDs* compact discs, *DVDs* digital video discs, *URLs* uniform resource locators, *KPIs* key performance indicators

An example of an online digital library available for KSU faculty is the Saudi Digital Library [5]. The library provides to all Saudi universities one umbrella, through which students and researchers can have free access to more than 300 international publishers, and more than (310,000) full e-books in various scientific specialization including other commercially available resources such as the Education Resources Information Center [6], composed of more than 1.3 million bibliographic records. It is the world's largest educational database that is used by teachers, researchers, education professionals, and policy makers around the world. It contains more than 1.4 million records from all areas of education and links to more than 337,000 full-text documents. Many documents, from research reports to curriculum guides, pamphlets to conference papers, are also included. Another database resource is EBSCO Health [7], which is one of the leading providers of evidence-based clinical decision support solutions, healthcare business intelligence, and peer-reviewed medical research information for the healthcare industry. Also, Ovid [8] is one of the world's leading medical, academic, and corporate institutions that help librarians, clinicians, researches, students, instructors, and other healthcare professionals find the information they need to make critical decisions that improve patients' care. In addition to the SDL, each academic institute will choose resources that match their needs and source for their financial support. Another useful resource is called MedEdPORTAL [9], founded in 2005. It is a MEDLINE-indexed, open-access journal of teaching and learning resources in the health professions published by the Association of American Medical Colleges (AAMC), in partnership with the American Dental Education Association. MedEdPORTAL publications are stand-alone, complete teaching or learning modules that have been implemented and evaluated with medical or dental trainees or practitioners. Each submission is reviewed by editorial staff and external peer reviewers using a standardized review instrument grounded in the tenets of educational scholarship. It is a great resource of toolkits, courses, and modules that were largely applied in HSCs. Such resources would expand faculty members' knowledge of the profession, broaden their teaching horizons, and give them a lifelong resource for improving professional competence.

In order to facilitate the execution of this initiative, the responsible bodies should formulate a task force committee consisting of expert educationists, librarians, and IT personnel who will make a sharing and unifying core educational resource for all HSCs.

13.5 Objective (Initiative) 5.3: To Provide a Listing of Courses

This initiative's strategy is presented in Table 13.3. Coinciding with previous initiatives to provide faculty members with learning resources, this initiative focuses on giving them list of courses on the best practices of teaching. In KSU, the Deanship of Skills Development provides the faculty members each semester with full list of various courses that can be a great opportunity for faculty members to enhance their skills in different aspects such as teaching, leadership, and management. However, each HSC might also provide their faculty members with needs-based list of courses. So, it can gather all available courses (national and international) and make lists to be sent to faculty members for subscription. Also, HSCs can provide courses that add specific skills to the faculty members needed for their roles in college. The action plan for this initiative starts with needs assessment data. Based on the results, a list of selected courses—offered by authoritative national and international institutions—will be presented to faculty members. A general needs assessment study was

Table 13.3 Strategic plan for providing a listing of courses

Goal 5: Promoting and supporting distinguished and innovative educational excellence and scholarship among faculty			
Objective (5.3): To provide a listing of courses			
Initiative (5.3) Provide a listing of relevant courses on educational scholarship	**Responsible** T&L steering committee and T&L units (medical education departments) in HSCs	**Accountable** VRHS and deans of HSCs	**Partners** Deanship of skills development and CELT
Initiative description Identifying and prioritizing (based on needs assessment) a list of high-quality courses on educational scholarship			
Requirements and interdependencies 1. Listings of courses related to educational scholarship offered by authoritative national and international institutions 2. Needs assessment data		**Stakeholders** Faculty staff	
Action plan 1. Needs assessment 2. Analyzing data of needs assessment 3. Providing a list of courses relevant to educational scholarship		**Estimated time** Phase II	
KPIs 1. List of courses available to faculty		**Estimated budget** Phase II	

T&L teaching and learning, *HSCs* Health Sciences Colleges, *VRHS* vice-rector for health specialties, *CELT* Center of Excellence in Learning and Teaching, *KPIs* key performance indicators

conducted in HSCs to evaluate faculty perception and readiness to engage in initiatives toward excellence revealed emphasis on teaching, learning and assessment, research and development, and graduate education [10].

13.6 Objective (Initiative) 5.4: To Foster the Utilization of Online Courses

The strategy for this initiative is summarized in Table 13.4. Continuing with the pervious initiative, there are more resources in online learning, e.g., providing useful links to improve skills through self-study and practice. Currently, there are online courses provided by prestigious institutions such as Harvard, MIT, Johns Hopkins, and Stanford. The courses are provided free and through online learning platforms such as edX [11], Coursera [12], and Stanford Online—Stanford Center for Professional Development [13]. Also, there is a Saudi Arabian online learning platform named "Rwaq" [14], an Arabic platform for open education. It is a personal project founded in (2013) that provides courses in all educational fields. KSU can make its own platform for all online courses provided that this initiative is supported and executed for this program through the center of excellence in interprofessional education (CEIPE), Chap. 1.

Table 13.4 Strategic plan for fostering the utilization of online courses

Goal 5: Promoting and supporting distinguished and innovative educational excellence and scholarship among faculty			
Objective (5.4): To foster the utilization of online courses			
Initiative (5.4) Provide links to relevant online courses on educational scholarship	**Responsible** T&L steering committee and T&L units (medical education departments) in HSCs	**Accountable** VRHS and deans of HSCs	**Partners** Deanship of e-learning and CELT
Initiative description Identifying and prioritizing (based on needs assessment) a list of high-quality online courses on educational scholarship			
Requirements and interdependencies 1. Listings of online courses related to educational scholarship offered by national, regional, and international institutions of repute 2. Needs assessment data			**Stakeholders** Faculty staff
Action plan 1. Needs assessment 2. Analyzing data of needs assessment 3. Providing a list of online courses relevant to needs 4. Developing local online courses			**Estimated time** Phase II
KPIs 1. At least 80% of faculty are aware of the availability of such courses list 2. At least 3 online courses are established 3. At least 30% of the faculty participated in at least one online course			**Estimated budget** Phase II

T&L teaching and learning, *HSCs* Health Sciences Colleges, *VRHS* vice-rector for health specialties, *CELT* Center of Excellence in Learning and Teaching, *KPIs* key performance indicators

13.7 Objective (Initiative) 5.5: To Train Faculty in Educational Scholarship

This initiative's strategy is presented in Table 13.5. It highlights the need for informing faculty members of the concept of scholarship and its importance on their career path. To be a scholar, it means to be able to produce creative work that has value, and its integrity is measured by the ability to think, learn, and communicate [15]. Previously, the concept of scholarship on the academic field was based on research and publication. However, in 1990 Ernest Boyer—President of the Carnegie Foundation for the Advancement of Teaching—called for the need to reform the concept of scholarship. He argues, "what we now have is more restricted view of scholarship, one that limits it to a hierarchy of functions" [15]. Educational scholarship refers to any material, product, or resource originally developed to fulfill a specific educational purpose that has been successfully peer-reviewed and is subsequently made public through appropriate dissemination for use by others. It must be made public, peer-reviewed, reproduced, and built on by others. The Boyer's paradigm includes the following four overlapping and interdependent domains of scholarship: Discovery, Integration, Application, and Teaching. Basic research has come to be viewed as the first and most essential form of scholarly activity, with other

Table 13.5 Strategic plan for training faculty in the concept of scholarship

<table>
<tr><td colspan="4">Goal 5: Promoting and supporting distinguished and innovative educational excellence and scholarship among faculty</td></tr>
<tr><td colspan="4">Objective (5.5): To train faculty in educational scholarship</td></tr>
<tr><td>Initiative (5.5)
Provide interprofessional workshops on educational scholarship</td><td>Responsible
T&L steering committee and T&L units (medical education departments) in HSCs</td><td>Accountable
VRHS, deans of HSCs, and KSU scientific council</td><td>Partners
KSU scientific council and CELT</td></tr>
<tr><td colspan="4">Initiative description
Conducting workshops on the new form of educational scholarship by affirming the value of faculty's educational activities</td></tr>
<tr><td colspan="2">Requirements and interdependencies
1. Collaboration between medical educationists, experts in educational scholarship both within and outside the university</td><td colspan="2">Stakeholders
Faculty staff</td></tr>
<tr><td colspan="2">Action plan
1. Identifying experts in the educational scholarship both across and outside the university who can serve as resource persons and facilitators
2. Workshops planning
3. Workshops implementation and evaluation</td><td colspan="2">Estimated time
Phase II</td></tr>
<tr><td colspan="2">KPIs
1. More than 80% increase in knowledge "post-workshops"
2. At least 25% increase in scholarly educational output of faculty</td><td colspan="2">Estimated budget
Phase II</td></tr>
</table>

T&L teaching and learning, *HSCs* Health Sciences Colleges, *VRHS* vice-rector for health specialties, *CELT* Center of Excellence in Learning and Teaching, *KPIs* key performance indicators

functions flowing from it. Scholars are academics who conduct research, publish, and then perhaps convey their knowledge to students or apply what they have learned. The latter functions grow out of scholarship, and they are not to be considered part of it. However, knowledge is not necessarily developed in such a linear manner. The arrow of causality can, and frequently does, point in both directions. Theory surely leads to practice, but practice also leads to theory. And teaching, at its best, shapes both research and practice. Viewed from this perspective, a more comprehensive, more dynamic understanding of scholarship can be considered, one in which the rigid categories of teaching, research, and service are broadened and more flexibly defined [15]. By 1992, numerous medical and dental schools had announced their acceptance of the new form of educational scholarship [16]. They even encouraged faculty members to provide evidence of their educational scholarship in portfolio-like documents. As of 2000, more recognition is shown to this concept with linking it to academic promotion [17].

This initiative aims to provide faculty members with training and detailed advice on the new concept of scholarship and how to utilize it to build up their professional career. To train faculty, collaboration between medical educationists, experts in educational scholarship both within and outside the university is needed.

13.8 Objective (Initiative) 5.6: To Provide Support for Educational Research

This initiative's strategy is presented in Table 13.6. Research is a major part of academic development. In the Lancet Commission Report for Health Professionals for a New Century [18], it is stated that expenditures for health professional education

Table 13.6 Strategic plan for supporting educational research

Goal 5: Promoting and supporting distinguished and innovative educational excellence and scholarship among faculty			
Objective (5.6): To provide support for educational research			
Initiative (5.6) Support a culture of educational research at KSU	**Responsible** T&L steering committee and T&L units (medical education departments) in HSCs	**Accountable** VRHS and deans of HSCs	**Partners** Scientific publishing center, CELT, king Abdullah Institute for research and consulting studies, and KACST-GDRG
Initiative description Supporting a culture of educational research at the university by improving research environment and increasing support services for researchers			
Requirements and interdependencies 1. Professional educational research support for all HSCs			**Stakeholders** Faculty staff
Action plan 1. Prioritizing the university's educational research agenda based on published educational research and new research needs assessment 2. Building individual and institutional capacity to access, use, and conduct research 3. Fostering research collaboration through networking and partnerships between and among faculty researchers and educators across university to address priority research needs 4. Communicating information about existing and new research activities and findings 5. Contributing to the national and international body of research knowledge about educational policies, programs, and practices 6. Supporting, recognizing, and rewarding scholarship of educational research through grants, fellowships, awards, and promotions based on educational research publications and contributions 7. Developing an active peer review system 8. Creating an educational research support unit within the program "the center" 9. Organizing annual educational research symposia and regular journal clubs (e.g., monthly), etc.			**Estimated time** Unlimited for ongoing research
KPIs 1. University educational research output increased by 30% over 5 years' time			**Estimated budget** Phase II

T&L teaching and learning, *HSCs* Health Sciences Colleges, *VRHS* vice-rector for health specialties, *CELT* Center of Excellence in Learning and Teaching, *KACST-GDRG* King Abdul-Aziz City for Science and Technology—General Directorate for Research Grants, *KPIs* key performance indicators and related research are less than 2% of the total health expenditures worldwide, which explains much of the glaring educational deficiencies that do so much harm to health system performance. Therefore, expenditures for health professions education and research should be at least doubled over the next 5 years of any new educational initiative. This initiative targets the culture of educational research at KSU by improving research environment in education and increasing support services for researchers, e.g., assistance in identifying and preparing of research proposals and grant applications. This requires availability of digital and non-digital library resources, faculty development and consultations regarding research methods, data collection and analysis, support for publication and dissemination of research results, and recognition of research achievements. This also includes providing incentives and rewards for publishing in professional educational, and not to be only limited to basic and clinical sciences research. Ready facilities and support for conducting professional education research in each HSC are required for this initiative.

The proposed action plan is to: start prioritizing the university's educational research agenda based on published educational research and new research needs assessment; ensure individual and institutional capacity to access, use, and conduct research; encourage research collaboration through networking and partnerships between and among faculty researchers and educators across KSU to address priority research needs; communicate information about existing and new research activities and findings; contribute to the national and international body of research knowledge about educational policies, programs, and practices; and support, recognize, and reward scholarship of educational research through grants, fellowships, awards, and promotions based on educational research publications and contributions. Developing an active peer review system within the academic community would be another useful step, in addition to creating an educational research support unit that aids researchers in writing grant proposals, finding literature, analyzing data, and proofreading of manuscripts. Organizing annual educational research symposia, regular journal clubs (e.g., monthly), would be an ideal faculty support as well.

13.9 Objective (Initiative) 5.7: To Develop and Suggest Ways to Recognize Innovation in Teaching

This initiative's strategy is presented in Table 13.7. It focuses on the necessity of innovation in education. Being an innovative teacher is about looking beyond what we currently do well, identifying new ideas in teaching and learning environments and putting them into practice. Development of new and evidence-based ways to facilitate and assess learning as education is in constant change. In addition, today's students are different and want learning that meets their individual needs and ambitions. They challenge the educational organization to be innovative and to make learning environments more challenging, fulfilling, and rewarding [19].

Table 13.7 Strategic plan for suggesting ways of identifying innovative ideas in teaching

Goal 5: Promoting and supporting distinguished and innovative educational excellence and scholarship among faculty			
Objective (5.7): To develop and suggest ways to recognize innovation in teaching			
Initiative (5.7) Promote, support, recognize, and reward innovation in education at the university	**Responsible** T&L steering committee and T&L units (medical education departments) in HSCs	**Accountable** VRHS, leadership committee, and deans of HSC	**Partners** CELT
Initiative description Devising an innovation strategy that not only encourages and supports educational innovation across the university but also rewards innovators. Innovation in teaching, learning, and assessment should be a strategic goal of the institution			
Requirements and interdependencies 1. Existing system that would support innovation		**Stakeholders** Faculty staff	
Action plan The strategies to support innovation in professional education include: 1. Aligning innovations in education with the strategic goal of the university 2. Determining priorities, budgets, and reward systems and including a set of policies and actions to facilitate and support the development and transference of innovation 3. Identifying a set of criteria to assess the success of an innovation 4. Investing in resources to improve usability of innovations 5. Supporting, recognizing, and rewarding innovation in education through grants, fellowships, awards, and promotions		**Estimated time** Ongoing	
KPIs 1. Innovations in education increased by 20% over 5 years from implementation of this initiative		**Estimated budget** Phase II	

T&L teaching and learning, *HSCs* Health Sciences Colleges, *VRHS* vice-rector for health specialties, *CELT* Center of Excellence in Learning and Teaching, *KPIs* key performance indicators

Therefore, the role of an organization in supporting innovation is vital by providing the opportunities and resources to innovate. Moreover, recent research highlights the role of organizational culture in facilitating organizations to transform innovative activity into tangible performance and routine practice [20].

The proposed action plan that would support innovation in professional education starts with aligning innovations in education with mission and strategic goals of the university. This is followed by identifying the priorities, budgets, and reward systems that would enhance the culture of innovation. Another step is following up innovative ideas by improving its usability and setting policies and actions to support continuous development and transference of innovation. Finally, there is evaluation of the success of innovative ideas against a set of criteria.

13.10 Summary

Excellence in teaching, learning , and assessment requires faculty who are motivated and well prepared for their tasks. At KSU, our goal is to promote educational excellence among faculty members. This can be accomplished by providing them with educational resources and lists of courses, training them on educational excellence and scholarship, supporting their educational research and innovations, and collaboration with the Deanship of Skills Development.

References

1. Wilkerson L, Irby DM. Strategies for improving teaching practices: a comprehensive approach to faculty development. Acad Med. 1998;73:387–96.
2. Steinert Y, Mann K, Centeno A, Dolmans D, Spencer J, Gelula M, et al. A systematic review of faculty development initiatives designed to improve teaching effectiveness in medical education: BEME guide no. 8. Med Teach. 2006;28(6):497–526.
3. Chalmers R. Faculty development: the nature and benefits of mentoring. Am J Pharm Educ. 1992;56:71–4.
4. Gruppen LD, Frohna AZ, Anderson RM, Lowe KD. Faculty development for educational leadership and scholarship. Acad Med. 2003;78(2):137–41.
5. Saudi Digital Library, 2010. https://sdl.edu.sa/SDLPortal/Publishers.aspx.
6. Education Resources Information Center (ERICTM,1966). http://eric.ed.gov/edXTM, 2012. https://www.edx.org/.
7. EBSCO HealthTM, 1984. https://health.ebsco.com.
8. OvidTM, Walter Kluwer, 1984. https://www.ovid.com/about-ovid.html.
9. AAMC. MedEdPORTAL. J Med Libr Assoc. 2016;104(3):250–2; https://www.mededportal.org/.
10. Zahedi M, Alshehri M, Al-Hadlaq SM, Jarallah N, Alnaami M, Alzahrani AM. Faculty perception and readiness to engage in initiatives towards excellence. South East Asian J Med Educ. 2015;9:35–40.
11. Harvard and Massachusetts Institute of Technology—MIT. edX—online courses and classes from the world's best, 2012. https://www.edx.org/.
12. Coursera™, Stanford University, 2012. https://www.coursera.org/.
13. Stanford OnlineTM. Stanford center for professional development, 1995; http://online.stanford.edu/.
14. Rwaq. http://www.rwaq.org/.
15. Boyer EL, Moser D, Ream TC, Braxton J. Scholarship reconsidered: priorities of the professoriate. San Francisco, CA: Jossey Bass; 2015.
16. Simpson D, Hafler J, Brown D, Wilkerson L. Documentation systems for educators seeking academic promotion in U.S. medical schools. Acad Med. 2004;79(8):783–90.
17. Hafler JP, Lovejoy FH Jr. Scholarly activities recorded in the portfolios of teacher-clinician faculty. Acad Med. 2000;75(6):649–52.
18. Frenk J, Chen L, Bhutta ZA, Cohen J, Crisp N, Evans T, et al. Health professionals for a new century: transforming education to strengthen health systems in an interdependent world. Lancet. 2010;376(9756):1923–58.

19. Banerjee B. Why innovate? Understanding innovation. In: Banerjee B, Ceri S, editors. Creating innovation leaders: a global perspective. Cham: Springer; 2016. p. 3–24. https://doi.org/10.1007/978-3-319-20520-5_1.
20. Salge TO, Vera A. Benefiting from public sector innovation: the moderating role of customer and learning orientation. Public Adm Rev. 2012;72:550–9.

Leadership and Management Qualities 14

Basil Amarneh and Mohammed Yahya Alnaami

14.1 Introduction

Leadership is a function of knowing yourself, having a vision that is well communicated, building trust among colleagues, and taking effective action to realize your own leadership potential [1]. Leadership influences people by providing purpose, direction, and motivation while operating to accomplish the mission and improve the organization. Thus, it is an activity, an influential persuasive process in which an individual gains trust and commitment of others with or without reliance on formal position or authority and moves the group into the accomplishment of one or more tasks. Leaders in professional education need to be good advocates of health. Health advocacy can be described as purposeful actions by health professionals to address determinants of health, which negatively impact individuals or communities by either informing those who can enact change or by initiating, mobilizing, and organizing activities to make change happen, with or on behalf of the individuals or communities with whom health professionals work [2]. Yet for many, providing such leadership is difficult! Why?

Adaptive change is distressing for the people going through it. They need to take on new roles, relationships, values, and approaches to work; many employees are ambivalent about the sacrifices required of them. In this complex world, and an increase in accountability to survive as a leader and pull the institutional development from the gutter, the leader should understand the complexity of contemporary organization as well as potentially self-adapting [3]. The principles for the leader to practice in order to be successful in leading adaptive work and change include:

B. Amarneh
College of Nursing, King Saud University, Riyadh, Saudi Arabia

M. Y. Alnaami (✉)
Department of Surgery, College of Medicine, King Saud University, Riyadh, Saudi Arabia

M. Y. Alnaami et al. (eds.), *Novel Health Interprofessional Education and Collaborative Practice Program: Strategy and Implementation*,
https://doi.org/10.1007/978-981-99-3420-1_14

- Getting on the balcony to perceive what is going on and have an overview of the organization and reflecting on a daily basis.
- Identifying adaptive challenges to have a clear picture or understanding of how the organization operates in order to address the challenges.
- Maintaining disciplined attention to be able to focus the staff's attention on the task.
- Giving the work back to the people involved to empower the staff to carry out the tasks needed related to achieving the goals.
- Protecting the voices of leadership from below to ensure the voices of heads of departments and units are heard.

Developing a leader is a process that requires learning new behaviors and skills through experience. It requires experimentation, application, and deliberate practice. It requires experiential learning (experience/activity). This allows the student to apply the lesson learnt in the class to their leadership development. In this chapter, we will discuss a set of goals and objectives with action plans and KPIs to implement leadership and management qualities/skills among health professionals.

14.2 Strategic Goal 6: Promoting Leadership and Management Qualities Among Healthcare Faculty to Cope with the Rapidly Changing Global Educational Environment

Leadership and management are often used interchangeably, and they are practically considered overlapping in necessary concepts. Both leadership and management involve influence, working with people, and working to achieve common goals. However, the fields of leadership and management are different [4]. Unlike management, which is a one-way authority relationship, leadership is a multidirectional influence connection. The majority of authors attempted to pinpoint discrepancies by contrasting management and leadership in terms of definition and competencies. There are many diverse definitions of management and leadership. Robert Katz defines management as exercising direction of a group or organization through executive, administrative, and supervisory positions [5]. He adds that management responsibilities are usually tasked-oriented, and they involve developing staff, mentoring persons with high potentials and resolving conflicts while maintaining ethics and disciplines. As a result, management as a whole is a process utilized to accomplish organizational goals. Managers concentrate on the formal leading and management of their staff, resources, systems, and structures. A manager works to achieve short-term objectives, minimize risks, and create standardization to boost productivity. On the other side, leaders prioritize inspiring and motivating others. Creating a passion for their vision, long-term goals, and taking risks to meet obstacles is a leadership ambition. People follow the leader freely because leaders are always mindful of the benefits to their followers [6]. To adapt and cope with the twenty-first century's health care reforms and challenges, health professionals need to be engaged at all levels—local, national, and global—to lead educational transformation to strengthen health systems in an interdependent world [7].

14.3 Objective (Initiative) 6.1: To Provide Forums for the Exchange of Ideas in Educational Developments

This initiative is summarized in Table 14.1. Educational transformation and development are of paramount necessity in health professions education in order to graduate health professionals well equipped with knowledge, skills, and high professional

Table 14.1 Strategic plan for providing forums to exchange ideas in educational developments

<table>
<tr><td colspan="4">Goal 6: Promoting leadership and management qualities among healthcare faculty to cope with the rapidly changing global educational environment</td></tr>
<tr><td colspan="4">Objective (6.1): To provide forums for the exchange of ideas in educational developments</td></tr>
<tr><td>Initiative (6.1)
Provide forums for the exchange of ideas in educational developments</td><td>Responsible
T&L steering committee and T&L units (medical education departments) in HSCs</td><td>Accountable
VRHS, leadership committee, and deans of HSCs</td><td>Partners
Deanship of e-learning and distance learning, CELT, and deanship for skills development at KSU</td></tr>
<tr><td colspan="4">Initiative description
Improving faculty awareness of new trends in education</td></tr>
<tr><td colspan="3">Requirements and interdependencies
1. Special purpose rooms outfitted to host health science forums on educational developments
2. Creating a virtual learning environment for health colleges to facilitate online participation in the forums small-group discussions, etc.</td><td>Stakeholders
Faculty staff</td></tr>
<tr><td colspan="3">Action plan
1. Organizing monthly health science faculty forums/clubs to discuss global trends and developments in education
2. Establishing guidelines to run these activities
3. Establishing an annual reward system for the best innovative approaches to education among health sciences faculty
4. Establishing the guidelines for issuing such awards
5. Archiving these activities should be for future reference</td><td>Estimated time
Phase II</td></tr>
<tr><td colspan="3">KPIs
1. More than 20% attendance of each forum
2. More than 70% satisfaction of forum participants
3. More than 70% of randomly sampled staff agree with the choice of recipient of an award for a particular academic year
4. The forums for a particular academic year are verified in the archives</td><td>Estimated budget
Phase II</td></tr>
</table>

T&L teaching and learning, *HSCs* Health Sciences Colleges, *VRHS* vice-rector for health specialties, *CELT* Center of Excellence in Learning and Teaching, *KSU* King Saud University, *KPIs* key performance indicators

attitudes in the complexity of ever-changing health care systems. This requires well-educated and trained faculty to lead this notion of educational reforms for the twenty-first century. In order to achieve this objective, KSU should promote and support faculty development programs across HSCs. Qualified educators representing all HSCs should form a team that plans and conducts progressive faculty programs to improve HSE. The initial forum should involve policy and decision makers, to present and discuss published research and reports on the importance of educational reforms and needs assessment results that involve students and faculty and other stakeholders, current trends in educational development, strategic planning, ways for implementation and evaluation, and other educational matters. This will hopefully result in opening the support and funding gate by KSU administration. The next step is to nominate a leadership panel of qualified and expert educators representing all HSCs that will be responsible for strategic planning, establishing guidelines for educational development and reforms, and formulation of teams who will educate and train faculty in new trends for promoting HSE at all levels as a joint program [8]. This can be achieved onsite by providing common educational facilities such as well-equipped conference halls, small-group rooms, and clinical skills labs for demonstration and training. Nevertheless, virtual and online faculty development programs proven as effective as onsite education and training especially in knowledge domain, as most faculty nowadays are computer literate and prefer to do these faculty development exercises at their free time off the working hours. However, combining both onsite and online activities may achieve the educational development and reform goals. Estimated timeframe and budget outline of this and other initiatives in this chapter will be studied and decided later as a second phase.

14.4 Objective (Initiative) 6.2: To Coordinate Educational Offerings to Faculty Across HSCs

This initiative (Table 14.2) discusses one of the leadership panel's responsibilities, which is to coordinate all educational development activities across HSCs. In order to achieve this objective, the leadership panel needs to establish a central body (e.g., VRHSs) supported by qualified secretaries and equipped with computer desktops and intranet system. Faculty educational development needs may vary from a college to another. Therefore, each HSC should submit corresponding needs (based on needs assessment) few months before the beginning of each academic year, so the leadership expert panel would arrange and coordinate the FD program for all HSCs. Once the program for all is ready, it can be posted on the central body website, sent as brochures, faculty e-mails, and to the education unit in each HSC. According to research by Lucas et al. [9] on the characteristics of faculty leadership development

Table 14.2 Strategic plan for coordinating educational offerings to faculty across colleges

Goal 6: Promoting leadership and management qualities among healthcare faculty to cope with the rapidly changing global educational environment			
Objective (6.2): To coordinate educational offerings to faculty across HSCs			
Initiative (6.2) Coordinate educational offerings to faculty across colleges	**Responsible** The T&L steering committee, vice-deans academic affairs of HSCs, and the T&L units (medical education departments) in HSCs	**Accountable** VRHS, leadership committee, and deans of HSCs	**Partners** All departments and IT units in HSCs
Initiative description Coordinating educational offerings across HSCs to use and benefit from available resources			
Requirements and interdependencies 1. T&L units (medical education departments) in HSCs 2. IT subunits in HSCs 3. VRHS		**Stakeholders** Faculty staff	
Action plan 1. Establishing a body at the VRHS in charge of coordinating educational offerings across HSCs 2. Designated body should enforce the presentation at the beginning of each academic year with all the educational activities scheduled to take place at all HSCs for that year. Such presentations (ideally in printed and online brochures) should state the plans, etc., of each educational offering		**Estimated time** Ongoing	
KPIs 1. A proper coordinating body has been established at the VRHS 2. In the academic year following the establishment of the aforementioned body (and in the subsequent academic years), all educational offerings across HSCs for an academic year can be found online and in printed brochures, with detailed descriptions stating the goals, objectives, etc.		**Estimated budget** Phase II	

HSCs Health Sciences Colleges, *T&L* teaching and learning, *VRHS* vice-rector for health specialties, *IT* information technology, *KPIs* key performance indicators

programs in HSCs in North America, lectures and case discussions were the most common teaching methods. They concluded in their study that programs can improve by basing content on a leadership competency model, incorporating multiple approaches to teaching, and implementing more rigorous program evaluation. Further details about this initiative are presented in Table 14.2.

14.5 Objective (Initiative) 6.3: To Develop and Conduct Surveys for Faculty Staff Concerning the Use of Up-to-Date Teaching Methods to Achieve Excellence

This initiative is presented in Table 14.3. Faculty opinions and needs are usually appreciated through qualitative research using surveys, interviews, reflections, feedback, etc. Designing proper and valid surveys requires experienced workers and

Table 14.3 Strategic plan for developing and conducting surveys for faculty concerning the use of up-to-date teaching methods

<table>
<tr><td colspan="4">Goal 6: Promoting leadership and management qualities among healthcare faculty to cope with the rapidly changing global educational environment</td></tr>
<tr><td colspan="4">Objective (6.3): To develop and conduct surveys for faculty staff concerning the use of up-to-date teaching methods to achieve excellence</td></tr>
<tr><td>Initiative (6.3)
Develop and conduct surveys of faculty concerning the use of up-to-date teaching methods</td><td>Responsible
T&L steering committee and T&L units (medical education departments) in HSCs</td><td>Accountable
VRHS, leadership committee, and deans of HSCs</td><td>Partners
Deanship of skills development and CELT</td></tr>
<tr><td colspan="4">Initiative description
Developing annual online surveys to be conducted on a randomly selected, predetermined, sample of actively teaching faculty for that year to determine and improve how faculty are coping with the changing global environment</td></tr>
<tr><td colspan="3">Requirements and interdependencies
1. Professional survey development and analysts
2. T&L units in all HSCs
3. IT deanship and its subunits in HSCs</td><td>Stakeholders
Faculty staff</td></tr>
<tr><td colspan="3">Action plan
1. Designing surveys on the use of best educational practices
2. Selecting a small random sample of teaching faculty (perhaps 15%) from the database of teaching staff to survey
3. Using survey results to plan for improvements in leadership and management qualities and ensure that faculty are using up-to-date teaching skills
4. Establishing an annual reward system for the best innovative approaches to education among health sciences faculty. Establish the guidelines for issuing such awards
5. Conducting workshop on teaching style surveys</td><td>Estimated time
Phase II</td></tr>
<tr><td colspan="3">KPIs
1. More than 70% response of randomly sampled staff to survey
2. Concrete plans set in motion to use results of surveys to improve leadership and management qualities of faculty as well as improve the use of up-to-date teaching methods
3. More than 70% of randomly sampled staff agree on the choice of recipient of an award for a particular academic year
4. Surveys and responses to them are verified in the archives
5. More than 70% satisfaction of teaching style survey workshop participants</td><td>Estimated budget
Phase II</td></tr>
</table>

T&L teaching and learning, *HSCs* Health Sciences Colleges, *VRHS* vice-rector for health specialties, *CELT* Center of Excellence in Learning and Teaching, *IT* information technology, *KPIs* key performance indicators statisticians who can generate appropriate and relevant research questions, analyze data, and make valid conclusions and recommendations. It is necessary to generate additional initiatives, such as seminars, workshops, courses, etc., to conduct teaching style surveys. Our study on faculty perspective and readiness to participate in initiatives for teaching excellence involved a sample of academic faculty from all HSCs (medicine, dentistry, applied medical sciences, nursing, pharmacy, and Emergency Medical Services) [10]. Our recommendations included a stronger focus on enhancing graduate education, research and development, teaching, learning, and assessment. It is interesting to see that they had the least concern for academic writing, paper publications, simulation applications in health research, leadership and administration, and mentorship. These conclusions were a good example to base leadership faculty development programs on needs assessment, which might differ from one institute to another and may change from time to time. As teaching excellence was ranked first of all faculty concerns, we developed and conducted a 3-day program on "teaching how to teach," involving more than thirty academic faculty leaders/educators representing all HSCs at KSU.

This program included best practices in microteaching (interactive lecturing), small-group tutoring, clinical skills and simulation, and assessment. Faculty feedback was excellent that this course should be repeated twice a year at the beginning of each academic, especially new staff. Nonetheless, the Deanship of Faculty Development at KSU adopted a similar program done once a year for all new joining academic faculty in all departments as a requirement for the assistant professor title. Another strategy for achieving teaching excellence is the rewards for best teachers in each department. The Quality Department in HSCs conducts and analyzes results of surveys of students' evaluation for each individual faculty at the end of each academic year. The percentage of each individual faculty ranking in each HSC will be confidentially sent to the faculty staff for their information only, without any tenure actions taken accordingly.

Unfortunately, no rewards for teaching excellence are yet in action at KSU, when compared to research excellence. However, there are grants to faculty for innovative projects in educational development, and currently the center for educational development at KSU is planning to make awards for teaching excellence, similar to the awards currently awarded to best research projects at KSU. These awards play major roles to encourage faculty to do more in developing own educational skills and KSU reputation [10]. Lee et al. [11] raised the concerns that the dependence of faculty on research and research grants for their promotion and tenure decisions and salary increments may negatively and indirectly affect teaching excellence. They indicate that while research and its resulting publications are vital to universities, teaching excellence must be, too. Guidelines for teaching excellence awards must be developed; otherwise, universities will be accused for bias and payback favors, especially when companies are sharing in this endeavor. Developing such guidelines by expert educators is crucial for universities to help faculty on achieving their goals on best educational practices [12]. An example for such guidelines can be extrapolated from the ASPH/Pfizer Award for Teaching Excellence [13].

14.6 Objective (Initiative) 6.4: To Provide Support as Well as Training and Modeling the Use of Online Courses

This initiative describes the importance of online leadership faculty development (FD) programs. Onsite participation is considered the norm for most FD programs in most universities [9]; however, some FD programs are increasingly adopting online-FD courses and programs. The majority of faculty could attribute this to many factors including its proven efficacy [14], faculty preference to do such online programs during their non-working hours' free time, busy daily schedules, and the increasing dependence on computers and laptops for work. Such online courses, however, require IT and educationists' expertise and collaboration to develop such courses based on scientific means and robust evaluation methods. Chan et al. [15] published a very good model to create, assist, and share in online faculty development resources.

Their approach is to recruit expert faculty to write a monthly complex and realistic case scenario featuring a nonclinical medical education dilemma and to publish online with accompanying discussion questions answered by clinical faculty. College of Medicine at KSU with the collaboration of its Medical Education and IT departments is establishing an online-FD programs. This can be extrapolated to a leadership IPE-FD programs, involving all HSCs faculty in the near future. Also, collaborating with international universities in this and other FD development programs would seem to be prudent, especially during the early experience of training and developing such programs. The strategic aspects to achieve this objective are highlighted in Table 14.4.

Table 14.4 Strategic plan for providing support/training and model the use of online courses

Goal 6: Promoting leadership and management qualities among healthcare faculty to cope with the rapidly changing global educational environment			
Objective (6.4): To provide support and training and to model the use of online courses			
Initiative (6.4) Provide support and training and model the use of online courses	**Responsible** T&L steering committee and T&L units (medical education departments) in HSCs	**Accountable** VRHS, leadership committee, and deans of HSCs	**Partners** Deanship of skills development and deanship of e-learning and distance learning
Initiative description Engaging local and/or international experts to train and support faculty in the use of online courses, to help them cope with the rapidly changing educational environment			
Requirements and interdependencies 1. Professional developers and trainers on the use of online courses 2. Resources for workshops/forums on online course design			**Stakeholders** Faculty staff
Action plan 1. Designing an interprofessional course on "how to design online courses" and make HSCs adopt it as a regular course 2. Evaluating the success of this course with the ultimate aim of getting other HSCs to adopt it as a regular course 3. Exploring local and international expertise in online course design			**Estimated time** Ongoing

Table 14.4 (continued)

KPIs	Estimated budget
1. Up to 80% limited-seat capacity filled per course run in the pilot at HSCs 2. Up to 70% satisfaction of faculty attending each course 3. Up to 70% satisfaction of faculty with the support services (following the course) offered by professional trainers/experts over the course of the academic year	Phase II

T&L teaching and learning, *HSCs* Health Sciences Colleges, *VRHS* vice-rector for health specialties, *KPIs* key performance indicators

14.7 Objective (Initiative) 6.5: To Promote Leadership and Management Qualities Among Healthcare Faculty

Healthcare professions' faculty need to improve their leadership and managerial skills to cope with the rapidly changing environment in healthcare and health sciences education (HSE). Programs that integrate non-physician and physician professionals are lacking, more interactive learning and feedback are rarely used to help people become more self-aware, and there is an excessively narrow focus on individual-level outcomes rather than system-level outcomes, according to a systematic review of published literature on leadership development programs for doctors [16]. The Lancet Commission Report [7] emphasizes the need to generate healthcare professionals who can lead the integration of health professions' education with the changing healthcare systems to cope with the twenty-first century healthcare needs. Leadership and managerial qualities among health professions faculty not only make changes in healthcare systems but can influence policy and decision makers to prioritize healthcare problems and issues according to their importance and public needs. For example, Road Traffic Accidents (RTAs) are considered the highest among other causes of mortalities and morbidities in Saudi Arabia [17]. As a national priority, leaders in healthcare professions were able to convince the Minister of Health and his administration to adopt a new system to deal with trauma in Saudi Arabia [18]. Consultants and experts in this field can be recruited locally or from abroad, and resources are mobilized to promote this initiative.

Currently, the Deanship for Skills Development at KSU are running a regular leadership and management program for all faculty throughout the academic year, which has excellent short courses on management and leadership. However, participants are usually those who are leaders and managers interested to promote and improve their own leadership and managerial skills. We need to widen this individualized-level to system-level outcomes where all concerned FD departments in KSU work together to integrate such efforts under one umbrella (e.g., Deanship of Skills Development) to run courses in leadership and management at all levels. To produce such healthcare professional leaders and managers in the community, universities should take the lead and responsibility to train and certify some faculty educators to prepare and conduct interprofessional leadership and management courses at the university, college, department, graduate, and undergraduate levels. College of Medicine at KSU took this initiative and adopted interactive lectures in leadership and management under the professionalism course for undergraduate students. Leadership and management programs should not be limited to courses only. They can be done as annual or bi-annual forum where all consultants and experts in this field convene and discuss updated research and methods on how to teach and train faculty and students in leadership and managerial skills. Best evidence practices have shown that these skills are best taught as small-group sessions, where a limited number of participants' exchange ideas and have more interactive learning and feedback to develop greater self-awareness [16]. Details on how to achieve this strategic objective are presented in Table 14.5.

Table 14.5 Strategic plan of promoting leadership and management qualities among health faculty

<table>
<tr><td colspan="4">Goal 6: Promoting leadership and management qualities among healthcare faculty to cope with the rapidly changing global educational environment</td></tr>
<tr><td colspan="4">Objective (6.5): To promote leadership and management qualities among healthcare faculty</td></tr>
<tr><td>Initiative (6.5)
Promote leadership and management qualities among healthcare faculty</td><td>Responsible
T&L steering committee and T&L units (medical education departments) in HSCs</td><td>Accountable
VRHS, leadership committee, and deans of HSCs</td><td>Partners
CELT, deanship for skills development, and HSCs</td></tr>
<tr><td colspan="4">Initiative description
Familiarizing health sciences faculty with (and encouraging the application of) best practice principles and skills in leadership and management so that they can better cope with the rapidly changing environment in healthcare and HSE</td></tr>
<tr><td colspan="3">Requirements and interdependencies
1. Internal/external consultants to run courses
2. Resources to develop and run leadership and managerial skills courses
3. Collaboration with the deanship for skills development</td><td>Stakeholders
Faculty staff</td></tr>
<tr><td colspan="3">Action plan
1. Running overlapping, limited-seat courses for health sciences faculty on essential skills of good leadership and management
2. Running regular, small-group discussions (within and between HSCs faculty) to allow for the exchange of ideas on leadership and management skills
3. Running forums for HSCs faculty to discuss successful applications of leadership/management principles (skills) to their jobs as lecturers, clinicians, surgeons, researchers, mentors, etc.</td><td>Estimated time
Ongoing</td></tr>
<tr><td colspan="3">KPIs
1. More than 70% attendance of each limited-seat course
2. More than 70% satisfaction of course participants
3. At least 30% of randomly sampled health science faculty have participated in at least one leadership or management course during the course of one academic year</td><td>Estimated budget
Phase II</td></tr>
</table>

T&L teaching and learning, *HSCs* Health Sciences Colleges, *VRHS* vice-rector for health specialties, *CELT* Center of Excellence in Learning and Teaching, *HSE* Health Science Education, *KPIs* key performance indicators

14.8 Discussion

Most of the current leadership and management development programs target individuals' skills, but lack a more comprehensive system-outcome, which should encompass individuals, teams, organizations, and national level leadership. Although the development of leadership and management abilities at the individual level is vital, research suggests that the development of groups' and organizations' capacities for leadership as a shared and communal process is much more valuable [19]. The majority of the data, however, emphasizes the value of group leadership and calls for striking a balance between the development of personal abilities and that of organizations. Also, there is an obvious, compelling, and urgent need for cross-organizational leadership cooperation (another essential component of collective leadership). More and more, a network of institutions that are dependent on one another must provide healthcare. Leadership at the national level is also very important in influencing people, groups, and organizations.

Many publications have urged the national leadership organizations to create a single integrated system approach that is characterized by uniformity in its demands, processes, and demands. When a national leadership body takes a supportive, developmental, appreciative, and sustainable approach, when health service organizations are viewed as partners in the development of health services, and when health service organizations are supported and given the tools they need to provide continuously improving, high-quality patient care, these characteristics are most likely to be present. This calls for executives to collaborate across organizational boundaries both within and between organizations, putting the success of overall patient care ahead of the performance of their individual component. To achieve collective leadership at the system level, leaders must collaborate and create an integrative, cooperative culture. The responsibility of leadership is to guarantee that teams and organizations have direction, alignment, and commitment [20]. Direction ensures that everyone is on board with the organization's goals and is proud of them, in line with its vision, values, and strategy. Effective coordination and integration of the work are referred to as alignment. Everyone in the organization must accept responsibility for the organization's success and make it a personal priority. This is how commitment is shown.

Conversely, providing services to the community in a way that is appropriate, effective, equitable, and sustainable is the goal of good management. Only by carefully bringing together and synchronizing the essential resources for service provision, such as personnel, funds, hardware, and process elements of care delivery, can this be accomplished [21]. Management and leadership are crucial for the provision of high-quality healthcare services. Although there are some similarities between the two, there may also be differences in terms of mindset, abilities, and actions. Effective managers must have management abilities because good managers should aspire to be good leaders. Leaders will develop methods for achieving the vision after developing a vision of what can be accomplished. They inspire others and have the negotiating skills to secure funds and other forms of assistance to further their objectives. Managers make sure that the resources are used efficiently and effectively to get the best results. To obtain the best outcomes in the resource-constrained and challenging conditions seen in many low-to-middle income countries, a manager must also be a leader. In conclusion, many challenges will face healthcare leaders, managers, organizations, and community as a whole to nurture and sustain high-quality, safe, and compassionate care. In order to cope with the changing healthcare systems in the twenty-first century, universities should strive for robust leadership and management programs based on the evidence of what, why, where, and how it works.

14.9 Summary

The health care and educational systems of the twenty-first century will increasingly need to promote leadership and management skills in health professional education and collaborative practice. This objective will be accomplished through five efforts. Initially, to offer discussion forums for new educational innovations. To organize faculty education opportunities across HSCs, second. Finally, to create and administer surveys to faculty members about the usage of cutting-edge teaching techniques to attain greatness. Fourth, to assist, train, and set an example for how to use online courses. Finally, to encourage healthcare professors to possess leadership and management skills. Each initiative's strategic specifics were laid out. Each initiative's budgetary information and anticipated completion time are determined by studies, meetings, and discussions held by key participants in the implementation process.

References

1. Bennis WG, Nanus B. Leaders: the strategies for taking charge. New York, NY: Harper Collins; 2007.
2. Oandasan I, Reeves S. Key elements for interprofessional education. Part 1: the learner, the educator and the learning context. J Interprof Care. 2005;19(Suppl 1):21–38.
3. Heifetz RA, Laurie DL. The work of leadership. IEEE Eng Manag Rev. 2009;37:49–59.
4. Kotterman JP. What leaders really do? Harv Bus Rev. 2007;79(11):85–96.
5. Katz RL. Skills of an effective administrator. Harv Bus Rev. 1955;33(1):33.
6. Bennis W, Goldsmith J. Learning to lead: a workbook on becoming a leader. 4th ed. Boston, MA: Addison Wesley; 2010.
7. Frenk J, Chen LC, Bhutta ZA, Cohen J, Crisp N, Evans T, et al. Health professionals for a new century: transforming education to strengthen health systems in an interdependent world. Lancet. 2010;376:1923–58.
8. Schönwetter DJ, Hamilton J, Sawatzky JA. Exploring professional development needs of educators in the health sciences professions. J Dent Educ. 2015;79(2):113–23.
9. Lucas R, Goldman EF, Scott AR, Dandar V. Leadership development programs at academic health centers: results of a National Survey. Acad Med. 2018;93:229–36.
10. Zahedi M, Alshehri M, Al-Hadlaq SM, Jarallah N, Alnaami M, Alzahrani AM. Faculty perception and readiness to engage in initiatives towards excellence. Southeast Asian J Med Educ. 2015;9:35–40.

11. Lee JM, Kleinbaum D, Diener-West M, Grimley DM, Hellerstedt WL, Sullivan L, et al. Teaching excellence in public health: a call to action. Public Health Rep. 2008;123(3):405–7.
12. Schunemann HJ, Wiercioch W, Etxeandia I, Falavigna M, Santesso N, Mustafa R, et al. Guidelines 2.0: systematic development of a comprehensive checklist for a successful guideline enterprise. CMAJ. 2014;186(3):E123–42.
13. Association of Schools of Public Health. ASPH/Pfizer award for teaching excellence. http://www.asph.org/document.cfm?page=992.
14. Johnstone-Dodge V, Bowen DM, Calley KH, Peterson TS. A faculty development course to enhance dental hygiene distance education: a pilot study. J Dent Educ. 2014;78(9):1319–30.
15. Chan TM, Thoma B, Lin M. Creating, curating, and sharing online faculty development resources: the medical education in cases series experience. Acad Med. 2015;90(6):785–9.
16. Frich JC, Brewster AL, Cherlin EJ, Bradley EH. Leadership development programs for physicians: a systematic review. J Gen Intern Med. 2015;30(5):656–74.
17. Mansuri FA, Al-Zalabani AH, Zalat MM, Qabshawi RI. Road safety and road traffic accidents in Saudi Arabia. A systematic review of existing evidence. Saudi Med J. 2015;36(4):418–24.
18. Al-Naami MY, Arafah MA, Al-Ibrahim FS. Trauma care systems in Saudi Arabia: an agenda for action. Ann Saudi Med. 2010;30:50–8.
19. West M, Armit K, Loewenthal L, Eckert R, West T, Lee A. Leadership and leadership development in health care: the evidence base. London: The King's Fund; 2015. p. 1–36.
20. Drath WH, Mccauley CD, Palus CJ, Velsor EV, O'Connor P, McGuire JB. Direction, alignment, commitment: toward a more integrative ontology of leadership. Leadersh Q. 2008;19:635–53.
21. WHO. Leadership and management. 2008; www.who.int/hiv/pub/imai/om_10_leadership_management.pdf. Accessed 7 Dec 2020.

15 Faculty Policies and Career Pathways

Dalal Abdullah Alqahtani, Eiad Abdelmohsen Alfaris, and Naghma Naeem

15.1 Introduction

Motivating our students to learn is a critical component of effective education, motivating faculty members to excel as teachers is an essential component as well. Many faculty members enter the academic world with an interest in teaching. Nevertheless, as their clinical research and administrative duties accumulate, their commitment to teaching and learning how to be better teachers usually fades with time [1]. Therefore, universities should motivate and reward their faculty with incentives and recognition to be better teachers. Supporting faculty members to excel as educators is important by providing the needed attention and public recognition to teaching responsibilities. This is achieved by overcoming the obstacles of research and publication as the only indicator of good faculty [2]. Thomas Cech, president of the Howard Hughes Medical Institute said at his editorial in Science in 2003, "In universities across the United States and in many other parts of the world, the biological sciences continue to enjoy a wonderful revolution. Everything has changed in the research laboratory, but it is likely that far less has changed in the classroom. The same detachment of professor from student that frustrated university education 25 years ago is just as pervasive today. Although each course is now likely to have

D. A. Alqahtani (✉)
Oral Medicine and Diagnostic Sciences, College of Dentistry, King Saud University, Riyadh, Saudi Arabia

E. A. Alfaris
Department of Family and Community Medicine, College of Medicine, King Saud University, Riyadh, Saudi Arabia

N. Naeem
College of Medicine, King Saud University, Riyadh, Saudi Arabia

M. Y. Alnaami et al. (eds.), *Novel Health Interprofessional Education and Collaborative Practice Program: Strategy and Implementation*,
https://doi.org/10.1007/978-981-99-3420-1_15

its own website, with class schedule, lecture notes, and assignments, the professoriate still struggles with how to use technology to achieve a greater impact on student learning and how to communicate the genuine excitement surrounding today's discoveries" [3].

Guidelines and instructions for promotion and tenure vary from university to another within or outside the country's boundaries, based on policies and social context. In general, faculty promotion and tenure in health professions are basically judged by faculty performance in three tracks: academic, laboratory/clinical, and research activities with variable percentages. There are no hard or universal rules on how faculty get promoted or tenured; this depends on the nature of the work and activities performed. Therefore, ideally each institute should formulate a promotion and tenure committee, within a department or unit sharing similar responsibilities. This committee will decide on guidelines and conditions for promotion and tenure. These need to be aligned with general policies and rules of the university or institute with some variations that need to be approved further by higher education. Some faculty excel in administration or education more than clinical or research works; these variations also need to be considered for faculty promotion and tenure purposes.

At KSU, our goal is support faculty to excel as teacher by providing the needed recognition and incentives in professional education. The following sections discuss the strategic steps and initiatives proposed to achieve this goal.

15.2 Strategic Goal 7: Developing Faculty Policies, Career Paths, and Incentives that Support the Essential Role of Teaching in the Light of Competing Priorities

In the early stages of this program, this goal was developed through a planned process that involved conducting multiple meetings and workshops among the key faculty members, educators, consultants, and other relevant stakeholders. They discussed the need to provide faculty with regulations and incentives that would promote teaching excellence among faculty members. Among the specific initiatives are development of models for faculty incentives that promote teaching and the support for the teacher-researcher track. They are described in the following section.

15.2.1 Objective (Initiative) 7.1: To Study and Compile Models for Faculty Incentives that Support Teaching

According to the KSU designed strategic plan, the strategy of this initiative has been planned as shown in Table 15.1. It proposes to study the appropriate models for faculty incentives that would engage faculty in teaching excellence. Research has shown that with increased responsibilities and competing opportunities, faculty's time and effort for teaching decrease [4]. Given the new era of change in health professional education curricula and emphasis on new ways of teaching with

Table 15.1 Strategic plan for developing faculty incentives for teaching

<table>
<tr><td colspan="4">Goal 7: Developing faculty policies, career paths, and incentives that support the essential role of teaching in the light of competing priorities</td></tr>
<tr><td colspan="4">Objective (7.1): To study and compile models for faculty incentives that support teaching</td></tr>
<tr><td>Initiative (7.1)
Develop a contextual model for faculty incentives (monetary and non-monetary) that support teaching at KSU</td><td>Responsible
T&L Steering Committee, Incentive Policies Review Committee, Human Resources Department, and Leadership Committee in HSCs</td><td>Accountable
VRHS and Deans of HSCs</td><td>Partners
Scientific Council, KSU</td></tr>
<tr><td colspan="4">Initiative description
Developing teaching incentives through recognition of faculty excellence in the following key areas: course quality, course performance, course content, innovative teaching methods, advising, supervision, and mentorship. Rewards can include: (1) Monetary compensation (salary and merit raise), (2) Recognition (with tangible and intangible benefits), (3) Acknowledgment (at departmental, unit, college, and university levels), (4) Recognition in a newsletter or an annual event, (5) Mentoring or professional development opportunities, and (6) Availability of professional development funds</td></tr>
<tr><td colspan="2">Requirements and interdependencies
1. Faculty policies of national and international HSCs
2. Faculty policies of KSU</td><td colspan="2">Stakeholders
Faculty staff</td></tr>
<tr><td colspan="2">Action plan
Phase I: development
1. Seeking the faculty incentive policies of national and international HSCs through online searching and requests to faculty affairs representatives
2. Developing work-based assessment models for better evaluation and feedback to teachers
3. Compiling a faculty incentive policy committee to re-examine the current state of faculty incentives at KSU
4. Developing a summary of new policy requirements compared with current practices for addressing identified gaps
5. Developing a contextual model for incentive policies and career paths that support teaching
6. Getting approval from the VRHSs and Deans' Board
Phase II: implementation, monitoring and evaluation
1. Implementing, monitoring, and evaluating the model</td><td colspan="2">Estimated time
Phase II</td></tr>
<tr><td colspan="2">KPIs phase I
1. Contextual Faculty Incentive Model developed
KPIs phase II
1. Incentive policy implemented
2. At least 80% faculty satisfied with the new system of incentives at the time of evaluation</td><td colspan="2">Estimated budget
Phase II</td></tr>
</table>

KSU King Saud University, *T&L* teaching and learning, *HSCs* health sciences colleges, *VRHS* vice-rector for health specialties, *KPIs* key performance indicators

required update from faculty, it would be difficult to motivate them to implement and incorporate the new educational strategies. Hence, new forms of rewards and incentives for teaching should be developed [5]. Rewards may vary; they can be internal or external. Internal rewards include a feeling of fulfillment as a teacher through interacting with students and refining skills by attending faculty development activities [6]. External rewards include academic acknowledgment and recognition by colleagues or patients as educators. However, Dahlstrom et al. [7] found that internal factors such as intellectual satisfaction, altruism, personal skills, and truth seeking are the main motivators for senior clinicians to teach medical students. Conversely, the reasons for not to be involved in teaching were no strong involvement in course design, a heavy clinical load, or feeling it was a waste of time. Selecting what the best motivators for faculty is context-based and depends on the school culture, which should be built upon short- and long-term plans [8].

The responsible for implementation of this initiative are the Teaching and Learning Steering Committee, the Incentive Policies Review Committee, and the Human Resources Department and Leadership Committee for HSCs. The Accountable are VRHSs and Deans of HSCs. The suggest partner is the Scientific Council at KSU. This initiative would mutually depend upon the availability of faculty policies of KSU, national and international HSCs. Stakeholders are the faculty. Regarding the proposed action plan, it would be in two phases: phase I, development; and phase II, implementation, monitoring, and evaluation. The estimated timeframe and budget allocation for this and other initiatives in this section will be considered later as a second phase.

15.2.2 Objective (Initiative) 7.2: To Support and Help Develop Teacher-Researcher Track

This initiative's strategy is presented in Table 15.2. It highlights the need for developing a track system that emphasizes the teaching role of faculty and facilitates educational excellence. This can be achieved by establishing clear standards of academic productivity and professional accomplishment for promotion on a career track by establishing a faculty promotion system that is realistic and achievable to enhance academic productivity. A track system provides a framework for an integrated and comprehensive approach that regulates and coordinates the process of faculty development and promotion in educational, clinical, research, and administrative duties. It gives the faculty the freedom to excel in areas that they like. Generally, faculty in health profession schools have three major roles: as academic teacher, scientist/clinician, and researcher. However, the promotion and tenure systems have focused mainly on the research role. Nieman et al. [9] described a strategy for making and implementing changes in faculty roles, rewards, and professional development in the era of health care reform. They designed a track system based on expanded categories of faculty academic activity and scholarship. Conversely, less attention and recognition are directed to other important roles such as clinical or laboratory duties, academic or educational skills, and administrative or community services. In reality, each of those roles would need more attention and effort that not all faculty members can perform in a balanced way. But with the track system, faculty would have the choice to select based on the career aspirations and

Table 15.2 Strategic plan for promoting the track system that would support teaching role of faculty

Goal 7: Developing faculty policies, career paths, and incentives that support the essential role of teaching in the light of competing priorities			
Objective (7.2): To support and help develop teacher-researcher track			
Initiative (7.2) Develop a faculty track system at KSU that enhances the value of teaching as a core mission of health-related colleges and which appropriately recognizes, honors, and facilitates faculty excellence in teaching	**Responsible** The T&L Steering Committee and Deans and Departments' Heads in HSCs	**Accountable** VRHS and Leadership Committee	**Partners** Scientific Council, and Human Resources Department
Initiative description Faculty members generally serve a primary role in research, teaching, or clinical care/service. Choice of track is primarily based on the career aspirations and potential of each individual. No single track or faculty role should be perceived to carry greater prestige or incentives or offer more opportunities for promotion. The track system should be designed as a career pathway for faculty who are involved in Scholarship. "Scholarship" should be defined and understood in its broader meaning to include both basic and applied research (discovery), and other domains of intellectual and academic activity (integration and application), in addition, of course, to teaching scholarship			
Requirements and interdependencies 1. Reviewing track systems of national and international HSCs 2. Reviewing faculty policies for promotion and tenure	**Stakeholders** Faculty staff		
Action plan **Phase I: development** 1. Seeking the track system documents of national and international HSCs through online searching and requests to faculty affairs representatives 2. Creating a task force to develop a new policy on "track system" faculty of health-related colleges at KSU. The policy should balance research, teaching, and service loads of faculty in to increase productivity 3. Getting approval from the VRHSs and Deans Board for the aforementioned policy 4. Implementing the policy **Phase II: implementation, monitoring, and evaluation** 1. Implementing, monitoring, and evaluating the model	**Estimated time** Phase II		
KPIs 1. Tracking system establishment 2. All new faculty hired or promoted using the track system	**Estimated budget** Phase II		

KSU King Saud University, *T&L* teaching and learning, *HSCs* health sciences colleges, *VRHS* vice-rector for health specialties, *KPIs* key performance indicators

potentials. No single track or faculty role should be perceived to carry greater prestige or incentives or offer more opportunities for promotion. The track system should be designed as a career pathway for faculty. "Scholarship" should be defined and understood in its broader meaning to include both research (discovery), and other domains of intellectual and academic activity (integration and application), in addition, of course, to education as described by Boyer [2]. Papaconstantinou and Lairmore [10] suggested four career tracks for promotion and tenure of surgeons in their corresponding departments: *Clinical Surgeons* who will devote 80–90% of their time focused on clinical activities, when the clinical load is high, while incorporating remaining times in faculty development programs, teaching undergraduate and postgraduate students, and research activities such as providing samples and tissues for basic sciences and clinical research; *Clinical Scholars* who are interested in performing clinically based research with less clinical duties, ranging from 60 to 80%, allowing substantial time to develop and perform clinical trials and other research projects; *Surgical Educators* looking for the development of excellence in clinical teaching and the advancement of the field of surgical education through research while devoting about 50–75% of their time in clinical activities; and *Surgical Scientists* who have usually completed 2–3 years of investigative laboratory training during their residency, devoting about 60% of their time to basic research, while remaining times incorporate clinical and academic activities. In order to develop a new track system at KSU, there is a need to study other track systems of national and international HSCs and policies for faculty promotion and tenure as a guide.

15.3 Summary

At KSU, our goal is to develop faculty policies, career paths, and incentives that support the essential role of teaching in the light of changing education. This can be accomplished by using an appropriate rewards system and developing the track system that would support faculty potentials. By taking this a proactive stand, gaining faculty interest, and promoting teaching role, we expect to see the emergence of a new faculty culture with new ways of defining faculty roles, incentives, and professional career development. Guidelines and instructions for promotion and tenure vary from one university to another within or outside the country's boundaries, based on policies and social contexts. In general, promotion and tenure of faculty in health professions are basically judged by the institutional policies on faculty performance divided among academic, clinical, and research activities with variable percentages.

References

1. Wiese A, Kilty C, Bennett D. Supervised workplace learning in postgraduate training: a realist synthesis. Med Educ. 2018;52(9):951–69.
2. Boyer EL, Moser D, Ream TC, Braxton J, editors. Scholarship reconsidered: priorities of the professoriate. San Francisco: Jossey Bass; 2015.
3. Cech TR. Rebalancing teaching and research. Science. 2003;299(5604):165.
4. Goldberg J. Doctor's earnings take a nosedive. Med Econ. 1994;71(17):122–32.

5. Bland CJ. Beyond corporate-style downsizing: a better way for medical schools to succeed in a changing world. Acad Med. 1997;72(6):489–95.
6. Kumar A, Loomba D, Rahangdale RY, Kallen D. Rewards and incentives for nonsalaried clinical faculty who teach medical students. J Gen Intern Med. 2007;14(6):370–2.
7. Dahlstrom J, Dorai-Raj A, McGill DA, Owen CA, Tymms K, Watson DA. What motivates senior clinicians to teach medical students? BMC Med Educ. 2005;5(1):27.
8. Ceriani PJ. Compensating and providing incentives for academic physicians: balancing earning, clinical, research, teaching, and administrative responsibilities. J Ambul Care Manage. 1992;15(2):69–78.
9. Nieman LZ, Donoghue GD, Ross LL, Morahan PS. Implementing a comprehensive approach to managing faculty roles, rewards, and development in an era of change. Acad Med. 1997;72(6):496–504.
10. Papaconstantinou HT, Lairmore TC. Academic appointment and the process of promotion and tenure. Clin Colon Rectal Surg. 2006;19(3):143–7.

Implementing Interprofessional Education and Collaboration

16

Mohammed Yahya Alnaami, Anand R., Ciraj Ali Mohammed, Saleena Velladath, Sunitha Calvin, and Abhishek Chaturvedi

16.1 Introduction

Health professional education underwent major changes over the last century through four stages of innovation. In a significant shift from the scientific approach to health professional education commonplace in Europe at the end of the nineteenth century,

M. Y. Alnaami (✉)
Department of Surgery, College of Medicine, King Saud University, Riyadh, Saudi Arabia

A. R.
Pulmonary Medicine, Kasturba Medical College, Mangalore, India

C. A. Mohammed
Medical Education, College of Medicine and Health Sciences, National University of Science & Technology, Sohar, Oman

S. Velladath
College of Medicine and Health Sciences, National University of Science and Technology, Sohar, Oman

S. Calvin
Manipal College of Nursing, Manipal Academy of Higher Education, Manipal, India

A. Chaturvedi
Department of Basic Medical Sciences, Manipal Academy of Higher Education, Manipal, India

M. Y. Alnaami et al. (eds.), *Novel Health Interprofessional Education and Collaborative Practice Program: Strategy and Implementation*, https://doi.org/10.1007/978-981-99-3420-1_16

the Flexner era at the beginning of the twentieth century [1] was noted for the idea of teaching basic sciences as the basis of clinical sciences and practice. In the 1970s, problem-based learning was strongly promoted in an attempt to integrate basic, clinical, and social sciences through the use of problem scenarios [2]. Competency/outcomes based curricula became popular around the turn of this century [3]. Key competencies focus on demonstrable professional outcomes guided by local and global needs [4, 5]. Globally, many health profession educational programs have not kept pace with changes and challenges of the twenty-first century; curricula have remained static, and faculty often work in silos instead of promoting interprofessional or interdisciplinary approaches to teaching. The potential and actual consequences of outdated approaches are that we produce graduates under-equipped for the increasingly linked and complex world of healthcare. The fourth significant innovation was put forward in 2010 in the Lancet Commissions Report [5]. This report promotes health professional education and health care systems appropriate for the complex needs of the twenty-first century (echoing the Flexner Report of the twentieth century); it advocates reforms in health profession curricula guided by two outcomes: interdependence in education and transformative learning. KSU is taking up the challenge of enacting these recommendations and actually began the reforms even before the Lancet Commissions Report. Our key aim is to develop new leaders who can affect meaningful and sustainable change in health professional education and healthcare systems. In addition to the influence of external international drivers, our main internal drivers for health professional education reform include preparedness for the NCAAA accreditation; making the appropriate response to students' dissatisfaction and mismatch of their learning styles with current curricula; and meeting public demand for better health professional education and graduates. There is mounting evidence that interprofessional care improves patient outcomes [6, 7] and that there are positive experiences with IPE [8–10]. The Interprofessional Education Collaborative Expert Panel [11] clearly defined the competency domains for interprofessional practice and the recommendations from a conference sponsored by the Josiah Macy Jr. Foundation [12] outline the need to align IPE with clinical practice redesign. The health care environment today is characterized by the presence of a good proportion of patients who are distressed with complex health problems. It is exceedingly difficult for a single health-care professional to handle all aspects of the medical treatment and care for such patients [13]. Through this approach, students from different professions aim to learn and collaborate interdependently with a common goal toward providing the best health care for patients with difficult problems that cannot be solved only from the standpoint of a single profession [13, 14]. For the same reason, it is important to consider students learn to work together across different professions right from their formative years of training. Hence, IPE as an essential educational strategy is being advocated and justified in the health professions curricula [15, 16]. The World Health Organization (WHO) is a strong proponent of patient-centered collaborative approach to care. The Centre for the Advancement of IPE outlines it as learning that occurs when students from two or more professions learn about, from and with each other to improve collaboration and the quality of care [17]. IPE is a necessary step in preparing a "collaborative practice ready" health workforce that is better prepared to respond to local health needs [18].

Our goal is to improve health professional education programs and their products through collaborative, interprofessional co-education and to share this experience with other local universities. The following sections highlight the strategic steps and initiatives to achieve this goal.

16.2 Strategic Goal 8: Promoting IPECP to Develop Insights, Shared Knowledge, and Teamwork Skills that Promote Effective Collaboration to Deliver High and Efficient Quality Care

This goal and subsequent related initiatives were written early in this phase of the program after few workshops combining key faculty and educators, students' representation, external consultants, and other relevant stakeholders. The consensus was to promote IPECP that already exists at KSU in and among some HSCs, but in a rather small scale. After analyzing the present status of IPECP in HSCs, we found some experiences including courses taught by faculty from another HSC; for example, some basic science courses of the dental college are taught by faculty from College of Medicine. There are courses that combine students from different HSCs, e.g., the optometry course taught to medical and applied medical sciences students. There are also courses that combine both faculty and students from different HSCs, e.g., the epidemiology and communicable diseases integrated course combining both faculty and students from nursing and applied medical sciences colleges. Also, a unified course exists in professionalism between colleges of medicine and pharmacy involving both faculty and students. To build on and develop this experience further, we propose the following initiatives:

16.3 Objective (Initiative) 8.1: To Develop Core and Common Competencies for Health Sciences Professionals

Four Core competencies for interprofessional collaborative practice put forward are Values/Ethics, Roles/Responsibilities, Interprofessional Communication, and Teamwork and Teams based practice [19]. *The ethical values and codes of ethics* for both students and faculty, with its implications to IPECP, are highlighted in "Chap. 12*: Professionalism, under the objective* (4.2)".

The second competency addresses the topic *"Role Clarification and Collaborative Practice."* As a fundamental element of interprofessional collaboration and practice, clear insights into interprofessional team members' professional roles are vital for the success of interprofessional care. Hence, role clarification is an essential competency identified in every competency framework on IPE and collaborative practice. It is one of the pillars on which interprofessional collaboration stands. It also complements other competencies like communication and teamwork. Differences among team members are both an opportunity and a challenge in interprofessional teams [20]. In today's ever-changing health scenario with the emergence of newer diseases, compounded by ever-rising patient expectations, resource constraints, and varied healthcare delivery, effective collaboration and coordination are the only strategies certain to successfully attain the desired patient outcomes [21]. Interprofessional collaboration requires effective teamwork. The success of the initiative is mainly dependent on how well the team performs. Hence, for any collaboration to succeed, the team must function well. There are many ingredients for effective team functioning. One of the crucial elements is the team members getting to understand each other better and realizing the strengths of fellow team members, and more importantly, complementing and supplementing one another's skills. This can happen only with role clarification.

For interprofessional teams to be effective, healthcare professionals need to be aware of their own roles and other team members [22]. The role here represents "a set of anticipations what one is expected to do" [23]. These perceptions on the roles of themselves and others in the team should be translated into real actions in clinical practice for enhanced patient care [24, 25].

To prepare health professional students for interprofessional practice, the curriculum should provide them with suitable learning opportunities to enable them to work with other team members from different professions and to gain knowledge about their roles, professional values and cultures, and contributions [22, 23]. Generally, clarity on the roles or responsibilities and contributions of the team members from other professions is important to overcome professional barriers as well as understanding one's own function and professional role.

16.4 What Is Role Clarification?

A team is made up of different members. An interprofessional team has members from different professions. A healthcare interprofessional team may also have members with a non-healthcare background. These teams are created to ensure better health outcomes, be it for the patient, the community, or the population. Since members are drawn from diverse backgrounds, there is a strong possibility of other members being unaware of what a particular team member brings to the team [26]. While the team members understand their own roles, they also need to consider the roles of other members of the healthcare team. It is not sufficient that they know their roles, but they should also be able to describe the roles of other team members. This understanding will ensure that gaps in the skills set are filled and, importantly, avoid duplication. It will facilitate team members to use the knowledge gained to develop the optimal strategy to achieve the goal [27].

16.5 Why Role Clarification?

The critical purpose of role clarification is to assist individual team members in understanding their own role and the roles of fellow team members (especially those from other professions). It should help establish the unique role of each member of the healthcare team. This will help identify overlapping skills/expertise and go a long way in preventing conflicts. It would assist in reducing role ambiguity. In many instances, the roles and responsibilities of the profession are defined by statutory norms. The scope of practice is not constant, and it keeps evolving. Further, depending on the specific care situation, the roles and responsibilities change. By articulating the roles and responsibilities of one's own and other profession's role, the team will deliver safe and effective care. The second purpose of role clarification is to improve working relationships. Boundaries between professional roles can become blurred because it is not an easy task to understand one's own role and then supplement it with an understanding of other professionals' roles and responsibilities. This could result in potential confusion of which profession should perform a particular task and result in strained relationships. The dissolution of professional boundaries and clarity on each member's strengths helps in building trusting relationships. Over time, healthcare professionals develop a range of beliefs and attitudes about not just their profession but also other professions. These are often set on false beliefs and assumptions because of lack of clarity on other professions' role. Hence, when working in interprofessional teams for the first time, they tend to carry some of these false beliefs and assumptions and develop their biases. Role clarification helps team members develop an understanding of other professions' boundaries and how they may interact with others to achieve the goal of better patient/community/population outcomes.

While team members' individual professional expertise helps in achieving the team's goals, it has its limitations when it comes to efficiency and effectiveness. The final purpose is increased cooperation and better team effectiveness. This is derived from the first two purposes and is the end result of role clarification. The result of role clarification would be division of tasks into yours, mine, and ours!

16.6 What Does Role Clarification Entail?

As stated in the Interprofessional Education Collaborative (IPEC) updated competencies list of 2016, role clarity is all about using "the knowledge of one's own role and those of other professions to appropriately assess and address the health care needs of patients and to promote and advance the health of populations" [19, 28]. The IPEC document outlines ten sub-competencies. The key sub-competencies are listed below:

1. Clear communication of roles.
2. Recognition of limitation of one's knowledge, skill, and abilities.
3. Involving different professionals to complement one's professional expertise.
4. Explanation of the roles and responsibilities of other team members, and how this helps the team to work together.
5. Utilizing the unique and complementary abilities of all professionals in the team to provide patient-centric care and optimize the health of the population.

It also entails that team members recognize, appreciate, and respect the diversity of various professions. While deciding one's role, the team members also need to consider fellow team members' expertise and consider their roles. It is all about seamless integration for effective care delivery.

16.7 How to Go about it?

A simple strategy is first to list one's professional role and then read it out for everyone's benefit in one of the early team meetings. A checklist could ensure that there is standardization in the way the roles are listed, and that it is relevant to the task. During the team meeting, clarifications should be sought, and complementary skill sets should be identified. A consensus has to be arrived at regarding each team member's role. The initiative's success depends on approaching the team meeting with an open mindset and being ever willing to listen to other viewpoints.

Examples: Developing a pulmonary rehabilitation program for patients suffering from obstructive airway disease entails working together of medical, physical therapy, and dietetics personnel. There is also an opportunity to involve other professionals like a counselor who will help in counseling these patients and an IT professional who will develop an easy-to-use app for home monitoring. Each of these professions can individually deliver part of the pulmonary rehabilitation program, but collectively they can provide a patient-centric program and lead to better outcomes. Though the clinician and physical therapist are well-versed with the treatment, when they sit together and start the discussion, they will realize that the clinician's strength is in prescribing the pharmacologic treatment, and the physical therapist will ensure that the patient is put on the right exercise regimen. Rather than prescribe a diet based on jargon (for example, a protein-rich diet), the dietician will work together with the team and consider the patient's preferences, the exercise regimen, and the clinician's concerns to come up with the right diet for the patient. Though this sounds very simple, in clinical practice, most professionals are not aware of how patient care would improve by leaps and bounds by involving other professionals and following the tenets of role clarification.

Nurses are a major component of the healthcare delivery system and often have performed in high performing care teams with power struggles and resistance issues. The nurses' role in the practice context is analyzed as per the patients' needs in a particular setting and the practice settings framework. The intricacies of a given clinical situation play a significant role where the interaction between the team members concerning their expectations makes it possible for teamwork without overstepping into each other's boundaries yet working together for the patient's benefit.

The crucial issue in having good team interaction and performance is having clarity in the partners' role. For this to happen, nurses should be able to describe their own role in the given situation and understand the roles of other team members. Support from the team members to explain their role would also improve team effort. Another team member can identify strengths in nurses, beneficial to the team, which may not have been identified by the nurse. Consequently, considering the diversity of the roles will also give a positive perspective into the overall care, considering the various cultural and professional legalities that might be encountered in due course. By encouraging team consultations, communication is enhanced, knowledge and understanding are improved, and gray areas of functioning can be discussed and clarified for the client and the team's benefit. Nurses also utilize this knowledge to understand the other team members' roles, which will enable smooth functioning within the teams, thereby integrating all the competencies developed into interprofessional collaboration and practice [29].

Likewise, laboratory professionals represent another important but often neglected segment of healthcare professionals. They experience a lack of autonomy and are professional hierarchy victims in clinical services. Healthcare professionals who are unaware of lab professionals' roles and contributions are likely to face problems while working with them in a team. Activities that focus on interprofessional collaborative practice serve as facilitators for organizing and promoting collaborative practices that will prepare lab professionals in clearly identifying their roles, and how it intersperses with the roles of other health care professionals. This, in turn, can foster a higher degree of responsibility and decision-making within the healthcare team, leading to enhanced patient outcome [30].

The third core competency addresses "*interprofessional communication*" as a major pillar for effective and safe IPECP. We converse every day with colleagues, students, patients, friends, and family and at times with strangers too. After having these conversations, seldom do we think about the way the conversation went and the way we communicated with others. We often fail to reflect on whether our communication was effective, and if not, how to change the way we communicate. Both verbal and non-verbal modes of communication are complex. They may be subject to misunderstandings and misinterpretations if not done appropriately and, either or both of these can pose issues during a conversation. Therefore, communication is the key component needed for a healthy workplace culture. It refers to how we communicate in a team, and with one another we determine the outcomes of the shared goals.

Issues with Spoken Language: What will you think of when you hear the word "mouse"? You could think of a mouse, as a pointing device used with computers, or a rodent. Therefore, the manner in which we communicate makes a difference between putting the points across or letting someone infer for themselves. One of the biggest issues we face relates to acronyms. An acronym is the abbreviation of the initial letters of the word and pronounced as a word, e.g., ICU: Intensive Care Unit. Such acronyms are heavily used in all forms of communication, and it is often assumed that people would comprehend what is being conveyed. Ambiguity is another issue. It is admired and deemed fit in a creative writing piece in order to give the reader an opportunity to infer based on their thoughts. But in healthcare, ambiguity or ambiguous communication could be disastrous. It can lead to medical errors, prolong hospital stay, and can increase the monetary burden on the patient, which in turn can lead to poor patient satisfaction and health outcomes [31]. Hence, it is vital to have non-ambiguous communication in a healthcare team. It should have only one meaning and no other interpretation [32]. Another issue is gender, as it influences the way we communicate and comprehend. In the past, the male workforce dominated the health care system, but today women account for almost half of the health workforce. They are involved in diverse healthcare teams and assume leadership roles in many organizations. In spite of a balanced number, the conversation often gets entangled in communication knots on the pretext of the gender of the persons involved in that conversation. The main reason for such obstacles can be attributed to the style of communication, which is governed by the genders in play. It has been documented in the literature that patients perceive a difference in the way a male and female physician and the specialty physician communicate with them [33, 34]. This difference could be due to the way they communicate in the teams as well. Therefore, in order to provide balanced patient care where the patient perceives no bias, communication within and outside a team should be gender-neutral.

A mis-communicated or an ineffectively communicated piece of information often embodies the elephant in the room. No one wants to bring it up to discuss. It leads to disputes, disagreements, procedural error, lack of rapport building, misdiagnosis, and even medical error [35]. This results in sub-standard patient care and that snowballs to reduce patient's trust toward the profession, demotivates the patient, and thus finally resulting in poor treatment compliance [36]. Thus, by being clear, confident, non-ambiguous, gender-neutral, and respectful, one can avoid the possibility of communication failure.

Spoken language is multivariate, and each of these variables is important for effective team communication. Let us look at a few of them. For example:

Intonation: It is a variation in the pitch of the voice used to express meaning. In a clinical practice environment, if one speaks robotically or mechanically, then it is very difficult to be empathetic. It is important that we be prosodic in a conversation, especially while in a team, to place emphasis on a specific and important piece of information like task, dosage, timing, or the clinical test. The tone we use conveys the feeling, emotion, and a specific meaning. Careful usage of intonation in doctor–patient communication or team communication can help in effectively conveying the necessary information [37].

Interjection: One would come across as being impolite if they were to interrupt their fellow conversationalist from speaking any further only because a point had to be made and could not wait till the sentence saw the period. When in conversation with a team or a patient, interjecting is considered very rude. One has to hold their urge to interject, be patient, and wait for the other to finish their sentence. The longest pause one can take within an ongoing conversation is about 13–15 s. One should not get weary of a pause taken by the speaker and allow them to finish putting their thoughts into sentences. It is natural to feel a sense of discomfort during such a pause and the urge to speak anything to fill in the pause. We should quell such an urge and listen and let the other person complete the conversation. This is especially important while talking to patients and in history taking. Listening is central to communication in a doctor–patient relationship. It helps in gathering important clinical data, acts as a therapeutic agent, and most importantly it fosters and strengthens the relationship between the persons involved in the conversation [38, 39].

Turn taking: We have to allow each other to take turns in a conversation. This again means listening carefully, and checking that what was heard and understood is the same as what was intended and said. It is vital that the message which is passed on by the sender is received in the same form by the receiver and this transfer of information may be validated by feedback. If the receiver gives feedback of the content which he/she received and the same is acknowledged by the sender that "yes that's the message I sent," then the conversation is deemed successful and complete. This is important in every team communication and very pertinent in healthcare teams with diverse groups of professionals.

Laughter and applause are two other variables of communication that need to be expressed based on the situation at hand. Laughter helps in reducing stress and tension in a conversation and accords the strength to deal with a difficult or an unpleasant situation, and more importantly, foster an amicable relationship and strengthen the human connection [40, 41]. Pause and silence are also interconnected with all the above elements, especially when you are trying to understand your patient. Compassionate silence is important in a clinical setting [42].

Body Language: The non-spoken words in a spoken language: There are various elements to non-verbal communication, and as a team working on patient care, we should be aware of our body language that constitutes about 80% of the language we use with patients. However, it is often neglected during doctor–patient or in team communication. Patients express their unhappiness in complaints, and facial expression, eye contact, and paralanguage (non-verbal communication) of a healthcare team are often reported as their primary complaint [43]. This unhappiness can result in a lack of trust in the healthcare team and may adversely affect the health outcomes of the patient. During COVID-19 pandemic, the mask drapes the beautiful smiles and facial expressions. Hence, in such times it becomes all the more pertinent to make sure that our body language is not a hindering factor in a conversation.

It is vital that we remember the multi-variant nature of the spoken language when we talk to people from different cultures (need not be indicative of a different country, between health science and social care professions itself there are many different cultures). One has to ensure that the words we use have equivalence. So, the best way to communicate is to be:

Open: balance listening time and talking time.

Accurate: use the best evidence about the topic, and.

Effective: best communicator can change the attitude of the person toward an issue and develop new behavior.

Communication as a process, not a data transfer: Data is information, and it is important to learn the way we transfer or present the data so that it is received and understood correctly. We assume that communication is very simple. I think something, I say it, and others should understand it.

Life would be much simpler this way. But in reality, it is not so. The thought has to be encoded by the sender in his/her style and transmitted via a medium (this medium being written, verbal, or non-verbal), the receiver then decodes this and tries to interpret the information and feel that he/she understood it [44]. It so happens most of the time that we assume we understood what is being said. But did we really understand? Hence, it is important to check with the sender whether your interpretation is correct or not. *Communication as a story:* Communication is indeed a great tool in terms of sharing information, getting the point across and convey the intended meaning. As a healthcare provider, we are telling our story as well as receiving the story from our patients and other stakeholders.

Listening is the first step. In order to be sure that you as a listener are able to understand what the person is saying, listen to their story, and then talk about it. So, we listen and then talk about it in order to ensure we understand it. And if we do not understand, then we have to reflect (quiet reflection is a good thing, reflect for few seconds) and then go back and confirm whether we got the message right by checking, "I think you were trying to tell me that" and if it is so, then the story continues and we sustain the conversation. And if we do not understand, we have to go back again and find out. We cannot just assume that we have understood it correctly. One should always make a check before proceeding further in the conversation so that later there is no room for error in understanding and in the task being carried out.

Interprofessional communication: a competency to improve health outcomes: It is one of the competencies laid down by Canadian Interprofessional Health Collaborative (CIHC) [45] and Interprofessional Education Collaborative [19] in a national interprofessional competency framework needed to improve team-based care to patients. This is one of the competencies which connects the other competencies to a common goal of interprofessional collaboration to improve health outcomes of patients and the community. The competency statement stated is "Learners/practitioners from different professions communicate with each other in a collaborative, responsive and responsible manner."

In healthcare, communication breakdowns or miscommunication often go unnoticed, when in actuality it can significantly influence the quality of care, patient safety, and overall health outcomes [46–48]. In any workplace, various teams come together and work toward a shared goal. During a team discussion, individual members put forth their thoughts which could be influenced by the culture, values, and thought process. Therefore, it is never easy to shift to a newer workplace, with different work culture, but it all boils down to one simple question. "Does the team communicate well?" With the evolution of in silo education to IPE, health professionals are accepting the differences in the training, culture, language, and education. In spite of this, the differences in communication still pose a threat to patient safety and patient health outcomes, and this has to be worked upon.

Miscommunication and Poor Patient Outcomes: In the process of healthcare delivery, there are many members who work collaboratively to improve the health of a patient. It is imperative that they communicate well in order to provide the best service without any negligence. Ineffective communication leads to delay in treatment, wrong diagnosis, misdiagnosis, medication error, patient injury, or even death [46–48]. In literature, there are pieces of evidence of miscommunication or ineffective communication among healthcare workers, which has adversely affected the health outcomes of a patient [49]. Physicians and nurses are taught and trained differently, and there is a contrast in their communication style and decision-making [50]. Physicians focus on the facts, and nurses focus on a holistic approach. This contrast in communication style and decision-making brings a structural hierarchy, hinders the relationship among the healthcare workers, and leads to miscommunication and misinterpretation. Miscommunication initiates a blame game where the poor patient outcome is handled like a baton and is passed on between physicians to nursing staff and other healthcare workers. Ego is another factor that hinders effective communication during healthcare delivery, which reduces the confidence and trust in the system. Improving communication in healthcare is taken as a global priority and IPECP is paving the way ahead for inculcating this competency among the health workforce.

Interprofessional Communication—A Competency to Improve Health Outcomes: The Canadian neuropsychologist, Donald Hebb used a sentence in 1949 "Neurons that fire together, wire together," and it holds good in IPE and collaborative practice too. This may be re-written as "Professionals that study/train together, work together." It is vital that health workers should study and train together in order to work effectively in a team aiming to improve collaborative practice and patients' health outcomes. When many members from different profession come together with their knowledge, experience, hierarchical structure, cultural background, language, ethnic difference, the conflict is bound to happen. This has been the highlight in the barriers of effective communication. These barriers are related to a lack of confidence and experience, fear of professional dilution, lack of standardization, lack of cultural competence, low consistency in communication technique, over expectations, lack of team structure or stability in the team, hierarchical differences, inconsistent technology, and the complex nature of healthcare delivery [51–56]. Interprofessional communication has been found to alleviate these barriers and create a positive workplace and organization culture [57] that fosters collaborative environment alongside a high level of satisfaction on teamwork [58]. It also helps sustain effective communication between the interprofessional team members, which promotes better functioning of the team and delivery of coordinated patient-centered care [59].

The first step toward improvement starts with accepting that communication failure is disastrous for collaborative patient care, and effective communication can improve patient safety and reduce medical errors. There are various approaches already being employed to teach interprofessional communication, which includes conducting workshops, case studies, and online modules. It has been indicated that training, simulation, and use of standardized communication tools can bring positive change in the young health workforce and can significantly improve interprofessional communication skills [52, 60–62]. Use of simulation is weighed to be a more effective approach to learning communication in a clinical setting than a traditional classroom approach [63, 64].

The available tools such as Team Strategies and Tools to Enhance Performance and Patient Safety (Team-STEPPS) [56], SBAR [51], closed-loop communication: Call-out and check back [65], Two Challenge rule [66], Checklist, and read back protocols [67, 68], Team Huddles [69] can be employed by the healthcare teams in clinical rounds, and they can also be used in medical education in a simulated environment to introduce and enhance interprofessional communication.

The healthcare system is dealing with a pandemic stricken world. This situation has called for coordination not just within the healthcare system but goes well beyond it to civic authorities, home affairs, volunteer organizations, and more. Professionals from various fields are working alongside healthcare professionals toward a single goal, the health of the community. In such a scenario, effective communication becomes crucial and will obviously determine the health curve of the community.

The fourth competency is about *"Interprofessional Teamwork."* This has been discussed in details in "Chaps. 3, 4".

The strategy for this initiative is presented in Table 16.1. The Leadership Committee of the program has already identified existing IPE experiences as mentioned before. The T&L Steering Committee of the program and T/L Units (Medical Education Departments) in HSCs will be responsible for developing common IPE core competencies. These will be derived mainly from the Interprofessional Education Collaborative Expert Panel Document [19] that highlights four

Table 16.1 Strategic plan for identifying and developing IPE competencies among healthcare professionals

<table>
<tr><td colspan="4">Goal 8: Promoting IPE to develop insights, shared knowledge, and teamwork skills to achieve effective collaboration and deliver high and efficient quality care</td></tr>
<tr><td colspan="4">Objective (8.1): To develop core and common competencies for health sciences professionals.</td></tr>
<tr><td>Initiative (8.1)
Developing important competencies for health sciences professionals</td><td>Responsible
T&L steering committee and T&L units (medical education departments) in HSCs</td><td>Accountable
VRHS and the leadership committee</td><td>Partners
Deans of HSCs, deanship of the preparatory year, and CELT</td></tr>
<tr><td colspan="4">Initiative description
1. Identifying existing IPE competencies among HSCs (formal IPE)
2. Identifying existing extracurricular activities that have some form of IPE (informal IPE)
3. Listing core skills (competencies) that are common for all health care providers</td></tr>
<tr><td colspan="3">Requirements and interdependencies
1. The leader of the T&L unit in each HSC will provide the leadership Committee for Health Sciences Education the educational plan and curriculum of a corresponding HSC, highlighting competencies suitable for IPE
2. Agreeing on common IPE competencies that are important and feasible to be adopted by health science programs</td><td>Stakeholders
Faculty staff and students</td></tr>
<tr><td colspan="3">Action plan
1. Developing core competencies for HSE
2. Developing a core curriculum for IPE
3. Conducting a workshop involving deans and vice-deans for academic and quality affairs, graduate students, some administrators, and community representatives on the implementation of IPE</td><td>Estimated time
To be decided later as Phase II</td></tr>
<tr><td colspan="3">KPIs
1. To adopt at least 7 core competencies
2. Measure qualities of these competencies using appropriate corresponding matrix</td><td>Estimated budget
To be studied and decided as phase II</td></tr>
</table>

IPE interprofessional Education, *T&L* teaching and learning, *HSCs* Health Sciences Colleges, *VRHS* vice-rector for health specialties, *CELT* center of excellence in learning and teaching, *HSE* Health Sciences Education, *KPIs* key performance indicators competency domains: values/ethics for interprofessional practice: roles, responsibilities, interprofessional communication, and teams and teamwork, with special emphasis on competencies matching our local needs. The VRHS and the Leadership Committee will be accountable for the success or failure of addressing and implementing these core competencies. The partners of course are the Deans of HSCs including Preparatory Year Deanship and the Center of Excellence in L&T (CELT). There is an ongoing debate about when it is the most effective time to implement IPE. However, evidence indicates that implementation of IPE during early years of professional education has a positive impact on students and their institutions. The first year of prequalification health science programs (the preparatory year in our case) was found to be the most effective if negative effects of professional socialization are to be prevented [70]. Also, students in the preparatory year need to develop insights and evaluate health science programs in some depth through IPE in order to choose their right future career.

Existing IPE competencies according to the strategic plans of some HSCs include quality and excellence, leadership and teamwork, freedom of inquiry, fairness and integrity, transparency and accountability, lifelong learning, confidence promotion, respect and responsibility for personal and professional behavior, social justice, altruism, autonomy, human dignity, compassion and understanding, cooperation, creativity, honesty, discipline, professionalism, etc. However, these were listed as values rather than competencies. Existing extracurricular and interprofessional activities include the International Diabetes Day arranged by the medical and nursing programs; a large contingent of dignitaries from universities and governments across the Gulf marked as the Gulf Nursing Day; and the smoking control campaign integrating the medical, nursing, and applied medical sciences as examples. Common competencies among HSCs will be segregated for further study and development. Stakeholders should agree on common IPE competencies that are important and feasible to be adopted by health science programs. Stakeholders include faculty and students. Of course, faculty and educators are key players for choosing the right IPE competencies. Students also play a major role in accepting these competencies as possible and applicable to their level of education and training. The Leadership Committee is responsible for studying and measuring the achievement and quality of these competencies. Selected and agreed upon competencies as well as a core curriculum for IPE will be developed and prepared for further discussion and approval by higher authorities at HSCs and KSU. The proposed strategy to achieve this initiative *"to develop core and common competencies for health sciences professionals"* is detailed in Table 16.1.

16.8 Objective (Initiative) 8.2: To Develop Core Interprofessional Courses

This initiative's strategy is presented in Table 16.2. As mentioned before, existing IPE courses are to be supported and developed further. This also involves expert faculty who have taught IPE or have some background in IPE competencies that will need to be identified and listed by members of the Leadership Committee

Table 16.2 Strategic plan for developing core interprofessional courses

<table>
<tr><td colspan="4">Goal 8: Promoting IPE to develop insights, shared knowledge, and teamwork skills to achieve effective collaboration and deliver high and efficient quality care</td></tr>
<tr><td colspan="4">Objective (8.2): To develop core interprofessional courses</td></tr>
<tr><td>Initiative (8.2)
Developing core interprofessional courses</td><td>Responsible
T&L steering committee and T&L units/medical education departments in HSCs</td><td>Accountable
VRHS and the leadership committee</td><td>Partners
Deans of HSCs, deanship of the preparatory year, and CELT</td></tr>
<tr><td colspan="4">Initiative description
1. Identify existing IPE courses among HSCs
2. Identifying consultants, experts, and facilitators for IPE
3. Designing interprofessional courses and seeing where they fit among the curricula of HSCs and deanship of the preparatory year</td></tr>
<tr><td colspan="3">Requirements and interdependencies
1. The leader of the T&L unit in each HCS will provide the leadership committee for HSE the educational plan and curriculum of corresponding HSC highlighting courses serving IPE
2. Agreeing on common, existing IPE courses to be supported and new courses to be implemented in HSE programs</td><td>Stakeholders
Faculty staff and students</td></tr>
<tr><td colspan="3">Action plan
1. Benchmarking with well-known IPE institutes/agencies (e.g., CAIPE, UK and CIHC, College of Health Disciplines, University of British Columbia, Vancouver, Canada)
2. Developing a core curriculum for IPE
3. Conducting pilot projects that support IPE in HSCs</td><td>Estimated time
Phase II</td></tr>
<tr><td colspan="3">KPIs
1. Conducting at least 50% of listed IPE courses
2. Stakeholders satisfaction surveys should score > 80% satisfaction rate in each group</td><td>Estimated budget
Phase II</td></tr>
</table>

T&L teaching and learning, *HSCs* Health Sciences Colleges, *VRHS* vice-rector for health specialties, *CELT* center of excellence in learning and teaching, *IPE* interprofessional education, *HSE* Health Sciences' Education, *CAIPE* center for the advancement of interprofessional education, *CIHC* Canadian interprofessional health collaborative, *KPIs* key performance indicators

representing their corresponding HSCs. Faculty will be employed as instructors for training and conduct of IPE faculty development activities. New core courses need to be added to emphasize IPE, improve collaboration among HSCs, and ultimately improve patient care. The T&L Steering Committee will be responsible for developing these new IPE courses based on needs assessment and a consensus with all relevant stakeholders. The accountable, partners, and stakeholders are the same as in initiative 8.1.

At this stage, benchmarking with other existing programs and agencies worldwide is of paramount importance to achieve this objective. The Center for the Advancement of Interprofessional Education (CAIPE) in UK was the first organization established in 1987 advocating IPE [17]. It aims to promote and develop IPE in the UK and overseas for the benefit of patients and clients. The Canadian Interprofessional Health Collaborative (CIHC) has been supported by the Canadian government to provide Canada and the International Community with leadership and support in IPE and collaborative practice [45]. A core curriculum for IPE will be developed by the T&L Steering Committee and the T&L Units (Medical Education Departments) in HSCs. Intended IPE courses include IPE, Professionalism and Communication, Social Accountability and Consciousness, Critical Thinking and Decision-Making, Teamwork, Ethics, Patients' Safety, and the IT/medical informatics course. Some of these courses are already taught in HSCs; however, they may need to be modified to address all health science disciplines. HSCs are volunteering to adopt one or more of the aforementioned new courses. For example, College of Medicine will manage the professionalism and communication course, College of Pharmacy will adopt the IPE course, and College of Applied Medical Sciences will adopt the IT and informatics course as they have the expertise and resources for that purpose. The KPIs were a bit realistic as at least 50% of intended IPE courses should be developed during 1 year keeping in mind the willingness and readiness of some HSCs to develop new or implement already existing IPE courses. Stakeholders' satisfaction surveys should score > 80% satisfaction rate in each group in order to measure the effectiveness of the IPE.

16.9 Objective (Initiative) 8.3: To Create a Database of Suitable Faculty with their Areas of Expertise in IPE

The strategy to develop this initiative is presented in Table 16.3. This initiative has already begun, and existing IPE courses have been identified with faculty staff. However, this process is still primitive in paper form and has not been transferred into a database. Therefore, a database consultant with expertise in computer sciences and programming needs to be hired. The initial step was the creation of a website for the program. The list of IPE courses and names of experts with their area(s) of expertise will be uploaded in the program website once completed. The Leadership Committee will be responsible for providing all courses and experts in IPE at all HSCs. Each head of the T&L unit in corresponding HSC will provide list of faculty experts and area(s) of expertise with their updated curriculum vitae (CV). Also, the Leadership Committee will send surveys to all HSCs faculty introducing IPE and find out about their knowledge, skills, and attitude toward IPE. Once surveys are completed and sent back to the program electronically, the T&L Steering Committee at the VRHSs will arrange for a 3-day workshop to address IPE and design the intended and related competencies and courses. The main aim of this workshop is to break barriers and enforce collaboration between health science disciplines. Reeves [71] identified six conditions that have to be addressed to achieve this goal: equality of status between the groups; group members working toward common goals; cooperation during the contact; positive expectations by participants; successful experience of joint working; and focus on understanding differences as well as similarities between themselves. After formulation of competencies and courses, the VRHSs and Deans of HSCs are deemed accountable for the success or failure of this initiative achievement. The partners are Preparatory Year Deanship, CELT, Deanship of e-Transactions and Communication, and Deanship of e-Learning

Table 16.3 Strategic plan for creating a database of participating faculty and their expertise in IPE

Goal 8: Promoting IPE to develop insights, shared knowledge, and teamwork skills to achieve effective collaboration and deliver high and efficient quality care			
Objective (8.3): To create a database of suitable faculty with their areas of expertise in IPE			
Initiative (8.3) •. Identifying existing IPE courses in HSCs, including the preparatory year and listing faculty experts • Identifying faculty who have experience with IPE	**Responsible** T&L steering committee and the leadership committee	**Accountable** VRHS and deans of HSCs	Partners Preparatory year deanship, CELT, deanship of e-transactions and communication, and deanship of e-learning and distance learning
Initiative description Establishing a database with a list of IPE courses and names of experts with their area(s) of expertise and uploading it in the program website			
Requirements and interdependencies 1. Each head of T&L unit in a corresponding HSC will provide a list of faculty experts and area(s) of expertise 2. Providing experts' CVs			**Stakeholders** Faculty staff and students
Action plan 1. Sending surveys to all health sciences faculty staff to introduce IPE and find out about their knowledge, skills, and attitudes toward IPE 2. Using this expertise to develop IPE core competencies and courses in a 3-day workshop at a suitable location outside KSU campus			**Estimated time** Phase II
KPIs 1. At least 75% of the experts should participate in designing IPHE core competencies and courses 2. > 80% of faculty participants are satisfied with the workshop results 3. Establishing a database for IPE			**Estimated budget** Phase II

IPE Interprofessional Education, *HSCs* Health Sciences Colleges, *T&L* teaching and learning, *VRHS* vice-rector for health specialties, *CELT* center of excellence in learning and teaching, *CV* curriculum vitae, *KSU* King Saud University, *KPIs* key performance indicators

and Distance Learning who will share directly or indirectly in the development of this initiative. Stakeholders include faculty and students. The estimated timeframe and budget necessary for this initiative will be studied and decided later as a second phase for the implementation process.

16.10 Objective (Initiative) 8.4: To Create Suitable Clinical, Laboratory, and Community Environments to Practice IPE

The strategy for this initiative is summarized in Table 16.4. The responsible, accountable, and partners are the same as in Initiative 8.3. This initiative emphasizes the application of IPE at workplaces not only in classrooms. This implies preparing

Table 16.4 Strategic plan for practicing IPE in various HSCs

Goal 8: Promoting IPE to develop insights, shared knowledge, and teamwork skills to achieve effective collaboration and deliver high and efficient quality care	
Objective (8.4): To create suitable clinical, laboratory, and community environments to practice IPE	
Initiative description Preparing clinics, skills labs, and community services to accommodate, facilitate, and monitor students' learning in IPE	
Requirements and interdependencies 1. Using space and resources available in HSCs for IPE 2. Employing facilitators to conduct, monitor, and assess IPE outcomes	**Stakeholders** Faculty staff and students
Action plan 1. Providing a suitable environment for IPE 2. Developing a system for delivering effective IPE	**Estimated time** Phase II
KPIs 1. At least 50% of IPE should be practiced in clinics, labs, and community	**Estimated budget** Phase II

IPE Interprofessional Education, *HSCs* health sciences colleges

clinics, skills labs, and community services to accommodate, facilitate, and monitor students' learning in IPE. This requires a system to deliver effective IPE in the form of providing spaces and resources that are already available in HSCs without exception and creation of new resources such as common simulation laboratories. The system will also encompass facilitators and trainers to conduct, monitor, and assess IPE outcomes. The attributes of facilitators and trainers of IPE include [72]:

- Experience of IP work (to draw upon when facilitating).
- In-depth understanding of interactive learning methods.
- Knowledge of group dynamics.
- Confidence in working with IP groups.
- Flexibility (to use professional differences within groups creatively).

Freeth [72] argues that immersion in the process of IPE is more important than assessment. However, most people perceive value in including some formative or summative assessment. In this case, assessment should reinforce the outcomes of IPE. Since IPE is extremely varied, we should expect that assessment associated with IPE would be equally varied. KPIs used by quality improvement initiatives, as listed in Tables 16.1, 16.2, 16.3 and 16.4 in this chapter, are considered the most useful and favored tools to assess IPE by many educators. The second important tool is formative assessment in the form of structured feedback from colleagues and supervisors representing the different disciplines. Summative assessment is a bit challenging like assessment of professionalism. However, if an institute chooses to give a real value for IPE, summative assessment must have clearly defined criteria.

16.11 Summary

Implementing interprofessional education and collaboration at health professions educational programs is highly encouraged by many reports and research data. However, this requires progressive efforts by both students and faculty educators. This usually starts by developing insights, shared knowledge, and teamwork skills that promote effective collaboration to deliver high and efficient quality care. At KSU, our goal is to improve health professional education programs and their products through collaborative interprofessional co-education. This can be achieved through some agreed upon initiatives that involve data collection and development of existing IPE courses and expertise, designing a core curriculum and competencies for IPE, and applying it at workplaces. Trained facilitators will conduct, monitor, and assess IPE outcomes.

References

1. Flexner A. Medical education in the United States and Canada: a report to the Carnegie Foundation for the Advancement of Teaching. New York: The Carnegie Foundation for the Advancement of Teaching; 2003.
2. Schmidt HG. Problem-based learning: rationale and description. Med Educ. 1983;17:11–6.
3. Albanese MA, Mejicano G, Mullan P, Kokotailo P, Gruppen L. Defining characteristics of educational competencies. Med Educ. 2008;42(3):248–55.
4. Zaini RG, Bin Abdulrahman KA, Al-Khotani AA, Al-Hayani AM, Al-Alwan IA, Jastaniah SD. Saudi Meds: a competence specification for Saudi medical graduates. Med Teach. 2011;33(7):582–4.
5. Frenk J, Chen L, Bhutta ZA, Cohen J, Crisp N, Evans T, et al. Health professionals for a new century: transforming education to strengthen health systems in an interdependent world. Lancet. 2010;376(9756):1923–58.
6. Reeves S, Perrier L, Goldman J, Freeth D, Zwarenstein M. Interprofessional education: effects on professional practice and healthcare outcomes (update). Cochrane Database Syst Rev. 2013;28(3):CD002213.
7. O'Leary KJ, Buck R, Fligiel HM, Haviley C, Slade ME, Landler MP, et al. Structured interdisciplinary rounds in a medical teaching unit: improving patient safety. Arch Intern Med. 2011;171(7):678–84.
8. Hammick M, Freeth D, Koppel I, Reeves S, Barr H. A best evidence systematic review of interprofessional education: BEME guide no. 9. Med Teach. 2007;29(8):735–51.
9. Hylin U, Nyholm H, Mattiasson AC, Ponzer S. Interprofessional training in clinical practice on a training ward for healthcare students: a two-year follow-up. J Interprof Care. 2007;21(3):277–88.
10. Pelling S, Kalén A, Hammar M, Wahlström O. Preparation for becoming members of health care teams: findings from a 5-year evaluation of a student interprofessional training ward. J Interprof Care. 2011;25:328–32.
11. Schmitt M, Blue A, Aschenbrener CA, Viggiano TR. Core competencies for interprofessional collaborative practice: reforming health care by transforming health professionals' education. Acad Med. 2011;86(11):1351.
12. Josiah Macy Jr. Foundation. Transforming patient care: aligning Interprofessional education with clinical practice redesign. Conference recommendations. Atlanta; 2013.
13. Jayasuriya-Illesinghe V, Guruge S, Gamage B, Espin S. Interprofessional work in operating rooms: a qualitative study from Sri Lanka. BMC Surg. 2016;16:61.

14. Brandt BF, Cerra FB, Delaney CW. The United States National Center for Interprofessional practice and education: integrating an informatics approach to interprofessional work. J Interprof Care. 2016;29:592–5.
15. Angel VM, Friedman MH, Friedman AL. Integrating bar-code medication administration competencies in the curriculum: implications for nursing education and interprofessional collaboration. Nurs Educ Perspect. 2016;37:239–741.
16. Bluteau P, Jackson A. Interprofessional education: making it happen. London: Palgrave Macmillan; 2009. p. 37–58.
17. Centre for the Advancement of Inter Professional Education (CAIPE) on the definition and principles of interprofessional education. CAIPE Bulletin; 2006.
18. Gilbert JH. Interprofessional education for collaborative, patient-centred practice. Nurs Leadersh. 2005;18(2):32–8.
19. Interprofessional Education Collaborative. Core competencies for interprofessional collaborative practice: 2016 update. Washington, DC: Interprofessional Education Collaborative; 2016. https://ipec.memberclicks.net/assets/2016-Update.pdf.
20. MacNaughton K, Chreim S, Bourgeault IL. Role construction and boundaries in interprofessional primary health care teams: a qualitative study. BMC Health Serv Res. 2013;13(1):486.
21. Wei H, Corbett RW, Ray J, Wei TL. A culture of caring: the essence of healthcare interprofessional collaboration. J Interprof Care. 2020;34(3):324–31.
22. Wang J, Guo J, Wang Y, Yan D, Liu J, Zhang Y, et al. Use of profession-role exchange in an interprofessional student team-based community health service-learning experience. BMC Med Educ. 2020;20(1):212.
23. Bochatay N, Muller-Juge V, Scherer F, Cottin G, Cullati S, Blondon KS, et al. Are role perceptions of residents and nurses translated into action? BMC Med Educ. 2017;17(1):1–9.
24. Bittner CA. The importance of role clarity for development of interprofessional teams. J Contin Educ Nurs. 2018;49(8):345–7.
25. Saxe JM, Balano K, Wamsley M, Nakajima M, Brock T. Promoting role clarity for health professional students participating in an interprofessional behavior change counseling workshop. J Allied Health. 2017;46(2):35E–7E.
26. Franke H, Foerstl K. Goals, conflict, politics, and performance of cross-functional sourcing teams-results from a social team experiment. J Bus Logist. 2020;41(1):6–30.
27. Orchard CA. Persistent isolationist or collaborator? The nurse's role in interprofessional collaborative practice. J Nurs Manag. 2010;18(3):248–57.
28. Liller KD, Pruitt Z, Burke SG. Interprofessional education: reaching health professionals with an interactive professional virtual/online event on advocacy and policy. Front Public Health. 2020;8:1–5.
29. Brault I, Kilpatrick K, D'Amour D, Contandriopoulos D, Chouinard V, Dubois CA, et al. Role clarification processes for better integration of nurse practitioners into primary healthcare teams: a multiple-case study. Nurs Res Pract. 2014;2014:1–9.
30. Behan KJ, VanDer LJ. Introducing interprofessional education to BSN and CLS students using a simulated healthcare setting. Am Soc Clin Lab Sci. 2017;30(4):224–7.
31. Kaelber D, Bate D. Health information exchange and patient safety. J Biomed Inform. 2007;40(6):S40–5.
32. Menkes DB. Ambiguous or faulty medical communication is responsibility of doctors to put right. BMJ. 2015;350:h310.
33. Kiss A. Does gender have an influence on the patient-physician communication? J Mens Health Gend. 2004;1(1):77–82.
34. Ruiz-Moral R, Pérez Rodríguez E, Pérula de Torres L, de la Torre J. Physician–patient communication: a study on the observed behaviours of specialty physicians and the ways their patients perceive them. Patient Educ Couns. 2006;64(1–3):242–8.
35. Almutairi A, Gardner G, McCarthy A. Perceptions of clinical safety climate of the multicultural nursing workforce in Saudi Arabia: a cross-sectional survey. Collegian. 2013;20(3):187–94.

36. Albahri AH, Abushibs AS, Abushibs NS. Barriers to effective communication between family physicians and patients in walk-in Centre setting in Dubai: a cross-sectional survey. BMC Health Serv Res. 2018;18(1):637.
37. Sikorski W. Paralinguistic communication in the therapeutic relationship. Arch Psychiatry Psychother. 2012;14(1):49–54.
38. Berman A, Chutka D. Assessing effective physician-patient communication skills: are you listening to me, doc? Korean J Med Educ. 2016;28(2):243–9.
39. Jagosh J, Donald Boudreau J, Steinert Y, MacDonald M, Ingram L. The importance of physician listening from the patients' perspective: enhancing diagnosis, healing, and the doctor–patient relationship. Patient Educ Couns. 2011;85(3):369–74.
40. Sousa L, Marques-Vieira C, Antunes A, Frade M, Severino S, Valentim O. Humor intervention in the nurse-patient interaction. Rev Bras Enferm. 2019;72(4):1078–85.
41. Strean WB. Laughter prescription. Can Fam Physician. 2009;55(10):965–7.
42. Back AL, Bauer-Wu SM, Rushton CH, Halifax J. Compassionate silence in the patient-clinician encounter: a contemplative approach. J Palliat Med. 2009;12(12):1113–7.
43. Kee J, Khoo H, Lim I, Koh M. Communication skills in patient-doctor interactions: learning from patient complaints. Health Prof Educ. 2018;4(2):97–106.
44. Weaver W, Shannon CE, Weaver W, editors. Recent contributions to mathematical theory of communication in the mathematical theory of communication. Urbana: University of Illinois Press; 1949.
45. Canadian Interprofessional Health Collaborative (CIHC). 2009. www.cihc.ca/resources-files/CIHC_Factsheets_CP_Feb09.pdf.
46. Australian Commission on Safety and Quality in Health Care. NSQHS Standards (first edition) fact sheet on clinical handover. 2012. www.safetyandquality.gov.au/publications-and-resources/resource-library/nsqhs-standards-first-edition-fact-sheet-clinical-handover.
47. The Joint Commission. Sentinel event Data. Root causes by event type: 2004-2014. 2015. http://www.jointcommission.org/assets/1/18/Root_Causes_by_Event_Type_2004-2014.pdf.
48. Weller J, Boyd M, Cumin D. Teams, tribes and patient safety: overcoming barriers to effective teamwork in healthcare. Postgrad Med J. 2014;90(1061):149–54.
49. Vermeir P, Vandijck D, Degroote S, Peleman R, Verhaeghe R, Mortier E, et al. Communication in healthcare: a narrative review of the literature and practical recommendations. Int J Clin Pract. 2015;69(11):1257–67.
50. Matziou V, Vlahioti E, Perdikaris P, Matziou T, Megapanou E, Petsios K. Physician and nursing perceptions concerning interprofessional communication and collaboration. J Interprof Care. 2014;28(6):526–33.
51. Boaro N, Fancott C, Baker R, Velji K, Andreoli A. Using SBAR to improve communication in interprofessional rehabilitation teams. J Interprof Care. 2009;24(1):111–4.
52. Liaw S, Zhou W, Lau T, Siau C, Chan S. An interprofessional communication training using simulation to enhance safe care for a deteriorating patient. Nurse Educ Today. 2014;34(2):259–64.
53. Nadzam D. Nurses' role in communication and patient safety. J Nurs Care Qual. 2009;24(3):184–8.
54. Pfaff K, Baxter P, Jack S, Ploeg J. Exploring new graduate nurse confidence in interprofessional collaboration: a mixed methods study. Int J Nurs Stud. 2014;51(8):1142–52.
55. Rice K, Zwarenstein M, Conn L, Kenaszchuk C, Russell A, Reeves S. An intervention to improve interprofessional collaboration and communications: a comparative qualitative study. J Interprof Care. 2010;24(4):350–61.
56. Keller KB, Eggenberger TL, Belkowitz J, Sarsekeyeva M, Zito AR. Implementing successful interprofessional communication opportunities in health care education: a qualitative analysis. Int J Med Educ. 2013;4:253–9.
57. Braithwaite J, Herkes J, Ludlow K, Testa L, Lamprell G. Association between organisational and workplace cultures, and patient outcomes: systematic review. BMJ Open. 2017;7(11):e017708.
58. Sargeant J, MacLeod T, Murray A. An Interprofessional approach to teaching communication skills. J Contin Educ Heal Prof. 2011;31(4):265–7.

59. Kim L, Giannitrapani K, Huynh A, Ganz D, Hamilton A, Yano E, et al. What makes team communication effective: a qualitative analysis of interprofessional primary care team members' perspectives. J Interprof Care. 2019;33(6):836–8.
60. Bays AM, Engelberg RA, Back AL, Ford DW, Downey L, Shannon SE, et al. Interprofessional communication skills training for serious illness: evaluation of a small-group, simulated patient intervention. J Palliat Med. 2014;17(2):159–66.
61. Brock D, Abu-Rish E, Chiu CR, Hammer D, Wilson S, Vorvick L, et al. Interprofessional education in team communication: working together to improve patient safety. BMJ Qual Saf. 2013;22(5):414–23.
62. Wagner J, Liston B, Miller J. Developing interprofessional communication skills. Teach Learn Nurs. 2011;6(3):97–101.
63. Barnsteiner JH, Disch JM, Hall L, Mayer D, Moore SM. Promoting interprofessional education. Nurs Outlook. 2007;55(3):144–50.
64. Roberts NK, Williams RG, Schwind CJ, Sutyak J, McDowell C, Griffen D, et al. The impact of brief team communication, leadership and team behavior training on ad hoc team performance in trauma care settings. Am J Surg. 2014;207(2):170–8.
65. Härgestam M, Lindkvist M, Brulin C, Jacobsson M, Hultin M. Communication in interdisciplinary teams: exploring closed-loop communication during in situ trauma team training. BMJ Open. 2013;3(10):e003525.
66. Pian-Smith M, Simon R, Minehart R, Podraza M, Rudolph J, Walzer T, et al. Teaching residents the two-challenge rule: a simulation-based approach to improve education and patient safety. Simul Healthc. 2009;4(2):84–91.
67. Pugel A, Simianu V, Flum D, Patchen DE. Use of the surgical safety checklist to improve communication and reduce complications. J Infect Public Health. 2015;8(3):219–25.
68. Prabhakar H, Cooper JB, Sabel A, Weckbach S, Mehler PS, Stahel PF. Introducing standardized "readbacks" to improve patient safety in surgery: a prospective survey in 92 providers at a public safety-net hospital. BMC Surg. 2012;12:8.
69. Aldawood F, Kazzaz Y, AlShehri A, Alali H, Al-Surimi K. Enhancing teamwork communication and patient safety responsiveness in a paediatric intensive care unit using the daily safety huddle tool. BMJ Open Qual. 2020;9(1):e000753.
70. Barr H, Koppel I, Reeves S, Hammic M, Freeth D. Effective interprofessional education: arguments, assumptions and evidence. Oxford: Blackwell; 2005.
71. Reeves S. Education in an interprofessional context. In: Dornan T, Mann K, Scherpbier A, Spencer J, editors. Medical education: theory and practice. London: Churchill Livingstone; 2011. p. 51–64.
72. Freeth D. Interprofessional education. In: Swanwick T, editor. Understanding medical education: evidence, theory and practice. 2nd ed. Wiley, Hoboken, NJ; 2010. p. 53–86.

A System Approach to Assessment 17

Mohammed Yahya Alnaami,
Hamza Mohammad Abdulghani, Salwa Elsobkey,
and Asma Faden

17.1 Introduction

The term *Assessment* has been described in the literature for centuries. However, the reason for its use varies according to the intended purpose. In the academic literature, assessment can be defined as "a systematic process of documenting and using empirical data on the knowledge, skill, attitudes, and beliefs to refine programs and improve student learning" [1]. *Evaluation* is the process of making judgments about the assessment information [2]. However, there are some differences and common aspects between assessment and evaluation [3] (Fig. 17.1).

Both assessment and evaluation require criteria, i.e., statements specifying the standards that must be met and the evidence that will be gathered to demonstrate the achievement of learning outcomes; both use measures and tools; and both are evidence-based. Assessment is usually used continuously to examine the progress of student's achievement, has positive impact on the learning process, usually is concerned with individual's performance not a group or a program, and provides positive feedback for good performance and areas for improvement. Evaluation

M. Y. Alnaami (✉)
Department of Surgery, College of Medicine, King Saud University, Riyadh, Saudi Arabia

H. M. Abdulghani
Department of Medical Education, College of Medicine, King Saud University, Riyadh, Saudi Arabia

S. Elsobkey
College of Applied Medical Sciences, King Saud University, Riyadh, Saudi Arabia

A. Faden
College of Dentistry, King Saud University, Riyadh, Saudi Arabia

M. Y. Alnaami et al. (eds.), *Novel Health Interprofessional Education and Collaborative Practice Program: Strategy and Implementation*,
https://doi.org/10.1007/978-981-99-3420-1_17

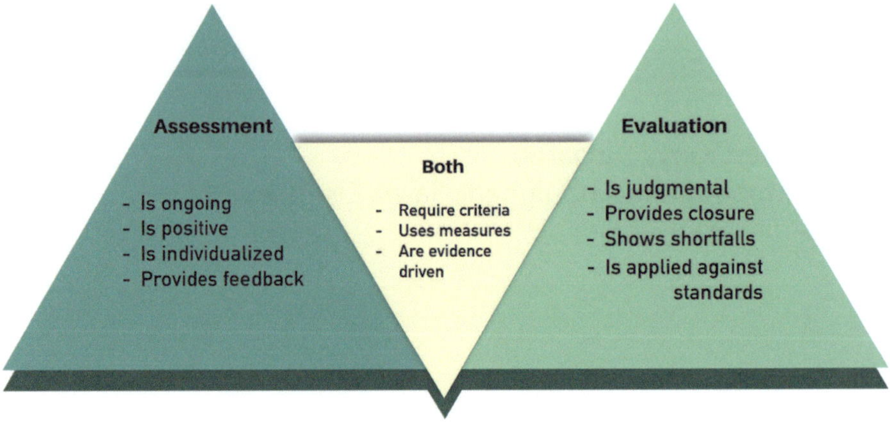

Fig. 17.1 Assessment and evaluation in educational psychology

usually provides closure statements at the end of the course or program (e.g., criterion-referenced for a whole group performance); usually as a judgment of a group of people; usually applied against standards compared to assessment that are less stressing on reference standards; and carries a decision making about the individual or a group of people at the end of a course or program.

17.2 Strategic Goal 9: Establishing a System Approach and "Culture of Assessment," in which Evaluation and Assessment in Health Sciences Education Encompass the Assessment of the Program and Resources; Students' Experience (Process) and Learning Outcomes; and Staff and Teaching

Assessment has been used for centuries in schools and universities to assure the quality and competency of their graduates. Many approaches are used to achieve these goals. However, most of these approaches lack comprehensiveness and system approach, leaving some gaps in the educational process, which are not addressed well by assessment at the student, teacher, and program levels. The system approach is a comprehensive assessment that addresses almost all components of the educational process assessment in health sciences education that encompasses the assessment of the program and resources, students' experience (process) and learning outcomes, and staff and teaching from the admission to graduation or even employment. In general, there are four types of assessment [4]:

1. *Screening tests that* measure the student's basic knowledge and skills to determine the most appropriate starting point for instruction and planning, e.g., admission and licensing examinations.
2. *Progress monitoring assessment* (which is also known as formative assessment) that assesses the effectiveness of teaching, learning, and curriculum

implementation. This would help educators to revise and improve areas of weakness in curriculum planning and instruction. The purpose of this type of assessment is to give feedback to trainees, tutors, and program coordinators to improve the deficiencies and gaps in learning outcomes achievement. Examples of progress monitoring assessment include progress, in-training, and continuous assessment tests.

3. *Diagnostic assessment* that pinpoints weaknesses to target necessary interventions to improve curriculum planning, instructions, and educational outcome, e.g., quizzes, national, and international exams.
4. *Outcome assessment* that is usually done at the end of the semester, year, or program outcomes to mass the number of students to validate the quality of the educational program and its implementation to take pass/fail decision about the students.

Data obtained from the aforementioned types of assessment would help all stakeholders to determine the achievements of the educational process at three levels as follows:

17.2.1 Students' Level

1. *Advanced students* who consistently exceed the targets and can handle advanced material. They need a further challenge, an extension of knowledge and skills, enrichment, and more in-depth work to continuously grow and avoid boredom. Assessment conducted two times a year is sufficient on the core materials and their advancement.
2. *Benchmark students* who are making good progress but may occasionally need further re-teaching, direction, and advice to upgrade to an advanced level. In such case, assessment conducted four times a year is sufficient on the core materials.
3. *Strategic students* are those not meeting benchmark targets on one or more indicators. They need direct instruction with a teacher in small groups (1:5–7) including adjustment of pace and material complexity by extending classroom instruction time to 60 minutes daily. They also need more frequent progress monitoring and diagnostic assessment to pinpoint problems and target interventions. Assessment is needed at least every 2–4 weeks on the core program with specialized and supplemental materials.
4. *Intensive students* who perform at chronically low levels far below benchmark in an otherwise effective program. They need intensive and specialized instruction in further smaller groups (1:3–5) focusing on their needs. They need frequent progress monitoring and testing every 1 or 2 weeks on the core and specialized supplemental materials and diagnostic assessment to pinpoint weaknesses and set up a specific instruction plan for remediation.

17.2.2 Teachers' Level

1. *Role-model teachers* who are exceeding benchmarks with more than 80% of the students. They may mentor other teachers and may need the help of educators and administration to challenge and extend material of benchmark students further. Also, they may need help to plan appropriate instruction and interventions for the remaining 20–25% of students who are below the benchmark target.
2. *Skillful teachers* achieving the benchmark target by 70–80% of the students. They may need to review their own videotaped classes for further improvement and the help of educators to plan appropriate instruction and interventions for the remaining 20–30% of students below the benchmark.
3. *Strategic teachers* achieving the benchmark target by about two-thirds (60–65%) of the students. They need strategic support through other peers, educators, and administration. This may include:
   (a) Review of the reading and instruction materials.
   (b) Review of the curriculum, preferably with a group of students with diverse levels.
   (c) Support for better instruction through strategic faculty development programs (FDPs), which may involve model lessons and constructive coaching.
4. *Intensive teachers* achieving the benchmark target with only one-half (~50%) of the students. They need intensive support by peers, educators, and administration in the form of:
   (a) Material support and FDPs.
   (b) Intensive small groups teaching with extended times.
   (c) Review of the curriculum content, instruction methods, and assessment. Generally, failures should not exceed 2–5%.

17.2.3 Program Level

1. *Benchmark level programs* are those with overall students achieving 75–80% and above of the benchmark target. These programs can have a greater degree of autonomy from higher authorities as long as they apply the assessment system at all levels.
2. *Strategic level programs* with overall students achieving 60–75% of the benchmark can have some degree of autonomy in educational planning and instruction, but with direct assistance by higher authorities (e.g., Ministry of Education).
3. *Intensive level programs* with overall students achieving 60% or lower of benchmark target should work closely with higher authorities with a minimal degree of autonomy in decision making and planning until they grow to higher levels.

Through several meetings and workshops during the construct of this program at the level of the Vice-Rector for Health Specialties (VRHS) in King Saud University (KSU), the Assessment Steering Committee was created along with other themes (the Leadership Committee and the T&L Steering Committee) to write the strategic plan for developing the assessment at all levels. The Assessment Steering Committee came up with the following initiatives to achieve this goal *"To establish a system approach and "culture of assessment" in which assessment in health sciences education encompasses the program and resources; students' experience (process) and learning outcomes; and staff and teaching."*

17.3 Objective (Initiative) 9.1: To Design a Comprehensive Quality Management System (QMS) that Dovetails with the University QMS

QMS is a formalized system that documents processes, procedures, and responsibilities for achieving quality policies and objectives. A QMS helps coordinate and direct organizational activities to meet standards and regulatory requirements and improve its effectiveness and efficiency on a continuous basis. It also entails improving processes, reducing waste, lowering costs, facilitating and identifying education and training opportunities, engaging staff, setting organization-wide direction, and assuring best outcomes/products. One can argue that QMSs should not be aimed for accreditation purposes only, but to raise institutional quality standards to match and benchmark with other international QMS standards (e.g., ISO 9001 QMS). Recently, KSU witnessed lots of development in its strategies and programs including a comprehensive QMS. The Deanship for Quality and Development produced the KSU–QMS Manual that consists of two handbooks. Handbook I (2012) addresses the "What" and "How" framework. The "What" aspects tackle the Standards, Criteria, and KPI, the audit, and assessment methodology. The "How" proposes the methodology KSU uses to develop its internal quality assurance (IQA) system to comply with the basic requirements and go beyond the expectations of the accreditation. While the first handbook of the KSU–QMS describes in detail the overall KSU–QMS approach, framework, and mechanisms, the KSU–QMS Handbook II (2012) concentrates on the evidence-based approach used in the KSU–QMS. The second handbook describes the Statistics, Information, and Documents (SID) System that has been established as part of the evidence-based approach underlying the mechanisms used to collate, collect, compute, disseminate, and use the Statistics, Information, and Documents to support the audit and assessment of the institution, college, or programs. In addition to these two manuals, KSU established a quality development unit in each college under the umbrella of KSU Deanship for Quality and Development. Accordingly, and as an example, College of Medicine took an initiative and published its Academic Quality Unit Manual in 2014. This manual outlines the College of Medicine strategic planning, Academic Quality Unit Functions, College's Policies and Procedures, Academic Job Description, Academic Terms of References, Key Performance Indicators, Accreditation, Evaluation Surveys, and the Annual Academic Activities Self Report [5]. The Assessment Steering Committee will study all these documents and other resources and try to design a common QMS for all HSCs.

To achieve the best of this initiative, the Assessment Steering Committee members will need to consider themselves as external evaluators. The committee will study available quality documents, policies, and procedures and assessment systems at KSU and HSCs. The committee will meet and communicate with all partners (through a one-day workshop), preferably with an external expert quality consultant to discuss quality aspects and issues (SWOT analysis) and come up with an agreement to make a common QMS outlines pertinent to HSCs programs. Once this common QMS is established, the committee can communicate and explain this new QMS and its relationship to assessment systems in HSCs to all stakeholders through another SWOT-workshop to consolidate the important relationship between QMSs and the Assessment Systems. This will make assessment goals and objectives (initiatives) to be developed and achieved on solid bases of information and data. Details of this initiative (design a comprehensive QMS that dovetails with the university system) are summarized in Table 17.1.

Table 17.1 Strategic plan for designing a comprehensive quality management system (QMS)

Goal 9: Establishing a system approach and "culture of assessment" in which evaluation and assessment in HSE encompass the assessment of the program and resources, students' experience (process) and learning outcomes, and staff and teaching			
Objective (9.1): To design a comprehensive QMS that dovetails with the university system			
Initiative (9.1) Revision of KSU-QMS	**Responsible** T&L steering committee and assessment units in HSCs	**Accountable** VRHS, leadership committee and vice-deans for quality in HSCs	**Partners** Deanship of quality, HSCs quality units, and deanship for admission and registration
Initiative description As long as the KSU deanship of quality has developed a comprehensive KSU-QMS, the assessment steering committee will revise this system			
Requirements and interdependencies 1. Survey forms 2. Letters for facilitation and cooperation with the KSU deanship of quality 3. Data collectors 4. Data entry 5. Statistician(s) 6. Computer with internet access, printer, copier, A4 paper, and the SPSS program 7. Workshops 8. An allocated group of 5–7 faculty to moderate the workshops 9. External quality consultant 10. Brainstorming meetings (2–3 sessions) for interpretation of collected data and the SWOT analysis 11. Proper time and place for the SWOT analysis 12. Reward for the consultant for the SWOT analysis 13. An allocated group with moderator for report 14. External consultant for report 15. Brainstorming meetings (2–4 sessions) for report 16. Proper time and place for report 17. Reward for the consultant for report 18. Other members as needed			**Stakeholders** Faculty staff, students, and deans of HSCs representing HSCs programs

Table 17.1 (continued)

Action plan	**Estimated time**
1. Organizing a workshop with the KSU quality consultant to represent the KSU-QMS 2. Collecting and sorting data of the following: (a) Colleges and programs using the KSU-QMS (b) Satisfaction of stakeholders regarding the KSU-QMS 3. SWOT analysis 4. Report including priorities for improvement	To be decided later as phase II
KPIs	**Estimated budget**
1. At least 75% of the required data are collected from each program of HSCs 2. Providing informative texts, tables, and graphs of the collected data 3. Providing clear, specified, and evidence-based SWOT matrix for 75% of programs of HSCs 4. Providing informative, realistic, prioritized, feasible, report with achievable actions for improvement for KSU-QMS	To be studied and decided later as phase II

QMS quality management system, *HSE* Health Sciences' Education, *KSU* King Saud University, *VRHS* vice-rector for health specialties, *T&L* teaching and learning, *HSCs* Health Sciences Colleges, *SWOT* strengths weaknesses Opportunities and threats, *KPIs* key performance indicators

17.4 Objective (Initiative) 9.2: To Establish Comprehensive Assessment Guidelines for all HSCs

This initiative discusses the general assessment guidelines to be established and standardized across all HSCs. This will facilitate a common ground on assessment based on evidence and best practices. The initial step to achieve this objective is to explore and discuss available assessment systems used by all HSCs. Then, we should contrast these systems with other national and international assessment guidelines for health science educational programs, for example, the National Commission for Academic Accreditation and Assessment (NCAAA) [6] and the Association for Medical Education of Europe (AMEE) [7], through a workshop that involves all stakeholders in HSCs. The established guidelines will be reviewed by an external reviewer for the pre-final version approval of the new guidelines for assessment of health science programs, students, and faculty. Also, these guidelines will need to be reviewed and get authorized by the "Legal Affairs Department" at KSU for final approval to avoid any legal issues in the future. Once these guidelines get the final authorization, the next step is to train each HSC assessment unit on how to implement such guidelines. This requires the assessment steering committee to conduct a half-day workshop in each HSC to be prepared for implementing the new assessment guidelines. One potential HSC will pilot the implementation process of the new guidelines over one semester. This may be witnessed and shared by the other HSC assessment units. These guidelines would help all stakeholders including faculty, students, and health science programs to facilitate effective assessment. The activities to achieve this objective are summarized in Table 17.2.

Table 17.2 Strategic plan for establishing comprehensive assessment guidelines for all HSCs

<table>
<tr><td colspan="4">Goal 9: Establishing a system approach and "culture of assessment" in which evaluation and assessment in HSE encompass the assessment of the program and resources, students' experience (process) and learning outcomes, and staff and teaching</td></tr>
<tr><td colspan="4">Objective (9.2): To establish comprehensive assessment guidelines for all HSCs</td></tr>
<tr><td>Initiative (9.2)
Establishing comprehensive assessment guidelines for all HSCs</td><td>Responsible
Assessment steering committee and assessment units in HSCs</td><td>Accountable
VRHS, leadership committee, and deans of HSCs</td><td>Partners
Deanship for skills development, deanship for quality and development, and CELT</td></tr>
<tr><td colspan="4">Initiative description
These guidelines will help in encompassing the assessment of the program and resources, student experience (process and learning outcomes), and faculty teaching</td></tr>
<tr><td colspan="3">Requirements and interdependencies
1. Workshop arrangements (place, agenda, and moderators)
2. Letters for facilitation and cooperation with HSCs
3. Survey forms
4. Data collectors and data entry personnel
5. Statistician
6. Computer with internet access, printer, copier, A4 paper, and the statistical program in use
7. Budget</td><td>Stakeholders
Faculty staff, students, and HSCs</td></tr>
<tr><td colspan="3">Action plan
1. Collect data samples of "assessment guidelines" of each HSC
2. Reviewing the literature and best practices for assessment guidelines and accreditations (national/international) bodies, e.g., NCAAA and AMEE
3. Establishing an initial draft of general guidelines
4. Performing a workshop for all stakeholders as pilot groups. At this stage, the guideline should answer all questions posed by the pilot study group. Workshops performed separately in different halls at the same day moderated by a steering committee member
5. External reviewer (benchmarking)—Pre-final version
6. Obtaining a legal review of the guidelines by "legal affairs," need legal implication, add personal modification and appropriate wordings
7. Orientation workshop to the leaders of teaching/learning and assessment units in each health college to implement the guidelines</td><td>Estimated time
To be decided later as phase II</td></tr>
<tr><td colspan="3">KPIs
1. At least 75% of the required data are collected from each HSC
2. Provision of the informative texts, tables, and graphs of the collected data
3. Establishing a database of the collected data</td><td>Estimated budget
To be studied and decided later as phase II</td></tr>
</table>

HSCs Health Sciences Colleges, *VRHS* vice-rector for health specialties, *T&L* teaching and learning, *CELT* Center of Excellence in Learning and Teaching, *NCAAA* academic accreditation and assessment, *AMEE* Association for Medical Education of Europe, *CELT* Center of Excellence in Learning and Teaching, *KPIs* key performance indicators

17.5 Objective (Initiative) 9.3: To Develop a Comprehensive Approach to Look at the Entire Students' Process (Input–Process–Outcomes) and Document Issues Arising during Studies

This initiative is about needs assessment. It consists of three parts: data gathering, analysis, and reporting. Through the VRHS, the assessment steering committee will request each HSC to provide details of courses' assessment blueprints against learning outcomes/competencies, students' assessment methods, courses' evaluation methods, and effectiveness of teaching and teachers' efficiency system. The assessment steering committee at the VRHSs will design surveys for program (course) director/coordinator, students/interns/alumni, and faculty to assess the quality of the programs mentioned in (Initiative 9.1), learning, and teaching experiences, respectively. Program evaluation involves making a value judgment about available information [8]. In other words, program evaluation is about understanding the program or a course through a routine, systematic, and deliberate gathering of information to uncover and/or identify what contributes to the "success" of the program and what actions need to be taken in order to address the findings of the evaluation process [9]. The Assessment Steering Committee will study commonly used theories and models for the program evaluation [10] and come up with models that match and serve each program needs. Assessment of learning outcomes involves studying the goals of the program, what students actually learn (curriculum blueprint), the evidence that students achieved institutional goals (performance measurements), and what needs to be changed [11]. Institutional goals can be reflected as outcome competencies or learning outcomes that depend on institutional environment and community needs. In North America, the Associated of American Medical Colleges [12] adopted certain competencies referred as the Medical Schools Objectives Project (MSOP), and the Canadians adopted what is known as the "CanMEDS" [13] competencies based on societal needs in 2000. In the UK, the General Medical Council [14] generated the "Tomorrow's Doctors" document in 1993, which has been modified to encompass new competencies and their assessment strategies in 2002. A similar experience was initiated in Saudi Arabia leading to the production of what is called the "Saudi MEDs" [15]. The Saudi MEDs competencies include a scientific approach to practice patient care, community-oriented practice, communication and collaboration, professionalism, and research and scholarship. The Saudi MEDs competencies have now been applied to all medical colleges in Saudi Arabia, and these are known as minimal criteria for Saudi doctors as well as for the accreditation by NCAAA [6]. The sum of data collected from surveys of programs, students and alumni, and faculty will be communicated to all HSCs by the assessment steering committee through discussion sessions for the SWOT. The quality management systems that are implemented in the programs to assure the appropriateness, effectiveness, and fairness of assessment as well as available assessment blueprints and resources will be discussed for the SWOT that will be analyzed by the assessment steering committee and reported back to HSCs for further improvement. Details of this initiative are summarized in Table 17.3.

Table 17.3 Strategic plan for developing a comprehensive approach looking at the entire students' process (input–process–outcomes) and documenting issues arising during studies

Goal 9: Establishing a system approach and "culture of assessment" in which evaluation and assessment in HSE encompass the assessment of the program and resources, students' experience (process) and learning outcomes, and staff and teaching			
Objective (9.3): To develop a comprehensive approach looking at the entire students' process (input–process–outcomes) and to document issues arising during studies			
Initiative (9.3) Revising characteristics and resources of evaluation and assessment systems for all HSCs (programs, courses, student experience, and learning outcomes and staff teaching)	**Responsible** Assessment steering committee and assessment units in HSCs	**Accountable** VRHS, leadership committee, and deans of HSCs	**Partners** Deanship for quality and vice-deans for quality in HSCs
Initiative description Revising the characteristics and resources of program evaluation and students' assessment systems for all HSCs, including programs, courses, students' experience, learning outcomes, and staff teaching			
Requirements and interdependencies 1. Survey forms 2. Course assessment mapping form 3. Letters for facilitation and cooperation with HSCs 4. Data collectors 5. Data entry 6. Statistician 7. Computer with internet access, printer, copier, A4 paper, and the SPSS program 8. Workshops 9. An allocated group of 5–7 expertise faculty with a moderator for SWOT 10. External consultant for SWOT 11. Brainstorming meetings, (2–3 sessions) for SWOT 12. Proper time and place for SWOT 13. Reward for the consultant for SWOT 14. Allocated group with moderator for report 15. External consultant for report 16. Brainstorming meetings (2–4 sessions) for report 17. Proper time and place for the report 18. Reward for the report consultant 19. Other members as needed		**Stakeholders** Faculty staff, students, and HSCs	

Table 17.3 (continued)

Action plan	Estimated time
1. Collecting and sorting data of the following: (a) Program's vision, mission, and objectives (b) Program's learning outcomes/competencies (c) Programs' courses and credit hour distribution (theoretical, practical, and clinical) (d) Course specifications and reports (e) Feedback of students' learning experiences including undergraduate students, internees, and alumni (f) Feedback of teaching staff teaching experiences (g) Feedback about the availability of the QMS that is implemented in the programs to assure the appropriateness, effectiveness, and fairness of assessment (h) List of resources available at each program regarding labs, virtual facilities, chances for simulation, optical mark recognition, etc. (i) Assessment blueprint 2. SWOT analysis 3. Report including the priorities for improvement	Phase II
KPIs	**Estimated budget**
1. At least 75% of the required data are collected from each HSC 2. Providing informative texts, tables, and graphs of the collected data 3. Establishing a database of collected data 4. Providing clear, specified, and evidence-based SWOT matrix for 75% of programs of HSCs 5. Providing an informative, realistic, prioritized, and feasible report with achievable actions for improvement for 85% of the programs of HSCs	Phase II

HSE Health Sciences' Education, *VRHS* vice-rector for health specialties, *HSCs* Health Sciences Colleges, *SWOT* strengths weaknesses opportunities and threats, *QMS* quality management system, *KPIs* key performance indicators

17.6 Objective (Initiative) 9.4: To Assess Staff and Teaching Quality

Teachers are having less didactic teaching roles in modern learner-centered curricula when compared to teacher-centered traditional curricula. However, they still play major roles as leaders and role models, which contributes to curriculum planning and development, research and publishing, administration, students' coaching and mentoring, and of course teaching/training and assessment. Staff development programs over the years were traditionally aimed to improve teaching staff knowledge, teaching skills, and areas of research and administration [16]. The teacher of the twenty-first century needs to be more equipped with additional important qualities such as leadership as a change agent adaptive to changes in technology, educational innovations and excellence, awareness of societal priorities, sharing with students and patients their needs and ideas, and personal development [17]. Therefore, staff assessment should encompass a multifaceted approach including review of teacher's profile, participation in CME activities, leadership qualities, participation in faculty development programs, research and publications, and administrative qualities. Conversely, teaching quality can be assessed by self-assessment, peer-assessment, and students' assessment. Areas of staff assessment may include the organization of subject matter and course, communication skills, knowledge of the subject matter, enthusiasm for the subject and for teaching, a positive attitude toward students, fairness in testing and grading, flexibility in approaches to teaching, and utilization of appropriate methods for students' learning outcomes assessment. Teachers' evaluation over the years has changed. In earlier years, teacher evaluations were based on personal characteristics of the teacher. However, starting in the early 1950s until the 1980s, teacher evaluation took a shift and started to focus on teachers' teaching, observed through students' outcomes. After the 1980s, teacher evaluation was measured based on increased professional development, accountability, and institutional improvement [18]. Teacher evaluation has followed numerous approaches of teaching practices. Measures of Effective Teaching (MET) [19], Danielson's Framework Model [20], and Classroom Assessment Scoring System (CLASS) [21] are some of the evaluation tools that aim to measure student achievement using teacher evaluation. The MET evaluates teacher effectiveness through five measures: students' gains in standardized testing, recorded classroom sessions and teacher reflections afterwards, teachers' knowledge in pedagogical content, students' views of the classroom and instruction of the teacher, and the teachers' own views on their working conditions and the support of the school [19]. The Danielson Framework Model evaluates teachers using four domains: planning and preparation, classroom environment, instruction, and professional responsibilities [20]. In this framework of evaluation, teachers are evaluated through a rubric that contains these four domains. They can either be ranked or measured as unsatisfactory, basic, proficient, or distinguished. In this rubric, teachers are being evaluated through critical attributes and examples when being observed. The CLASS approach, suggested by Pianta et al. [21], evaluates teachers based on their interaction with students. To do this, the CLASS model evaluates teachers' interactions using three domains: emotional support, classroom organization, and instructional support. This approach is much more flexible as the domains used within the approach vary based on students' grade levels. Institutions vary on their conditions for staff and teaching quality evaluations from simple portfolios to robust written and practice examinations such as the Centre for Teacher Accreditation (CENTA) [22] approach practiced in India. Further aspects of this initiative are summarized in Table 17.4.

Staff teaching quality assessment is one of the most sensitive issues in any health profession. Therefore, strategic planning of this aspect needs to be carefully

Table 17.4 Strategic plan for assessing staff and teaching quality

<table>
<tr><td colspan="4">Goal 9: Establishing a system approach and “culture of assessment” in which evaluation and assessment in HSE encompass the assessment of the program and resources, students’ experience (process) and learning outcomes, and staff and teaching</td></tr>
<tr><td colspan="4">Objective (9.4): To assess staff and teaching quality</td></tr>
<tr><td>Initiative (9.4)
Assessment of staff and teaching quality</td><td>Responsible
Assessment steering committee and vice-deans for quality in HSCs</td><td>Accountable
VRHS, leadership committee, and deans of HSCs</td><td>Partners
Deanship for quality and development and CELT</td></tr>
<tr><td colspan="4">Initiative description
Staff and teaching quality assessment is one of the most sensitive issues in any health professions education. Therefore, strategic planning of this aspect needs to be carefully designed and executed</td></tr>
<tr><td colspan="3">Requirements and interdependencies
1. Surveying current practice for staff and teaching assessment by HSCs
2. Reviewing all forms used for staff assessment and teaching quality by KSU quality deanship, supervisors, department heads, students, and others
3. Surveys of the willingness of academic staff to participate in staff and teaching assessment programs
4. Data collectors and data entry personnel
5. Data analyst
6. Computer with internet access, printer, copier, A4 paper, the SPSS program
7. Budget</td><td>Stakeholders
Faculty staff, students, and HSCs</td></tr>
<tr><td colspan="3">Action plan
1. Collecting and analyzing the data regarding current staff assessment methods and teaching
2. Examining staff assessment and teaching forms against national and international standards
3. Performing a workshop for faculty staff and student volunteers on methods of faculty and teaching assessment with their feedback
4. Informing quality deanship at KSU and vice-deans for quality in all HSCs about best practices for staff and teaching assessment in the form of manual document
5. Conducting repetitive workshops for staff and teaching assessment in each HSC to adopt the manual
6. Implementing best practices for staff and teaching assessment strategies (manual) with close monitoring and process evaluation at all HSCs</td><td>Estimated time
Phase II</td></tr>
<tr><td colspan="3">KPIs
1. At least, 75% of the required data are collected from all HSCs
2. Providing the best practice manual
3. Reporting the implementation process evaluation and staff feedback</td><td>Estimated budget
Phase II</td></tr>
</table>

HSE Health Sciences’ Education; *HSCs* Health Sciences Colleges, *VRHS* vice-rector for health specialties, *CELT* Center of Excellence in Learning and Teaching, *KSU* King Saud University, *SSPS* statistical package for the social sciences, *KPIs* key performance indicators designed and executed. Assessment of staff and teaching quality is the responsibility of each HSC and the different departments. However, the Assessment Steering Committee at the VRHS and Vice-Deans for Quality in HSCs are also responsible for overlooking the whole process and make common standards and guidelines to follow by each HSC and department. In order to do this, other partners should also be involved including the Deanship for Quality and the Center of Excellence in Learning and Teaching located at KSU headquarter. The VRHSs and Deans in all health colleges are deemed accountable for its execution and implementation. Of course, faculty staff and students are considered the most important stakeholders for this initiative.

The first step for this initiative requirements and interdependency is to survey current practice for staff and teaching assessment by HSCs. Needs assessment surveys should address both faculty and students, and on a larger scale community if feasible. The Assessment Steering Committee at the VRHSs is responsible for designing such surveys based on expected qualities of faculties with regard to their attitude, knowledge, and teaching skills. The second task for the Assessment Steering Committee is to review current practice of staff evaluation referring to their sources whether in the Deanship for Quality at the KSU or the Vice-Deans for Quality in all health colleges. These need to be revised and compared against local and international standards for staff and teaching assessment. Before finalizing the revised forms for the staff and teaching assessment, staff have to be aware and approve such forms through a one-day workshop arranged by the Deanship for Quality at the KSU and the Vice-deanship for Quality in all health colleges. Participants of the workshop should include both stakeholders, i.e., faculty and students' representatives from all HSCs. After this workshop, the Assessment Steering Committee will have a solid ground to write and publish the KSU manual for staff and teaching assessment. The way of using and implementing this manual requires repetitive workshops at each HSC through vice-deans for quality. The implementation process also needs monitoring and evaluation in order to improve the manual content with time. This manual needs to be revised following same steps and process every 5 years (timeframe for the Assessment Steering Committee change) based on monitoring and evaluation results as well as the feedback surveys from the faculty and students.

17.7 Summary

The Assessment Steering Committee along with other partners from Quality Departments at KSU suggested some initiatives to develop and achieve this goal. Based on the revision of current QMS at KSU, the first initiative is to "design a comprehensive QMS for HSCs that dovetails with the university system." The second initiative—a follow up on the first initiative—is to "establish comprehensive assessment guidelines" to standardize a comprehensive assessment practice across all HSCs. The third initiative is to "develop a system looking at the entire students' process (input–process–outcomes) and to document issues arising during studies," which will be reflected on the characteristics and resources of program evaluation and students' assessment systems for all HSCs including programs, courses, student experience, learning outcomes, and staff teaching. The fourth initiative is to conduct careful and strategic steps to "assess teaching staff and teaching quality," hoping that this will improve their performance further and give positive impact on themselves and students. Once this goal is achieved, even partially, HSCs will be looked at as role models for the implementation of QMS designed by the Deanship for Quality and KSU administration.

References

1. Allen MJ. Assessing academic programs in higher education. San Francisco: Jossey-Bass; 2004.
2. Airasian PW. Classroom assessment: concepts and applications. 3rd ed. Boston: McGraw Hill; 2005.
3. Wiley D, Thanos K. Lumen learning (founders, 2013). https://courses.lumenlearning.com/edpsy/.
4. Diamond L. Assessment-driven instruction: a system approach. Perspectives. 2005;31:33–7.
5. Kotterman JP. What leaders really do? Harv Bus Rev. 2007;79(11):85–96.
6. National Commission for Academic Accreditation and Assessment NCAAA. 2004. https://www.ncaaa.org.sa/en/Pages/default.aspx%20.
7. Association for Medical Education in Europe AMEE. 1972. https://amee.org/publications/amee-guides.
8. Cook DA. Twelve tips for evaluating educational programs. Med Teach. 2010;32:296–301.
9. Durning SJ, Hemmer P, Pangaro LN. The structure of program evaluation: an approach for evaluating a course, clerkship, or components of a residency or fellowship training program. Teach Learn Med. 2007;19:308–18.
10. Frye AW, Hemmer PA. Program evaluation models and related theories: AMEE guide no. 67. Med Teach. 2012;34(5):e288–99.
11. Shumway JM, Harden RM. AMEE Guide No. 25: the assessment of learning outcomes for the competent and reflective physician. Med Teach. 2003;25(6):569–84.
12. AAMC. Report I: learning objectives for medical student education. Medical Schools Objectives Project. Washington: AAMC; 1998.
13. CanMEDS. Project societal needs project group report. Med Teach. 2000;22(6):549–54.
14. General Medical Council. Recommendations on undergraduate medical education. London UK: GMC; 2002.
15. Meds S. A competence specification for Saudi medical graduates. Med Teach. 2011;33(7):582–4.
16. Stienert Y. In: Dent, Harden, editors. Staff development. London: Churchill Livingstone; 2013. p. 269–376.
17. Frenk J, Chen LC, Bhutta ZA, Cohen J, Crisp N, Evans T, et al. Health professionals for a new century: transforming education to strengthen health systems in an interdependent world. Lancet. 2010;376:1923–58.
18. Ellett Chad D, Teddlie C. Teacher evaluation, teacher effectiveness and school effectiveness: perspective from the USA. J Pers Eval Educ. 2003;17(1):101–28.

19. MET Project. Working with teachers to develop fair and reliable measures of effective teaching. Seattle: Bill & Melinda Gates Foundation; 2010. p. 1–12. https://usprogram.gatesfoundation.org/news-and-insights/articles/measures-of-effective-teaching-project.
20. Framework for Teacher Evaluation. The teacher evaluation process guide. 2019. https://www.nctq.org/dmsView/2018-2019_HCPSS_Guide_to_Teacher_EvaluationFINAL. Accessed 28 Nov 2020.
21. Pianta RC, La Paro KM, Hamre BK. In: Paul H, editor. Classroom assessment scoring system™: manual K-3. Baltimore: Brookes Publishing Company; 2008.
22. Center for Teacher Accreditation (CENTA), India. http://centa.org/centastandards.

Assessment of Learning Outcomes 18

Mohammed Yahya Alnaami,
Hamza Mohammad Abdulghani, Salwa Elsobkey,
and Hazar Yacoub

18.1 Introduction

Recently, health professional curricula have emphasized competencies that are pertinent to each country based on population nature and needs. Hence, such local competencies (learning outcomes) were published as the Saudi Meds [1]. The Saudi Meds is a national competence framework that has been developed by medical schools in the Kingdom of Saudi Arabia. The framework has seven domains: (1) approach to daily practice, (2) doctor and patient relation, (3) doctor and community, (4) communication skills, (5) professionalism, (6) doctor and information technology, and (7) doctor and research. The framework will guide curriculum development and assessment existing in all health professional education to ensure its adaptation to changing needs. The following sections address assessment and evaluation of the aforementioned domains.

M. Y. Alnaami (✉)
Department of Surgery, College of Medicine, King Saud University, Riyadh, Saudi Arabia

H. M. Abdulghani
Department of Medical Education, College of Medicine, King Saud University, Riyadh, Saudi Arabia

S. Elsobkey
College of Applied Medical Sciences, King Saud University, Riyadh, Saudi Arabia

H. Yacoub
College of Pharmacy, King Saud University, Riyadh, Saudi Arabia

M. Y. Alnaami et al. (eds.), *Novel Health Interprofessional Education and Collaborative Practice Program: Strategy and Implementation*,
https://doi.org/10.1007/978-981-99-3420-1_18

18.2 Strategic Goal 10: To Develop a Comprehensive Approach to Students' Assessment that Addresses All Educational Domains Including Knowledge, Skills, and Attitudes/Values

This goal, along with other goals in this manual, was developed through several meetings and workshops shared by an elite group of faculty educators and students representing almost all HSCs at KSU. Assessment of learning outcomes encompasses several issues including understanding of the principals of assessment, appropriate use of assessment methods and tools, and the comprehensive approach of assessment that covers the full range of educational domains. Effective assessment must consider the psychometric properties of the examination, i.e., to be valid, reliable, and feasible and to have a measurable impact on learning through quality indicators. There are several assessment methods and tools to measure learning outcomes. However, each tool is appropriate for the context to be measured. Therefore, no one method is appropriate for all domains of learning outcomes. Assessment methods include written examinations, practical and clinical, observational, portfolios, peer assessment, and self-assessment. Learning outcomes include knowledge, skills, attitudes, and values. These learning outcomes differ from one institute to another and from an environment to another depending on community needs [2]. The Miller's Pyramid explains the learning outcome domains and specific tools and methods utilized to assess those domains (Fig. 18.1). The following initiatives are proposed to achieve this goal:

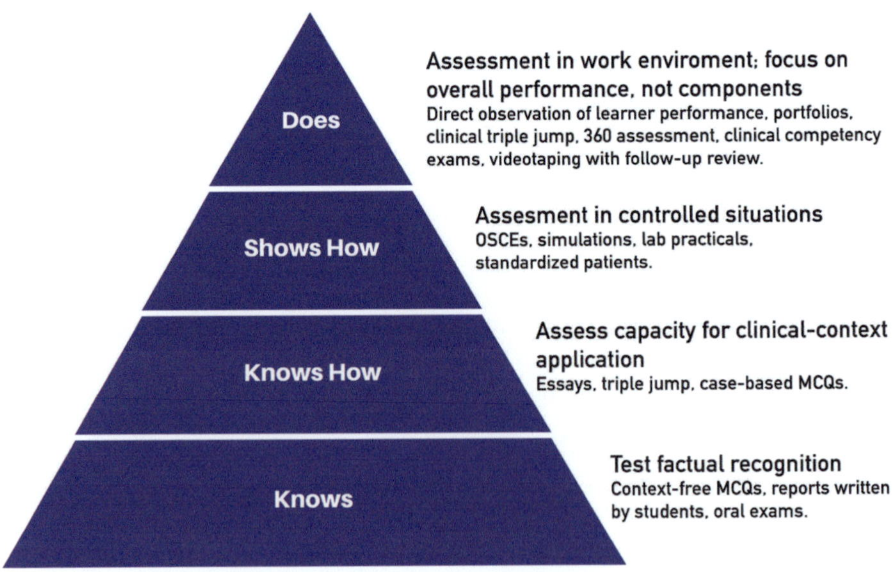

Fig. 18.1 Miller's pyramid to assess clinical competence

18.2.1 Objective (Initiative) 10.1: To Develop Comprehensive Assessment Approaches for Courses that Address All Learning Domains

This initiative is the core issue of assessment that addresses a product expressed as students' learning outcome. Most health professions educational programs adopt several methods that assess students' learning outcomes of their knowledge, skills, and attitudes/values. However, they vary in type and number of assessment methods used depending on staff experience in assessment methods, presence or absence of health professions educational departments or centers, and program accreditation requirements by higher authorities. Ideally, assessment methods should address the achievement of all learning objectives in a valid, reliable, and feasible manner with an impact on the learner and the educational program [3, 4]. *Validity* of an assessment tool is the degree to which the tool is measuring what it is supposed to measure. In other words, it assesses the validity of scores rather than the instrument itself. Validity can be further broken into three sub-types. The first type is *content validity*, which reflects the degree of sampling from different learning domains of the subject to be assessed. This is the most important type of validity, which could be achieved by appropriate assessment blueprint construction [5]. The second type is *criterion validity*, which compares test scores against a criterion or gold standard. The third type is *construct validity*, which is the ability of an instrument to measure what it purports to measure using additional information that supports this notion. *Reliability* refers to consistency, reproducibility, or stability of test scores upon repetition. When a group of experts agree or become in close agreement about an examinee is called *inter-rater reliability*. Therefore, reliability can be measured by test–re-test, equivalent forms, split-half, and item-to-total scores comparison *(internal consistency)*. Usually, reliability is measured by commercially available software, especially for multiple choice questions tests. *A reliability coefficient* value above 0.7 on regular exams or 0.8 and higher for high stakes exams is considered reliable. For a test to be valid, it has to be reliable as well, but not necessary the opposite (Fig. 18.2).

Feasibility refers to the practicality of the assessment method with regard to available resources and expertise and costs. The impact of assessment on the learner and educational programs varies from one system of assessment to another. Since assessment drives learning, learners will try to pass exams the way they are designed for, e.g., memorization, last moment studying, review of previous exams, and guessing or even cheating. In order to have positive impacts on learners, educators should ensure validity of the assessment content, the way it is conducted, what is asked (information is given), and the time and frequency of continuous assessment sessions. Once these concepts of psychometric properties for testing are understood, it has to be applied to all types of testing methods to ensure best assessment and learning outcomes. Learning domains include knowledge, skills, and attitudes/values.

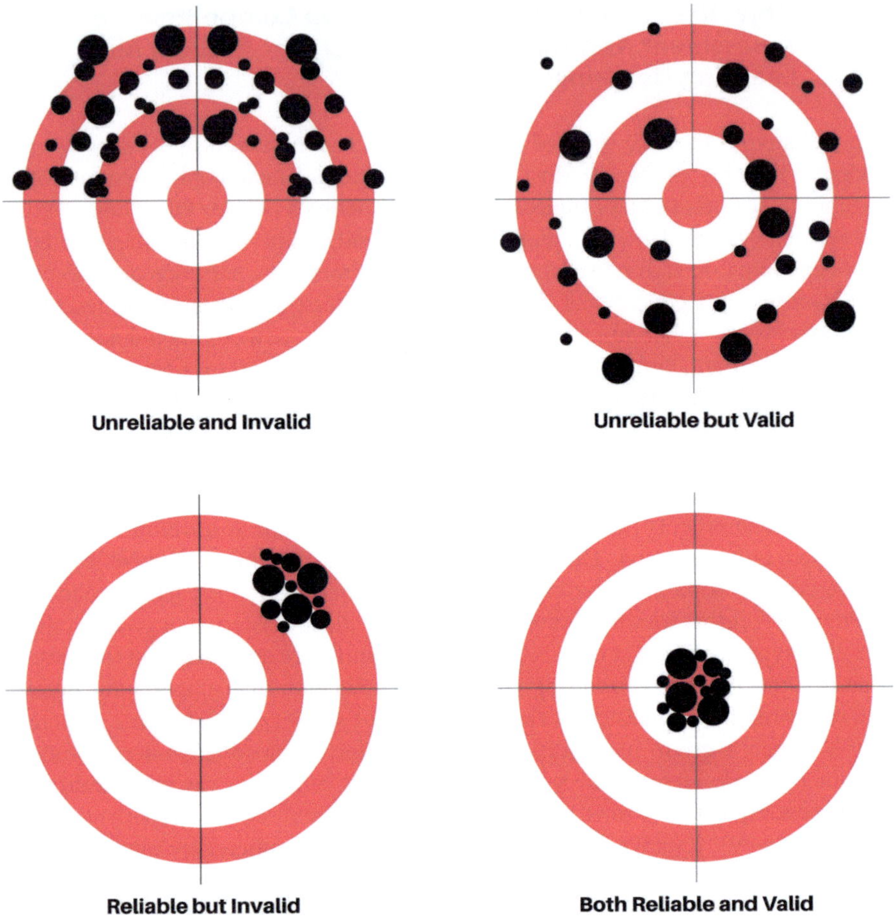

Fig. 18.2 Reliability and validity target

Details of this initiative are summarized in Table 18.1. Reports of the needs assessment from Goal 9, initiative 9.3 "*Develop a comprehensive approach looking at the entire students' process (input–process–outcomes) and document issues arising during studies*" are reviewed by the Assessment Steering Committee and areas for improvement in assessment systems are highlighted. Assessment systems are then benchmarked with best practices in assessment approaches in order to develop a comprehensive handbook for assessment approaches through several workshops and final workshop inclusive of all HSCs and stakeholders. The handbook assessment guide must be aligned with the NCAAA and similar international assessment guidelines. Once the final draft of the handbook is reviewed and approved, it can be implemented and monitored with supporting research studies to validate it.

Table 18.1 Strategic plan for developing comprehensive assessment approaches for courses

Goal 10: Developing a comprehensive approach to students' assessment that addresses all educational domains including knowledge, skills, and attitudes/values			
Objective (10.1): To develop comprehensive assessment approaches for courses that address all learning domains			
Initiative (10.1) Developing comprehensive assessment approaches for courses that address all learning domains	**Responsible** Assessment Steering Committee and Assessment Units in HSCs	**Accountable** VRHS, Leadership Committee, and Deans of HSCs	**Partners** Deanship of Development and Quality, Vice-Deans of Academic Affairs in HSCs, and Vice-Deans of Development and Quality
Initiative description Reviewing report of priorities for improvement, benchmarking best practices in assessment approaches, and developing workshop and handbook for assessment approaches			
Requirements and interdependencies 1. Workshop arrangements (place, agenda, and moderators) and members invited to the workshop are: (a) Members of the teaching, learning, and assessment unit from each HSC (b) Vice-dean for academic affairs from each HSC (c) Vice-dean for quality and development from each HSC (d) Senior students\interns (e) Representatives from faculty members (f) Alumni representatives 2. Letters for facilitation and cooperation with HSCs 3. Survey forms 4. Data collectors and data entry personnel 5. Statistician 6. Computer with internet access, printer, copier, A4 paper, the SPSS program			**Stakeholders** Faculty staff and undergraduate and postgraduate students
Action plan 1. Reviewing the report of 9.1.3 2. Benchmarking best practices in assessment approach for HSCs courses 3. Developing a draft of Comprehensive Assessment Approaches Handbook for HSCs courses, considering national and international accreditation requirements, and the matrix should combine NCAAA learning domains with professional bodies domains 4. Organizing a workshop for all stakeholders to review the drafted handbook in assessment approaches for HSCs courses 5. Distributing drafted handbooks for comprehensive assessment approaches for HSCs courses to all deans for internal review and feedback 6. Getting the approval of handbook for assessment approaches from the vice-rector for educational affairs			**Estimated time** To be decided later as phase II

(continued)

Table 18.1 (continued)

Goal 10: Developing a comprehensive approach to students' assessment that addresses all educational domains including knowledge, skills, and attitudes/values	
KPIs 1. Reviewing at least five top international assessment centers in HSE for benchmarking, e.g., Dundee UK, Singapore, Harvard USA, and Maastricht 2. Attendance of the workshop should be >80% of nominated members 3. >75% satisfaction of the effectiveness of the workshop 4. Developing a handbook for comprehensive assessment approaches for HSCs courses 5. Collecting internal feedback from each HSCs on the drafted handbook	**Estimated budget** To be studied and decided later as phase II

HSCs health sciences colleges, *VRHS* vice-rector for health specialties, *SPSS* statistical package for the social sciences, *NCAAA* National Commission for Academic Accreditation and Assessment, *HSE* health sciences education, *KPIs* key performance indicators

18.2.2 Objective (Initiative) 10.2: To Develop Guidelines for Comprehensive Assessment Across All Learning Domains

This initiative (Table 18.2) discusses how to implement the assessment handbook and guidelines by all HSCs. This requires tremendous efforts by responsible parties and partners of this initiative to train faculty and administration of HSCs in every step and detail of the assessment handbook in order to be ready for successful implementation. Once the approved guidelines manual is ready, it will be published by KSU press and distributed to all HSCs teaching and learning (medical education) units/departments as a reference. At this stage, the assessment guidelines manual will be ready to be implemented at all levels of health professional education. Before implementation, however, knowledgeable and experienced educators at all HSCs will start making a strategic plan to implement the assessment guidelines manual at all HSCs through a one-day workshop led by the assessment steering committee at VRHSs. Then, each T&L unit/medical education department at the corresponding HSC will conduct a half-day seminar introducing the assessment manual to all faculty, students, and administrative representatives who are actively involved in courses coordination and students' assessment. When the assessment manual needs to be implemented, the assessment, teaching, and learning unit (the medical education department) in each HSC needs to conduct short workshops for the various assessment tools along with course coordinators, faculty, students, and administrative representatives in each department. Monitoring and measuring the effectiveness of the implementation process is also of paramount importance to assure best learning outcomes. Assessment of the assessment methods is another issue that deserves more attention from educators and statisticians to analyze exam

Table 18.2 Strategic plan for developing guidelines for comprehensive assessment across all learning domains

Goal 10: Developing a comprehensive approach to students' assessment that addresses all educational domains including knowledge, skills, and attitudes/values			
Objective (10.2): To develop guidelines for comprehensive assessment across all learning domains			
Initiative (10.2) Providing HSCs with the handbook of comprehensive assessment approaches for implementation	**Responsible** Assessment Steering Committee and Assessment Units in HSCs	**Accountable** VRHS, Leadership Committee, and Deans of HSCs	**Partners** CELT, IT Deanship, and IT units in HSCs
Initiative description Providing HSCs with the handbook of the comprehensive assessment approaches for implementation			
Requirements and interdependencies 1. The HSCs comprehensive assessment approaches handbook that was developed and approved in initiative 10.3.1 2. Cover letter from the MEU/D of the HSCs to the colleges' deans. 3. Secretary 4. Computer with internet access, a printer, a copier, A4 paper, and a cartilage 5. An allocated assessment steering group to conduct the orientation workshops 6. An allocated group to moderate the orientation workshops 7. Proper time, place, audiovisual facilities, and catering 8. Rewards for trainers of the workshops 9. Budget for conducting workshops 10. Workshops equipment/materials 11. Feedback surveys to measure the satisfaction of workshops' participants 12. Internal and/or external experts to carry on the requested training workshops 13. An allocated group to moderate the requested training workshops 14. Proper time, place, audiovisual facilities, and catering for the requested training workshops 15. Rewards for the requested training workshops experts 16. Budget for the requested training and conducting workshops 17. Feedback survey to measure the effectiveness of implementation of comprehensive assessment approaches handbook on improving assessment strategies 18. An allocated assessment steering group to handle the survey 19. Data entry and statistician 20. SPSS program 21. Allocated assessment steering group to report on the statistical results 22. Independent opinion of expert on the report 23. Budget			**Stakeholders** Faculty staff, students, and HSCs

(continued)

Table 18.2 (continued)

Goal 10: Developing a comprehensive approach to students' assessment that addresses all educational domains including knowledge, skills, and attitudes/values	
Action plan 10.2.1. Providing HSCs with the approved handbook of comprehensive assessment approaches 10.2.2. Conducting workshops for the HSCs representatives for orientation about the Comprehensive Assessment Approaches Handbook 10.2.3. Facilitating and supporting training workshops (as needed) for HSCs programs to enhance and support the implementation of the Comprehensive Assessment Approaches Handbook 10.2.4. Measuring the effectiveness of implementing the Comprehensive Assessment Approaches Handbook on improving assessment strategies	**Estimated time** Phase II
KPIs 1. At least 75% of HSCs will receive a copy of the comprehensive assessment approaches handbook 2. At least 75% of HSCs representatives attend orientation workshops 3. HSCs representatives attended orientation workshops show 75% overall satisfaction of organized workshops 4. At least 75% of HSCs programs members attend different training workshops 5. HSCs members attended training workshops show 75% overall satisfaction of the organized workshops 6. At least 75% of the HSCs members respond to the survey 7. Statistical analysis of the survey shows overall 75% effectiveness of implementing the Comprehensive Assessment Approaches Handbook	**Estimated budget** Phase II

HSCs health sciences colleges, *VRHS* vice-rector for health specialties, *CELT* Center of Excellence in Learning and Teaching, *IT* information technology, *MEU/D* medical education units/departments, *SSPS* statistical package for the social sciences, *KPIs* key performance indicators

results and assure their reliability and validity. This will improve examination items writing, conduct, and results. Moreover, it will assure justice and equity among students who always look for evidence of their performance in examinations. Most health science programs have assessment centers where assessment training and workshops are conducted and examinations are revised before their conduct. In addition, assessment centers can monitor and supervise examinations, analyze and assess examination results, give feedback reports to various departments, and publish research on assessment and learning outcomes. The process of implementation may take one full academic year time depending on the degree of authority and support of the VRHSs, knowledge and skills of the personnel involved, and enthusiasm and cooperation of faculty. An estimated budget of 26,000 USD will be needed for the initiative resources, personnel incentives, and rewards for those who cooperate and compete for excellence. The KPIs of this initiative indicate that not all HSCs will be ready for the implementation of the assessment manual. Therefore, about (75%) of the HSCs are expected to participate in this initiative.

18.3 Discussion

Health professional education has undergone dramatic changes over the last century through four stages of innovation. In a significant shift from the scientific approach to health professional education commonplace in Europe at the end of the nineteenth century, the Flexner Era at the beginning of the twentieth century [6] was noted for the idea of teaching basic sciences as the basis of clinical sciences and practice. In the 1970s, problem-based learning was strongly promoted in an attempt to integrate basic, clinical, and social sciences through the use of problem scenarios [7]. Competency/outcome-based curricula became popular around the turn of this century. Learning outcomes vary from country to another and from an institute to another depending on societal and political needs [8]. In North America, broad learning objectives and learning outcomes were recommended by the American Association of Medical Colleges (AAMC) and the Accreditation Council for Graduate Medical Education (ACGME), respectively [9, 10]. Canadians also developed their own (CanMEDS) competencies [11]. The WHO—International Institute of Medical Education has produced a consensus of learning outcomes as minimal essential requirements for medical school graduate [12]. The Scottish Deans Medical Curriculum Group [13] adopted a framework of outcomes based on a three-circle model: what the doctor is able to do, his/her approaches to practice, and professional attributes (Table 18.3).

Table 18.3 Recommended assessment methods for the 12 learning outcomes in order of importance

What the doctor is able to do	
Learning outcomes	Assessment methods
1. Clinical skills OSCE	Observation; logbooks; mini-CEX
2. Practical procedures	OSPE; portfolios and logbooks; observation; DOPS
3. Patient investigations	Written examinations OSCE; observation; portfolios
4. Patient management	Written examinations OSCE; observation; portfolios
5. Health promotion and disease prevention	OSCE; portfolios and logbooks; observation; and written examinations
6. Communication	OSCEs; observation; peer/self-assessment; portfolios
7. Information management	Skills; portfolios; OSCE; observation; written exam
How doctors approach their practice	
1. Principles of social, basic, and clinical sciences	Written examinations; portfolios; observation; and OSCE
2. Attitudes, ethics, and legal responsibilities	Observation; portfolio; OSCE; peer/self-assessment; and written examinations
3. Decision making; clinical reasoning and judgment	Portfolio; observation; written assessment; OSCE; and peer/self-assessment
Doctors as professionals	
1. Role as a Professional	Observation; peer/self-assessment; OSCE; written
2. Personal development	Portfolio; observation; peer/self-assessment; OSCE; and written assessment

In the Kingdom of Saudi Arabia, the Executive Committee for SaudiMED Framework developed six learning domains or themes with seventeen learning outcomes which are adopted by all medical schools: scientific approach to practice; patient care; community-oriented practice; communication and collaboration; professionalism; and research and scholarship [14]. Assessment of such learning competencies/outcomes worldwide, however, did not develop well along with these innovations in curricular development [10]. Assessment of learning outcomes in fact encompasses several issues including an understanding of the principals of assessment, appropriate use of assessment methods and tools against the desired competency/outcome, and the comprehensive approach of assessment that covers the full range of educational domains. Effective assessment must consider the psychometric properties of the examination that is to be valid, reliable, feasible and has a measurable impact on learning outcomes through quality indicators. These metrics are important measures that guard appropriateness and quality of examination methods; otherwise, examinations will be of low quality and products are usually weak. Low performance in common placement testing such as the progressive testing [15] may indicate indirectly poor performance at health professional schools and/or low-quality examinations. There are several assessment methods and tools to measure learning outcomes; however, each tool is appropriate for the context to be measured. Therefore, no one method is appropriate for all domains of learning outcomes. Investment in good assessment is also an investment in teaching and learning [16]. Shumway and Harden [2] summarized the assessment tools against each assessment category in “AMEE’s Assessment Guide No. 25” (Table 18.4).

Written tests such as Long Essay Questions (LEQs) were a common assessment tool in health profession education at the begging of the nineteenth century. The

Table 18.4 Assessment tools (instruments) against each assessment category

Assessment category	Assessment tools
Written assessments	Essay: Short answer questions; completion questions; multiple choice questions (MCQs); extended matching items (EMIs); modified essay questions (MEQs); script concordance; key features; patient management problems (PMPs); and dissertation report
Practical assessments	Spot examination; objective structured practical examination (OSPE); practical examination
Clinical assessments	Long and short cases examination; objective structured clinical examination (OSCE); objective structured long examination record (OSLER); group objective structured clinical examination (GOSCE); mini clinical evaluation exercise (Mini-CEX), direct observation of practical skills (DOPS), etc.
Direct observation	Tutors report; checklists; rating scales; patient report; reflective and diary
Portfolios and other records	Logbooks; portfolios report; and procedural logs
Peer- and self-assessment	Peer report and self report

LEQs are reliable for in-depth assessment of a knowledge segment (e.g., Describe the process of fat digestion and absorption in the gut?); however, they are not content valid tool that can explore the knowledge domain of the gastrointestinal tract, for example. Therefore, long essays might be appropriate assessment tool for in-depth knowledge. LEQs are very easy to construct but time consuming to correct, and teachers will lose concentration and interest while reading many texts, which may affect concentration and compromise fairness in grading. This, of course, will affect its practicality and validity to some extent. To avoid these disadvantages of long essays, the modified essay questions (MEQs), completion questions, and short answer questions have emerged at the middle of the past century as reliable, valid, and practical assessment tools, which have replaced most LEQs in health professions education [17]. Over the last three decades or so, there has been a general move to MCQs over all types of essay questions as objective, reliable, content valid, practical, easy to administer/share/correct and analyze assessment tools with good impact on learning outcome in health professions education [2]. Not only that, MCQs nowadays are widely used in admissions, progress testing, promotion from one level to a higher level, licensing, and in high stakes postgraduate board examinations. MCQs, however, cannot assess in-depth knowledge like essays, difficult and costly to construct, and have some cuing and guessing effects. Patient management problems (PMPs) and Extended Matching Items (EMIs) are not popular assessment tools nowadays as they used to be at the end of the past century because of difficulties with question setting, marking, and standardization.

Practical and clinical examinations are very important tools to assess practical and clinical skills and attitude domains of the clinical practice. Practical assessment includes spot examination and practical observation. These are easy to construct and administer, but lack content validity, i.e., they cannot sample enough from the skills and attitudinal domains. In order to solve this problem, the Objective Structured Practical Examination (OSPE) came to improve this issue by increasing the number of practical encounters through multiple stations and by standardizing answer checklists for all stations. Similarly, the clinical assessment tools are used to include long and short cases, which lack content validity and fairness of distribution among students (the luck of the draw!). Therefore, Objective Structured Clinical Examination (OSCE), Objective Structured Long Examination Record (OSLER), and Group Objective Structured Clinical Examination (GOSCE) have emerged as more valid and reliable tools to solve these issues and drawbacks. The OSCE, however, gained popularity over other methods during the last three decades as a reliable, valid, and feasible tool to assess clinical competence [18]. For a reliable and valid OSCE, a minimum of 20 stations are required, with the use of checklist and standardized patients (SPs) [10, 19]. SPs need to be well trained to portray real patients' role in order to increase OSCEs' validity [16, 20]. Feasibility of OSCEs varies from one academy to another depending on available resources, SPs, and experienced educators. Also, cost of OSCEs varies from center to center [21]. These costs increase with recruitment and training of SPs, training of examiners, and maintenance of exam security. Positive impacts of OSCEs on students include increased learning, satisfaction due to fairness in evaluation, and increases of their experience for future OSCEs. However, OSCE has some drawbacks including fragmented learning, no time for in-depth assessment, and students know most OSCE stations beforehand. However, lots of modification in OSCE constructions have modified these drawbacks.

Other forms of learning outcome assessment include direct observation during attachment (global rating), reviewing written reports (portfolios), logbooks, and self/peer/360° feedback reports. These are best used for communication, interpersonal, and other attitudinal skills. Reliability of these assessment tools increases if done by a committee of expert faculty/examiners and decreases if done by a biased faculty. For positive impacts on learning, these forms of assessment are best used for formative feedback, improving communication and interpersonal skills, and must be revealed to the student as early as possible. Negative impacts on learning happen when students are informed late and/or if done by inexperienced or biased faculty. More research to assess the validity and reliability of these forms of assessment is needed to encourage educators and faculty to use them more frequently. Another important area in any assessment system is the practice of post-assessment test items analysis, which gives the function of each tool and gives valid and reliable results.

18.4 Summary

To develop a comprehensive approach to students' assessment requires faculty's knowledge and skills on assessment principles, use of appropriate assessment method(s) that matches the appropriate domain (i.e. knowledge, skills, attitude), analysis of the results, and their interpretation. The strategy to achieve this goal involves two initiatives. First, to develop comprehensive assessment approaches for courses that address all learning domains. Second, to develop guidelines for these domains. The strategic details for each initiative, the recommended assessment methods, and tools were outlined. The estimated time needed to complete each initiative and its budgetary details depends on studies, meetings, and discussions by relevant stakeholders involved during the implementation process.

References

1. Zaini RG, Bin Abdulrahman KA, Al-Khotani AA, Al-Hayani AM, Al-Alwan IA, Jastaniah SD. Saudi Meds: a competence specification for Saudi medical graduates. Med Teach. 2011;33:582–4.
2. Shumway JM, Harden RM. AMEE education guide No 25: the assessment of learning outcomes for the competent and reflective physician. Med Teach. 2003;25(6):569–84.
3. Schuwirth LW, Van der Vleuten CP. Programmatic assessment: from assessment of learning to assessment for learning. Med Teach. 2011;33(6):478–85.
4. Souza AC, Alexandre NMC, Guirardello EB. Psychometric properties in instruments evaluation of reliability and validity. Epidemiol Serv Saude. 2017;26(3):649–59.

5. National Board of Medical Examiners. Test blueprinting II: creating a test blueprint. 2019. https://www.nbme.org/sites/default/files/2020-01/Test-Blueprinting-Lesson-2.pdf.
6. Flexner A. Medical education in the United States and Canada: a report to the Carnegie Foundation for the Advancement of Teaching. New York: The Carnegie Foundation for the Advancement of Teaching; 2003.
7. Schmidt HG. Problem-based learning: rationale and description. Med Educ. 1983;17:11–6.
8. Alderson A, Martin M. Outcomes based education: where has it come from and where is it going? Issues Educ Res. 2007;17(2):161–82.
9. AAMC. Report I: learning objectives for medical student education. Medical Schools Objectives Project. AAMC Washington; 1998.
10. ACGME & ABMS. Toolbox of Assessment Methods. A product of the Joint Initiative. Accreditation Council for Graduate Medical Education (ACGME) Outcomes Project. American Board of Medical Specialties (ABMS). Version 1.1. September 2000. Accreditation Council for Graduate Medical Education and American Board of Medical Specialties, 2000.
11. CanMEDS. Extract from the CanMEDS 2000 Project Societal Needs Working Group Report. Med Teach. 2000;22(6):549–54.
12. IIME Core Committee. Global minimum essential requirements in medical education. Med Teach. 2002;24(2):117–20.
13. Harden RM, Crosby JR, Davis MH. An introduction to outcome-based education. Med Teach. 1999;21(2):7–14.
14. SaudiMED Framework. 2016. https://etec.gov.sa/en/productsandservices/NCAAA/AccreditationProgrammatic/Pages/Medical-Colleges.aspx.
15. René A, Schutte B, Meiboom A, Greidanus J, Dubois E, Bremers A. The progress test of medicine: the Dutch experience. Perspect Med Educ. 2016;5(1):51–5.
16. van der Vleuten CPM, Swanson DB. Assessment of clinical skills with standardized patients: state of the art. Teach Learn Med. 1990;2(2):58–76.
17. Feletti GI. Reliability and validity studies on modified essay questions. J Med Educ. 1980;55(11):933–41.
18. Norman G. Research in medical education: three decades of progress. Br Med J. 2002;342:1560–2.
19. Cushing A. Assessment of non-cognitive factors. 2002. https://doi.org/10.1007/978-94-010-0462-6_27.
20. Tamblyn R, Klass DJ, Schnabl GK, Kopelow M. Sources of unreliability and bias in standardized-patient rating. Teach Learn Med. 1991;3(2):74–85.
21. Carraccio C, Englander R. The objective structured clinical examination: a step in the direction of competency-based evaluation. Arch Pediatr Adolesc Med. 2000;154(7):736–41.

Measurement Criteria and Quality in Assessment

19

Mohammed Yahya Alnaami,
Hamza Mohammad Abdulghani, Olfat Salem,
and Eqbal Darandari

19.1 Introduction

Measurement criteria are the system of metrics that defines what program and project success is and how it should be measured. Certainly, measurement plays an essential role in research in health sciences as in other scientific disciplines [1]. However, measurement in health sciences education in general, and more specifically in assessment, was less considered until recently when more critiques of the reliability and validly of the assessment tools were questioned in every assessment result. Therefore, the advent of measurement in assessment tools has improved the quality of these measures, leading to more objective results. The shift from subjective to more objective assessment has also improved equity and justice among students as some of the old assessment methods were judgmental and sometimes unfair. Moreover, measurement in health professional education and assessment has stimulated the advent of more reliable and valid assessment tools (e.g., OSPE, OSCE, OSLER, GOSCE, etc.), which replaced or modified some of the old clinical

M. Y. Alnaami (✉)
Department of Surgery, College of Medicine, King Saud University, Riyadh, Saudi Arabia

H. M. Abdulghani
Department of Medical Education, College of Medicine, King Saud University,
Riyadh, Saudi Arabia

O. Salem
College of Nursing, King Saud University, Riyadh, Saudi Arabia

E. Darandari
College of Education, King Saud University, Riyadh, Saudi Arabia

M. Y. Alnaami et al. (eds.), *Novel Health Interprofessional Education and Collaborative Practice Program: Strategy and Implementation*,
https://doi.org/10.1007/978-981-99-3420-1_19

and practical assessment methods (e.g., long case, short cases, spot diagnosis, and some other practical examinations). The following sections will elaborate more on our strategic goal for improving the measurement criteria and quality in assessment.

19.2 Strategic Goal 11: To Enhance All Relevant Assessment Methods That Are in Use for Health Sciences Education, Establish Adequate Measurements Criteria, and Make Use of Assessment and Evaluation Results for Further Improvement

Measurement criteria usually include performance metrics, which provide insight into how well a program or project is performing. Assessment criteria may include, but not exclusively, the following:

1. Assessment of higher-order cognitive skills that allow students to transfer their learning to new situations and real problems. The Blooms' Taxonomy [2] explains higher-order cognitive domain (Fig. 19.1). Unfortunately, most of health profession schools lack assessment of students beyond the application stage of the knowledge domain. This will certainly lead to conventional, non-innovative graduates.

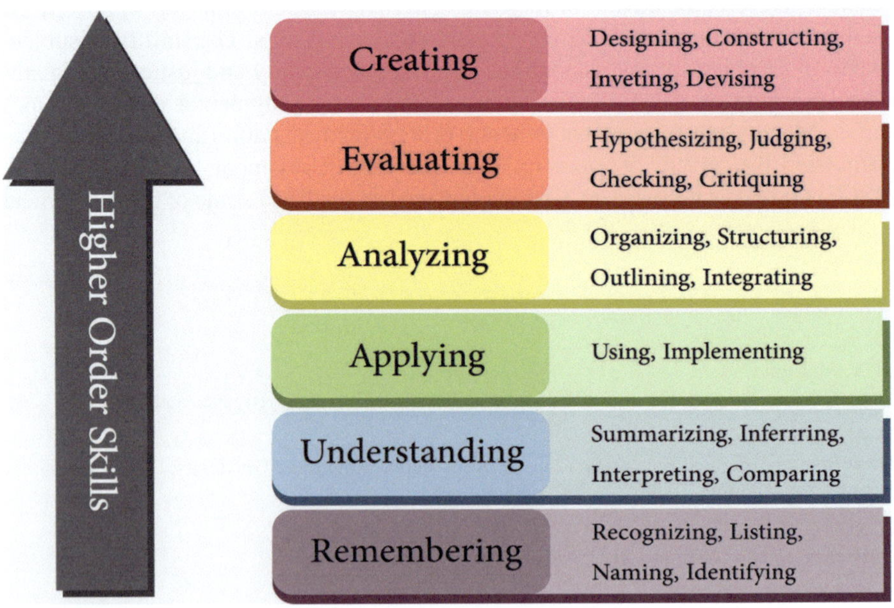

Fig. 19.1 Updated Bloom's taxonomy of the cognitive domain

2. Designing high-fidelity assessment of practical/clinical skills as they will be used in the real world, rather than through artificial alternates. This calls for tools that assess performance. As described by Miller initially [3], these tools directly evaluate such skills as they progress from novice to expert health professional practice (see Chap. 18).
3. Using tools that assess soft skills such as attitudes, values, communication, ethics, etc. Examples include the use of direct observation, portfolios, peer and self-reports, global rating scales, logbooks, patient report, feedback, and checklists.
4. Assessments that are valid, reliable, and practical should accurately evaluate students' abilities, appropriately assess the knowledge and skills they intend to measure, be free from bias, and be designed to reduce unnecessary obstacles to performance that could undermine validity. They should also have positive consequences for the quality of instruction and the opportunities available for student learning.
5. Assessments that are internationally benchmarked. Assessments should be evaluated against those of the leading health profession educational institutes and associations (e.g., NCAAA, AMEE, ASME, WAFME, AAMC, WHO, etc.) in terms of the kinds of tasks they present as well as the level of performance they expect.

Quality in assessment incorporates three main functions:

1. Defining the proposed quality. In this context, these are referred as assessment standards.
2. Improving quality by enhancing all relevant assessment methods that are in use for health sciences education.
3. Measuring quality of these assessment methods by studying validity, reliability, practicality, and their impact on students' learning.

19.2.1 Objective (Initiative) 11.1: To Set Standards for Assessment Tools to Increase the Quality of Students' Outcomes

This initiative is summarized in Table 19.1. The aim of this initiative is to establish standard guidelines for students' assessment tools that can be used by all HSCs. As shown in the table, there are multiple actors in this initiative, which require adequate communication and tactics to get all those involved working in an orchestrated manner. The *responsible* for the development of this initiative are the Assessment Steering Committee and the Assessment Units in HSCs. The *accountable* are the VRHS, Leadership Committee, and Deans of HSCs being the top authoritative and

Table 19.1 Setting standards for assessment tools to increase the quality of students' outcome

<table>
<tr><td colspan="4">Goal 11: Enhancing all relevant assessment methods that are in use for HSE, establishing adequate measurements criteria, and making use of assessment and evaluation results for further improvement</td></tr>
<tr><td colspan="4">Objective (11.1.1): To set standards for assessment tools to increase the quality of students' outcomes</td></tr>
<tr><td>Initiative (11.1.1)
Providing criteria for assessment tools, e.g., MCQs, OSCEs, OSPEs, and others</td><td>Responsible
Assessment Steering Committee and Assessment Units in HSCs</td><td>Accountable
VRHS, Leadership Committee, and Deans of HSCs</td><td>Partners
Deanship of Development and Quality, HSCs Quality Units, and Deanship for Admission and Registration</td></tr>
<tr><td colspan="4">Initiative description
Establishing standard guidelines for students' assessment tools that can be used by all HSCs</td></tr>
<tr><td colspan="3">Requirements and interdependencies
1. Group of 4–5 experts in assessment tools to establish the criteria (from inside of HSCs)
2. An expert consultant from KSU-QMS or from outside KSU
3. Brainstorming meetings (2–3 sessions) for the expert group
4. Computer with internet access, a printer, and A4 paper
5. Budget for the external consultant and also for the people in this special group</td><td>Stakeholders
Faculty staff, undergraduate and postgraduate students, and alumni</td></tr>
<tr><td colspan="3">Action plan
1. Assessing current criteria for assessment tools
2. Setting up rubrics to evaluate the current assessment tools
3. Browsing information regarding criteria for assessment tools
4. Establishing criteria for assessment tools
5. Establishing the manual for assessment tools with the following considerations:
(a) Format of the tool
(b) Purpose of the tool
(c) Advantages and disadvantages of each tool
(d) Development principle
(e) Training observers
(f) Scoring consideration
6. Performing an orientation workshop for course coordinators and the T&L Unit in each HSC about assessment tools</td><td>Estimated time
To be decided later as Phase II</td></tr>
<tr><td colspan="3">KPIs
• At least 75% of sample assessment tool gathered from each HSC
• Summary of a journal, an article, or any issues in assessment tools reported
• Development of assessment manual for HSCs
• At least 75% of course coordinators attend the workshop
• At least 75% of attendees satisfied with the workshop</td><td>Estimated budget
To be studied and decided later as Phase II</td></tr>
</table>

HSE health sciences education, *MCQs* multiple choice questions, *OSCEs* objective structured clinical examinations; *OSPEs* objective structured practical examinations, *HSCs* health sciences colleges, *VRHS* vice-rector for health specialties, *KSU* King Saud University, *QMS* quality management system, *T&L* teaching and learning, *KPIs* key performance indicators most influential bodies. The *partners* are the Deanship of Development and Quality in KSU and corresponding Development and Quality Units in HSCs, who will assist in explaining the university's Quality Management System (QMS) to align this initiative with the educational assessment components of this system. The *stakeholders* are faculty staff, undergraduate and postgraduate students, and alumni. This initiative starts by a robust assessment of the assessment tools that are currently in use in HSCs. A group of assessment experts from HSCs will be nominated by the Leadership Committee and tasks are assigned by the Assessment Steering Committee. Best rubrics available for this purpose include checking assessment blueprints, construct of MCQs and other written examinations, MCQs item analysis, construct of practical and clinical examinations, psychometric testing of these tests, and checking availability of other formal and informal assessment tools for values, attitudes, and other soft skills. After this task committee work is collected, it should be studied and discussed with all stakeholders in 2–3 days' workshop to establish a unified new guidelines manual for assessment tools to be used by all HSCs.

The NCAAA recommends the following general assessment standards [4]:

Standard 1: Student assessment mechanisms should be appropriate for the different forms of learning sought.

Standard 2: Assessment practices should be clearly communicated to students at the beginning of courses.

Standard 3: Appropriate, valid, and reliable mechanisms should be used for verifying standards of student achievement in relation to relevant internal and external benchmarks. The standard of work required for different grades should be consistent over time, comparable in courses offered within a program and college and the institution as a whole, and in comparison, with other highly regarded institutions. (Arrangements for verifying standards may include measures such as check marking of random samples of student work by teaching staff at other institutions, and independent comparisons of standards achieved with other comparable institutions within the Kingdom of Saudi Arabia and internationally.)

Standard 4: Grading students' tests, assignments, and projects should be assisted by the use of matrices or other means to ensure that the planned range of domains of student learning outcomes are addressed.

Standard 5: Arrangements should be made within the institution for the training of teaching staff in the theory and practice of student assessment.

Standard 6: Policies and procedures should include action to be taken to deal with situations where standards of student achievement are inadequate or inconsistently assessed.

Standard 7: Effective procedures should be used to ensure that work submitted by students is actually done by the students concerned.

Standard 8: Feedback to students on their performance and results of assessments during each semester should be given promptly and accompanied by mechanisms for assistance if needed.

Standard 9: Assessments of student work should be conducted fairly and objectively.
Standard 10: Criteria and processes for academic appeals should be made known to students and administered equitably.

Specific assessment standards include:

Standard 1: Assessment of higher-order cognitive skills. Currently, a large majority of items and tasks evaluate the conceptual knowledge and applied abilities that support transfer (i.e., tools that assess lower levels of the cognitive skills according to Bloom's Taxonomy starting from remembering (recall), understanding, and application skills of knowledge to practice). At least one-third of the assessment content should evaluate higher-order skills that allow students to become more critical and independent thinkers (i.e., tools that assess higher levels of the cognitive domain including analysis, synthesis, evaluation, and creative thinking). These may include research, experimentation, and evaluation and teaching a subject. Examples of tasks that assess different levels of the cognitive domain are presented in (Table 19.2).

Standard 2: High-fidelity assessment of practical and clinical skills that assess students' critical abilities not only application of knowledge to practice, as in most of programs, but also assessment of higher-order skills such as imitation, manipulation, precision, articulation, naturalization. Such tools may include moderate-high fidelity simulations, direct observation, video recording, and cautious use of real

Table 19.2 Levels of the cognitive domain and corresponding assessment tasks/objectives

Cognitive domain levels					
Increasing complexity					
Remember	Understand	Apply	Analyze	Evaluate	Create
Cite	Abstract	Apply	Analyze	Argue	Assemble
Choose	Associate	Carry out	Attribute	Assess	Build
Count	Categorize	Demonstrate	Deconstruct	Check	Combine
Define	Clarify	Determine	Differentiate	Conclude	Compose
Describe	Classify	Develop	Discriminate	Coordinate	Construct
Identify	Compare	Employ	Distinguish	Criticize	Create
Label	Conclude	Execute	Focus	Critique	Design
List	Contrast	Implement	Organize	Detect	Draft
Locate	Exemplify	Operate	Outline	Evaluate	Formulate
Match	Explain	Show	Parse	Judge	Generate
Memorize	Extrapolate	Sketch	Select	Justify	Hypothesize
Name	Illustrate	Solve	Structure	Monitor	Integrate
Outline	Infer	Use		Prioritize	Plan
Recite	Interpret			Rank	Produce
Record	Map			Rate	
Rephrase	Match			Recommend	
Restate	Paraphrase			Test	
Select	Predict				
State	Represent				
	Summarize				
	Translate				

Table 19.3 Levels of the psychomotor domain and corresponding assessment tasks/objectives

Psychomotor domain levels				
Increasing complexity				
Imitation	Manipulation	Precision	Articulation	Naturalization
Observing and copying another's skill	Reproducing skill through instruction	Accurately executing skill on own	Integrating multiple skills and performing it consistently	Naturally and automatically performing skills at high level
Copy Follow Repeat Replicate	Build Execute Implement Perform Recreate	Calibrate Complete Control Demonstrate Perfect Show	Adapt Combine Construct Coordinate Develop Formulate Integrate Master Modify	Design Invent Manage Project Specify

cooperative patients. Example of tasks that assess different levels of the psychomotor (practical/procedural/clinical skills) domains is presented in Table 19.3.

Standard 3: Use of tools that assess soft skills (affective domain) such as attitudes, values, communication, ethics, emotions, etc. Examples include the use of direct observation, portfolios, peer and self-reports, global rating scales, logbooks, patient report, feedback, and checklists. Tasks that assess different levels of the affective domain are presented in Table 19.4.

Standard 4: Quality of assessment tools should be appropriate for the tasks they are intended to be used for accurately (validly and reliability), fairly and practically, and with a positive impact on students' learning. These are referred as psychometric and qualitative properties of the assessment tools. Expert educators and statisticians are important persons who can be trusted to maintain the quality of this standard.

Standard 5: Assessments that are benchmarked to local and international standards. Assessment standards depend on several factors that guard the educational process. These factors may include the type of curriculum, teaching and learning methods, type of students and learning environment, experience of teaching staff, and available resources. These factors are important to consider in order to design and implement standards successfully. There are a couple of available assessment standards recommended by local and international educational authorities; however, not all of these standards are applicable or can be managed by all educational institutions but can be used as a guide to design and implement own assessment standards.

Table 19.4 Levels of the affective domain and corresponding tasks/objectives

Affective domain levels				
Increasing complexity				
Receiving	Responding	Valuing	Organization	Characterization
Openness to new information or experiences	Active participation in, interaction with, or response to new information or experiences	Attaching value or worth to new information or experiences	Incorporating new information or experiences into existing value system	Full integration/ internalization resulting in new and consistent attitudes, beliefs, and/or behaviors
Choose Follow Give Hold Identify Listen Locate Name Select Reply Use	Answer Assist Aid Compile Conform Describe Discuss Greet Help Label Perform Practice Present Read Recite Report Select Tell Write	Complete Demonstrate Differentiate Explain Follow Form Initiate Join Justify Propose Read Share Study Work	Adhere Alter Arrange Combine Compare Complete Defend Formulate Generalize Identify Integrate Modify Order Organize Prepare Relate Synthesize	Act Discriminate Display Influence Listen Modify Perform Practice Propose Qualify Question Revise Serve Solve Verify Use

19.2.2 Objective (Initiative) 11.2: Encouraging the Best Application of Assessment Tools

This initiative (Table 19.5) discusses how to implement the assessment handbook and guidelines by all HSCs. This requires tremendous efforts by responsible parties and partners of this initiative to train faculty and administration on every step to be ready for successful implementation. Students also will certainly benefit from regular training courses on understanding types of assessment tools and how to be successful in passing different exams. Once the approved guidelines manual is ready, it has to be published by KSU press and distributed to all HSCs departments as a reference. At this stage, the assessment guidelines manual will be ready to be implemented at all levels of health professional education. Before the implementation, however, the knowledgeable and experienced educators at all HSCs will start making a strategic plan for the implementation of the assessment guidelines manual at all HSCs through a one-day workshop led by the Assessment Steering Committee. Using the same plan of this workshop, an assessment sub-committee at each HSC, led by one or more members of the Assessment Steering Committee, will hold training for the implementation of the assessment guidelines handbook at any ready HSC as a pilot trial. Once the implementation process has been tried and evaluated in

Table 19.5 Strategic plan for encouraging the best application of assessment tools

Goal 11: Enhancing all relevant assessment methods that are in use for health sciences education, establish adequate measurements criteria, and make use of assessment and evaluation results for further improvement			
Objective (11.2): To encourage the best application of assessment tools			
Initiative (11.2) Supporting the application of best practices based on assessment tools criteria	**Responsible** Assessment Steering Committee and Assessment Units in HSCs	**Accountable** VRHS, Leadership Committee, and Deans of HSCs	**Partners** Deanship of Development and Quality, HSCs Quality Units, and Deanship for Admission and Registration
Initiative description • Facilitating the implementation of best practice of assessment tools that lead to high quality of students' outcomes			
Requirements and interdependencies 1. Best practice assessment tools from other top ranked health colleges 2. Feedback regarding the assessment tools from other teaching staff 3. External consultant 4. Survey from student evaluation			**Stakeholders** Faculty staff, students, and HSCs
Action plan 1. Training the trainers in applying the assessment manual considering the followings: (a) Assessing across all learning domains (cognitive, psychomotor, and affective) (b) Helping students succeed on assessment tasks 2. Piloting for implementation of assessment manual for a sample from the HSCs programs, courses for one semester and modifying based on their feedback 3. Establishing recognition and reward for the courses that apply best practice in assessment			**Estimated time** Phase II
KPIs 1. At least 75% of course coordinators are trained in items writing of different assessment tools 2. At least 75% of assessment manual tools are applied 3. Delivering a report of best practice in the administration of assessment tools			**Estimated budget** Phase II

HSCs health sciences colleges, *VRHS* vice-rector for health specialties, *KPIs* key performance indicators

piloted HSCs, then the assessment guidelines manual will be officially operational in all HSCs. At least 75% of all HSCs should implement the assessment guidelines manual completely, and the remaining 25% of HSCs at least partially. For a successful implementation of the assessment manual, preparations and training are essential, initial steps as mentioned above. However, monitoring and evaluation of the implementation process are also important to plan ahead of time and need to be considered as part of the strategic planning for this initiative. Monitoring involves scheduled site visits of the Assessment Steering Committee, faculty and students' surveys, administration interviews, and present annual report to the VRHSs. This report can be published locally and internationally as a whole report or a segmented report for each learning domain. Studies of validity, reliability, practicality, and impact on learning outcomes of the different assessment tools should be integral parts of the report. These studies can be published to benchmark with other international studies and for quality improvement as well. Recognition and reward for the courses that apply best practice in assessment need to be established to encourage positive competition and best assessment outcomes. The budget allocated for this initiative needs to be detailed based on number of workshops, participating faculty incentives, materials and other resources, report and writing costs, and external consultant expenses. Further details of this initiative are summarized in Table 19.5.

19.2.2.1 Objective (Initiative) 11.3: Establishing an Assessment System and Policies that Support Continuous Improvement at All Levels

This initiative discusses the establishment of systems and policies to use assessment and evaluation results for continuous improvement purposes at all levels starting from courses, programs, teaching/learning/assessment centers at individual HSCs, up to the VRHS (Table 19.6). As in the previous (Initiative 11.2), this initiative

Table 19.6 Strategic plan for establishing the assessment system and policies that support continuous improvement at all levels

Goal 11: Enhancing all relevant assessment methods that are in use for health sciences education, establish adequate measurements criteria, and make use of assessment and evaluation results for further improvement			
Objective (11.3): To establish the assessment system and policies that support continuous improvement at all levels			
Initiative (11.3) Establish a system to use assessment and evaluation results for continuous improvement at all levels (closing the loops)	**Responsible** Assessment Steering Committee and Assessment Units in HSCs	**Accountable** VRHS, Leadership Committee, and Deans of HSCs	**Partners** Deanship of Development and Quality, Deanship of Skills Development, IT Deanship, and IT Departments in HSCs
Initiative description Establishing a system to use assessment and evaluation results for continuous improvement purposes at all levels (closing the loops)			
Requirements and interdependencies 1. Best practice assessment tools from other top ranked health colleges 2. Assessment and evaluation centers 3. Data analysis and reporting center for HSCs 4. IT resources and software 5. Trainers, External Consultants, and E-assessment Experts 6. Periodic and annual reviews for assessment at course and program levels 7. Procedures and policies 8. Coordination with related deanships and committees (Quality, e-learning, university T&L committees, and Center for excellence in Learning and Teaching)			**Stakeholders** Faculty staff and students

Table 19.6 (continued)

Goal 11: Enhancing all relevant assessment methods that are in use for health sciences education, establish adequate measurements criteria, and make use of assessment and evaluation results for further improvement	
Action plan 1. Participating in reviewing university assessment and feedback policies to fit with the NCAAA standards 2. Developing a unified ongoing assessment cycle, with outcomes-based monitoring, feedback, and improvement plans "closing the loops," for HSCs. (This cycle works at 4 levels: courses, departments, colleges, and VRHSs) 3. Establishing a center for assessment and evaluation in each HSC to support staff and following up with assessment and evaluation results and improvement plans 4. Establishing a center for data analysis and reporting system for HSCs at the VRHSs level, which can be accessible for colleges and contain direct and indirect evidence of achieving student learning outcomes 5. Coordinating with KSU related deanships to implement an electronic system for assessment of student learning at all levels (courses, colleges/faculty, students/heads of departments, and deans) 6. Establishing a culture of data driven decisions and plans, self- and peer assessment, and reflections that encourage continuous improvements (e.g., portfolios for students, faculty, courses, and programs, and peer reviews)	**Estimated time** Phase II
KPIs 1. Percent of colleges establishing assessment centers (target 33% the first year, 66% the second year, and the 100% third year) 2. Percent of annual reviews for assessment results for courses and programs 3. Target 40% the first year, 60% the second year, and 70% the third year 4. Percent of courses responded to assessment feedback annually (target 40% the first year, 60% the second year, and 70% the third year 5. Approval of ongoing assessment and feedback system and procedures at several levels (courses, program, colleges, annual, or periodically if needed) 6. Approval of a review of assessment and feedback policies that fit the T&L strategic plan **Additional KPIs** 1. Establishment of a data analysis center for HSCs 2. Percentage of related decisions made based on assessment and feedback at each college level	**Estimated budget** Phase II

HSCs health sciences colleges, *VRHS* vice-rector for health specialties, *IT* information technology, *KSU* King Saud University, *KPIs* key performance indicators involves many parties, which requires tremendous communication and coordination efforts in order to be executed successfully. Establishment of an assessment and evaluation center as an integral part of the T&L unit/center, or as a separate unit/center, at each HSC is mandatory for managing examinations, analysis of results, training of faculty staff in assessment methods, and reporting of results. We have a good example of assessment and evaluation center at College of Medicine—KSU, which was established in the academic year 2008–2009, which made a real contribution and impact on assessment and evaluation at all courses and departments of the college. The center has been established as a centralized assessment system. In brief, the center was responsible only for first year at the beginning, and it took five years to cover all five years' academic courses assessment. All faculty members construct their assessment based on the evidence-based criteria published by the center, starting from the assessment blueprint, items construction, and review of all assessment items before examination and post examination analysis to look for any faulty item which may spoil the results. A similar center would be the ultimate goal to establish in each HSC at KSU. These assessment and evaluation centers/units will report their results of activities, results, and research work annually to the Dean and Vice-Dean for Academic Affairs of the HSC. In order to close the loop of this cycle, each HSC will report their achievements, results, and research studies to the VRHSs represented by the Assessment Steering Committee. At the VRHSs level, the Assessment Steering Committee consists of excellent experts' representation of all HSCs in Health Science Education, especially in Assessment and Evaluation. The leader and members of this steering committee will be nominated by the dean of each HSC, selected by the VRHSs, and will be appointed by the Rector of KSU as an administrative decision. Their term should not exceed five years and renewal would be for an additional term only when necessary as decided by the VRHSs. Main responsibilities of this assessment steering committee include strategic planning, policies and guidelines writing, monitoring of the implementation process at the HSC level, and research development. In order for this committee to succeed in its mission and gain trust of all parties, all of its procedures and policies should be done in coordination with related deanships and committees (e.g., Quality, e-learning, University T&L Committees, Center for Excellence in Learning and Teaching, etc.) to avoid duplications and people's resistance.

According to the NCAAA program evaluation and review processes [4], the quality of all courses and of the program as a whole must be monitored regularly through appropriate evaluation mechanisms and amended as required, with more extensive quality reviews conducted periodically. The level of compliance with this standard is judged by the extent to which the following good practices are followed:

1. Courses and programs should be evaluated and reported on annually and reports should include information about the effectiveness of planned strategies and the extent to which intended learning outcomes are being achieved.
2. When changes are made as a result of evaluation details of those changes and the reasons for them should be retained in course and program portfolios.

3. Quality indicators that include learning outcome measures should be established for all courses and the program.
4. Records of student completion rates should be kept for all courses and for the program, and they should be included among quality indicators.
5. Reports on the program should be reviewed annually by senior administrators and quality committees.
6. Systems should be established for central recording, analysis of course completion, program progression and completion rates, and student course and program evaluation, with summaries and comparative data distributed automatically to departments, colleges, senior administrators, and relevant committees at least once each year.
7. If problems are found through program evaluations, appropriate and timely action should be taken to make improvements.
8. In addition to annual evaluations, a comprehensive reassessment of the program should be conducted at least once every five years. Procedures for conducting these reassessments should be consistent with policies and procedures established for the institution.

The Assessment Steering Committee will participate along with the Quality Deanship in reviewing KSU assessment and feedback policies to fit with the NCAAA and similar international standards. It will develop a unified ongoing assessment cycle, with outcomes-based monitoring, and feedback and improvement plans for HSCs. This cycle starts at the level of courses, departments, deans, and vice-deans for academic affairs, and closes at the VRHSs (Assessment Steering Committee) with detailed procedures and timelines for:

1. Annual reviews and analysis of assessment results, assessment strategies, grading, and alignment with learning outcomes domains, etc.
2. Periodical reviews and analysis (every five years) of assessment results and trends with comparisons, assessment strategies, tools and criteria, and assessment processes and policies.

As mentioned above, the centers for assessment in HSCs are an essential development for all HSCs, with each center linked through an organizational structure to HSCs T&L Units or medical education department. At the level VRHSs, the Assessment Steering Committee should have a database center that contains all reports from all HSCs, references for assessment inquiries, and a statistician or data analyst to help the committee in their feedback to HSCs and related departments, partners, stakeholders, and also for research and publication purposes.

IT used for e-learning and e-assessment is increasingly becoming the norm in many academic institutions as it facilitates assessment of learning outcomes of mass students, and it is easy for teachers to deliver and give their feedback in a very short time and in a very cost-effective and secure way for the institute. However, e-assessment implementation in health professions education could face some challenges including students' inexperience in IT and lack of training, accessibility of computer and the internet, and errors and cut-offs of the internet during e-assessment. Also, teachers could have difficulties in entering, correcting, and analyzing questions and answers electronically, that is mostly due to lack of experience and training [5]. For a successful use and implementation of e-learning and e-assessment in health professions education, the responsible and accountable bodies should consider early involvement and coordination, even during strategic planning, with related partners and stakeholders.

Finally, in this initiative, the data generated from all HSCs at all levels, references, and reports available at the VRHSs website need to be available and transparently accessible by all KSU website portal users. Moreover, these data can also be used as evidence support for any further decisions and planning, modifications, and developments in assessment. Data sharing will also facilitate interprofessional education and collaboration among students, faculty, courses, and programs. This will eventually reflect on the culture of assessment, in which assessment in health sciences education encompasses the program and resources: students' experience (process) and learning outcomes as well as staff and teaching (see Chap. 17).

19.3 Summary

Assessment and evaluation of educational programs, students' learning process and outcome, and faculty and teaching are important general goals that require comprehensive planning, study of current assessment and evaluation practice, development and improvement efforts, and monitoring and evaluation of improved and developed assessment practice through educational research (closing the loop). This chapter highlighted the strategic planning and implementation processes of establishing the measurement criteria and quality assurance in assessment.

References

1. Streiner DL, Norman GR. Health measurement scales: a practical guide to their development and use. New York: Oxford Medical Publications; 1989.
2. Bloom BS, Engelhart MD, Furst EJ, Hill WH, Krathwohl DR. Taxonomy of educational objectives: the classification of educational goals. Handbook 1: cognitive domain. New York: David McKay; 1956.
3. Miller GE. The assessment of clinical skills/competence/performance. Acad Med. 1990;65(9):S63–7.
4. Standards for Program Accreditation, 2018. https://etec.gov.sa/en/productsandservices/NCAAA/AccreditationProgrammatic/Pages/insprogdeve.aspx.
5. Alruwais N, Wills G, Wald M. Advantages and challenges of using e-assessment. Int J Inf Educ Tech. 2018;8(1):34–7.

MIX
Papier aus verantwortungsvollen Quellen
Paper from responsible sources
FSC® C105338

If you have any concerns about our products,
you can contact us on
ProductSafety@springernature.com

In case Publisher is established outside the EU,
the EU authorized representative is:
Springer Nature Customer Service Center GmbH
Europaplatz 3, 69115 Heidelberg, Germany

Printed by Libri Plureos GmbH
in Hamburg, Germany